"An absolute delight! *Pre- and Perinatal Massage Therapy* is a gem of a book. The authors have managed to coalesce many years of clinical experience and research findings into a delightfully readable manuscript. Warning, readers: you, too, may lose sleep when you can't put it down! The layout is thoughtfully designed and the content excellent – all done with a sense of wonder and passion that is heart-warming and engaging. This is an important contribution to the field of massage therapy."

Douglas Nelson LMT, BCTMB, President, Massage Therapy Foundation

"This book has everything. Precise guidelines. Wise advice. Sensible, effective hands-on approaches. And a huge heart. The authors offer inspiration and encouragement and consider all that your pregnant, laboring, or postpartum client is going through. They guide you through clinical thinking, communication, massage precautions, and effective techniques. Their guidelines are clear, sensible, and impeccably researched. This comprehensive edition will benefit the profession – and our clients – for years to come. A must-have for every massage therapist's library."

Tracy Walton MS, LMT

"I love a reading experience – on any subject, in any form – where the author has anticipated where I might need an extra explanation, a specific image, or a mental detour. This book did that for me. *Pre- and Perinatal Massage Therapy* possesses my three essential qualities of an educational text: it is eminently readable, effortless to navigate, and possesses an experienced and compassionate voice. Students and practitioners will be in very good hands with this book at their side."

Andrew Biel, author of *Trail Guide to the Body: A hands-on guide to locating muscles, bones, and more*

"This is a welcome update to Carole's two previous editions. It broadens the scope to cover the increasingly relevant issues of working with assisted reproductive methods, a diversity of clientele, and other new topics. I admire Carole's willingness to constantly review her work and to collaborate with others, such as Michele and David. It is an important book for all those working in the maternity massage field."

Suzanne Yates, Shiatsu and massage therapist, childbirth educator and founder of Wellmother, UK

"Massage can be a w̶o̶n̶d̶e̶r̶f̶u̶l̶ g̶i̶f̶t̶ f̶o̶r̶ p̶e̶o̶p̶l̶e̶ w̶h̶o̶ are pregnant, but the topic is rife with myths and traditions that are well-meaning but inaccurate. This book dispels those myths by providing current, evidence-informed best practices for this important group of clients. Anyone who is interested in pre- and perinatal massage therapy will find value in this beautifully written and produced text."

Ruth Werner, author of *A Massage Therapist's Guide to Pathology*

"An empowering text that brings proper focus to stress management and therapeutic touch, not only for immediate benefit to the pregnant mother but for transgenerational health and resilience in her child and in her grandchildren yet to come; an integral part of every optimized pregnancy."

Leslie Stone MD, IFMCP, co-founder growbabyhealth.com and growbabylifeproject.org, and international lecturer in Developmental Programming of Health and Disease

"*Pre- and Perinatal Massage* is an excellent guide – both comprehensive and accessible – through a rich and complex field. It is brimming with both practical tips based on extensive experience and serious scientific references. This work goes far beyond simple anecdotes and stories through a logical order, deep correlations with the research literature and practical illustrations and diagrams. I recommend this book most highly to both students and practitioners."

Daniel J. Bressler MD, FACP

"For therapists wanting to work with pregnant and postpartum clients, this book is a must to help better understand all the complexities of this population. Its dynamic writing will assist in integrating concepts with hands-on skills. This comprehensive book gives manual therapists all the information needed to feel comfortable working with the pregnant and postpartum body."

Lynn Schulte PT, Institute for Birth Healing

"Your book leaves no stone unturned with your detailed explanations for massage therapists and all body workers. Even mothers-to-be will benefit by knowing the information you have shared in your third edition. I know many of my patients would have found "ease" in their stressful situations had they had your book as a resource! The

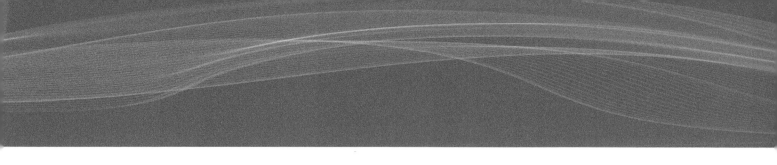

anatomy, physiology, patient-based information and functional approach, together with the overwhelming evidence about the importance of touch from a cellular perspective to an emotional perspective, makes this book imperative for those studying pre- and perinatal health."

Gail Wetzler PT, DPT, EDO, BI-D

"This book is a remarkable guide for how to use touch throughout pregnancy, birth, and the postpartum period. Many childbearing professionals could benefit from its insight and skills as they touch those in their care. The co-authors, Carole, Michele and David, are top authorities in the field. They teach and model the skills and compassionate understanding needed for safe and effective work. Let them guide you as you discover the joy and satisfaction of providing massage therapy during this unforgettable time of life."

Penny Simkin PT, CD (DONA), author of *The Birth Partner: A Complete Guide to Childbirth for Dads, Partners, Doulas, and Other Labor Companions* (5th Edition, with Katie Rohs)

"As a licensed midwife and former massage therapist I truly value the work that went into the creation of this textbook. In addition to comprehensive prenatal, labor and postpartum massage techniques, the authors, all seasoned massage therapists, offer research and additional online resources in an easy to read and enjoyable format. This is all accomplished with great sensitivity to and a deep understanding of the psychological state, and special circumstances, of the pregnant person. I highly recommend this book for massage students, practicing massage therapists, doulas, midwives, partners and anyone interested in supporting pregnant people. After all, if peace on earth begins with birth, what better way to facilitate this?"

Andrea Diamond MSN, CNM, LMT retired

"This is a thought-provoking collaborative textbook that outlines the benefits of massage and relaxation techniques applied throughout the perinatal cycle and validates their roles. Emphasis is placed on the importance of human touch for both the mother and infant to reduce stress and anxiety. Massage therapy safety is stressed throughout each perinatal phase with a variety of photos to demonstrate massage techniques. Features like *From the treatment room* and *What would you do?* allow for thoughtful responses on the part of the readers. These features link massage practice to the clients they serve. A highly impressive book!"

Susan Ricci, author of *Essentials of Maternity, Newborn & Women's Health Nursing* (5th edition) and (with T. Kyle) *Maternity & Pediatric Nursing* (4th edition)

"Masterfully written by experienced and well-known experts, this elegant book provides a clear, rational, and well-documented approach for practitioners of pre- and perinatal massage therapy. The authors' commitment, caring and compassion is evident on every page."

Raymond J. Hruby DO, MS, FAAO (Dist), author of *Exploring Osteopathy in the Cranial Field*

"I believe that smart movement is a vital tool in a healthy pregnancy and return to exercise postpartum, and that massage therapy is a must for optimizing the structural and musculature changes we see in this population. *Pre- and Perinatal Massage Therapy* is a deep dive into what you need to know when working with women during the pre and postnatal periods. Its pages provide an incredibly profound level of education and information that any pre and postnatal specialist would greatly benefit from. Every single massage therapist who works with pre- and perinatal clients should consider this book a must-have for truly understanding how to work with their bodies during this time."

Brooke Cates, Founder/CEO of The Bloom Method, Pre + Postnatal Health + Wellness Expert, Movement Content Creator for *Becoming Mama*, a Mother.ly book

"As a perinatal educator and LMT, I found this book to be an amazing tool! This is a wonderful and informative resource for massage therapists, healthcare professionals or anyone interested in perinatal bodywork. It balances beautifully, and in clear concise forms, perinatal physiology as well as the practical tools of bodywork."

Lara Kohn Thompson LMT, certified yoga teacher (ERYT-500/ PRYT), perinatal trainer, educator and mentor

Pre- and Perinatal Massage Therapy

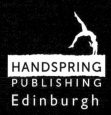

HANDSPRING
PUBLISHING
Edinburgh

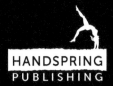

HANDSPRING
PUBLISHING

Third edition

Pre- and Perinatal Massage Therapy

A comprehensive guide to prenatal, labor and postpartum practice

Carole Osborne

Michele Kolakowski

David M Lobenstine

Forewords

Penny Simkin

Linda Hickey

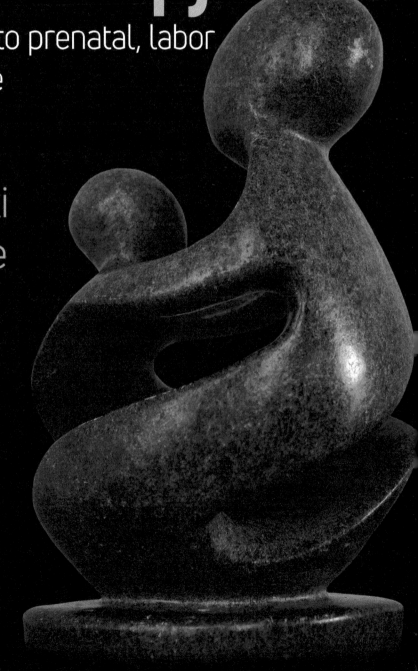

HANDSPRING PUBLISHING LIMITED
The Old Manse, Fountainhall,
Pencaitland, East Lothian
EH34 5EY, Scotland
Tel: +44 1875 341 859
Website: www.handspringpublishing.com

First published 2021 in the United Kingdom by Handspring Publishing Limited

First edition (1998) Body Therapy Associates ISBN 0-9665585-0-2
Second edition (2012) Lippincott, Williams & Wilkins ISBN 978-1-58255-851-6

Copyrighted materials used with the generous and kind permission of their owners include:
Ruth Ancheta (Figure 5.1); Wolters Kluwer (Figure 5.9 and 6.4); Edward Maupin (Figure 6.15); Benjamin and Sohnen-Moe
(Box 8.7); Anne Williams (online resource on foot zone therapy)

Photo credits
Al Gardner, Zachary Schulman, Elizabeth Beckmann, Ronnie Allan, Nanci Newton, Anne Gilbert, Kharisma Studios, Kyla Berry,
Julie Harris, AB Nevarez, Rick Raney

ISBN 978-1-912085-73-6
ISBN (Kindle eBook) 978-1-912085-74-3

British Library Cataloguing in Publication Data
A catalogue record for this book is available from the British Library

Library of Congress Cataloguing in Publication Data
A catalog record for this book is available from the Library of Congress

Notice
Neither the Publisher nor the Author assumes any responsibility for any loss or injury and/or damage to persons or property
arising out of or relating to any use of the material contained in this book. It is the responsibility of the treating practitioner,
relying on independent expertise and knowledge of the patient, to determine the best treatment and method of application for
the patient.

Commissioning Editor Mary Law
Project Manager Morven Dean
Copy Editor Wendy Lee
Designer and Cover Design Bruce Hogarth
Indexer Aptara, India
Typesetter DSM, India
Printer Melita, Malta

The
Publisher's
policy is to use
paper manufactured
from sustainable forests

CONTENTS

Dedication   vii
Acknowledgments   ix
About the Authors   xi
Subject Matter Reviewers   xii
Foreword by Penny Simkin   xiii
Foreword by Linda Hickey   xv
Preface   xvii

1   **Benefits:** Helping Our Clients and Their Babies   3

2   **Guidelines:** Massaging Safely and Effectively   39

3   **Practical Considerations:** Caring for Your Clients and Yourself   71

4   **Prenatal Techniques:** Nurturing Throughout Pregnancy   99

5   **Labor Techniques:** Supporting a Positive Birth Experience   153

6   **Postpartum Techniques:** Facilitating Restorative Healing   197

7   **Additional Considerations:** Working with Special Needs Clients   235

8   **Practice Considerations:** Growing a Satisfying Career   267

Glossary   293
Index   307

DEDICATION

To our families, clients and students, with deep respect and gratitude for all that you have taught us. May our work together help to create a more peaceful, connected world for all of us to thrive in.

ACKNOWLEDGMENTS

Every "gestation" and "birthing" of a textbook is humbling and exhilarating, and creating this third edition has certainly been that, and more. We are profoundly grateful for the "village" that it took to create this work. We are especially thankful to:

Our clients whose pregnancies, births and postpartum experiences have given us the context to explore and confirm the possibilities of this work.

The 5,000-plus therapists who have been our eager students, offering us innumerable lessons and refining our teaching and expressive skills.

Our earliest collaborators and colleagues, and all of those who helped create the foundations of this book, our careers and our fascination with nurturing the mother.

Carole personally thanks: From the beginning – Sandy Sara Karst, Ed Maupin, James Stewart, Bill Helm, Kate Jordan, Diana Panara, Ray Hruby DO, Barry Green and Andy Sheets, my children's father. And now – seldom has the stability and power of three been so palpable and essential to me. Thank you, Michele and David! You will keep this work potent for decades to come.

Michele personally thanks: My gracious co-authors Carole and David, my colleagues at Sanctuary Healing Arts, Joy Collective, Boulder College of Massage Therapy, Cortiva Institute, Longmont United Hospital's Health Center of Integrated Therapies, Birth Assistants of Boulder, Christine Caldwell, Rosita Arvigo, Suzanne Yates, Kate Jordan, Elaine Stillerman, Deanna Elliott, Carolyn Guenther-Molloy, Penny Stansfield and Melinda Ferguson.

David personally thanks: Linda Hickey, who was my introduction to prenatal massage, and whose passion was as infectious as it was inspiring.

Our former and current collaborators and fellow authorized instructors of Pre- and Perinatal Massage Therapy specialization workshops: Marjeanne Estes, Pam Guldi, Margi Hadorn and Sparrow Harrington, who help us to keep the work vibrant and current, and our esteemed former instructors Linda Hickey, Liz Ellis and Jennifer Hicks, who continue to nurture childbearing people, their families and communities.

Margi Hadorn, our stalwart and joyous research assistant, for her enthusiasm and perseverance in scouring resources for relevant, current research.

We are grateful beyond measure to others as well. They include:

Penny Simkin, for her wise and generous Foreword, our spirited discussions during brisk walks and leisurely meals, decades of support, and her example of a wise, humble and consummate professional and mother.

Linda Hickey, for her exuberant Foreword, brilliant reviewer's suggestions, crafting of sections of the second edition, her deep and abiding friendship, and the ultimate gift to a teacher: taking her learning to places beyond her teacher's reach.

Marjeanne Estes, for her steady presence and skilled management of Body Therapy Education's instructional projects, her stellar assistance in the classroom, and a fierce and real friendship.

Karen Lavelle, for many years of administrative assistance to various Body Therapy Education operations.

Cherie Sohnen-Moe, whose business consultations have helped ground and grow the bottom line more than once.

The various perinatal healthcare professionals who ensured technical and factual accuracy and infused a positive perspective to this book's earlier editions, particularly: James Webber, MD; Diane Smith, midwife; Penny Simkin, PT and doula trainer; Liz Smith, prenatal anatomy and physiology instructor; Ana de Vedia, licensed acupuncturist and instructor; Pamela Ferguson, Shiatsu instructor.

Our expert subject matter reviewers: Faith Davis, Yeliz Çakır Koçak, Penny Bussell Stansfield, Linda Hickey, Marjorie Johnson, Lynn Schulte and Ruth Werner, and our other consultants, Elizabeth Shrader,

Frances Reed and Dave Nimmons. This book would be a puny child without the enrichment of their knowledge and refinements.

The many scientists, researchers and scholars whose studies we have digested, cited and relied upon to elevate this third edition. The evidence-based techniques that we teach rest on the foundation of your work and are essential to clarifying and evolving what we feel with our hands.

Al Gardner, photographer and videographer, and Zachary Schulman, photographer, for capturing the facts and feelings of this work in appealing light and images, and having fun too. Rick Raney for our cover statue photo, and Julius Evans, videographer, whose creativity and focus complement the still images so well.

The other photographic contributors, and especially Ronnie Allan, Nanci Newton and Anne Gilbert for generously persevering to convey the progression of our work through photographing their excellent sessions with their clients for an entire childbearing cycle.

The Beckmann, Botting, Corwin, Dove-Alvarez, Lobenstine, Stumpf and Winter families who graciously shared sacred moments of their families' lives – birth, breath and death – shining a light on these profound personal experiences that sometimes remain in a memory, a scrapbook, behind closed doors or in the shadows.

All of our vibrant models for photos and video, especially our "marathoners": Elizabeth, Nick and Penelope Beckmann, Kenya Carmichael, Marjeanne Estes, Yazel Gerwe, Sparrow Harrington, Nicole Trombley, Angelica Villarruel, and Jenna Zamohi.

And the International Professional School of Bodywork (IPSB) in San Diego for space for the 2009 video shoot.

The remarkable team at Handspring Publishing, who gave this book new life, growing it in ways we only dared to imagine and during the unimaginable experiences of a global pandemic. Andrew Stevenson and Mary Law welcomed us into their exceptional author cohort and made us feel at home and exceptionally resourced, while offering grace and guidance at every step. Wendy Lee and Catherine Aitken word polished with care and an impressive precision. Bruce Hogarth tirelessly brought our illustrations and photos to vivid life within a design exponentially improved over prior editions. The ever-equanimous Morven Dean guided us and our "baby" through the (multiple) final stages of gestational production. And Stephanie Ricks and Hilary Brown ensured that the birth of this book will be properly acknowledged with robust sales.

And finally, we want to formally offer our deepest gratitude to those without whom this book's birth would be a hollow accomplishment: our families and friends. Their love and reminders of Truth took us through turmoil and transition into the completion of each edition, and especially this third edition. In addition to friends and family mentioned above, we thank:

Carole – those who lovingly sustained me while tolerating more neglect than they deserved: Josh, Elizabeth, Brandon, Connor and Penelope, Irene, Nick B and Nick G; Lee, Beth, Adam, Diana, Maela, Roger, Kate N, Lynn, Thom, Al, Peter, Marjeanne, my sister Lynn and her family. And my mother and father who rest in peace. My Heart is Your Heart. We are One.

Michele – dearest mother, Sarah Ann, who lost her mother too early, and despite this hardship, birthed and mothered me "without her map." And to my husband, Kyle, and my sons, Kyle and Jackson, in our enduring, transformational love now and always.

David – my mother, Amy March, who gave birth to me and continues to give me so much more; all three of my parents, who have shown me the possibilities that emerge from abiding love and care; my wife, Miranda Beverly-Whittemore, who is my heart and my home; and my children, Quentin and Kitsune, who give purpose and pleasure to every moment of every day.

ABOUT THE AUTHORS

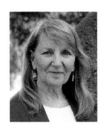

Carole Osborne BA, CMT, BCTMB is a pioneer of therapeutic massage and bodywork for childbearing. The previous editions of this book and her courses have paved the way for over 5,000 therapists working with this population. For almost 50 years, Carole has been in private practice in a variety of settings. She was the American Massage Therapy Association's 2008 National Teacher of the Year. For more on Carole, visit www.bodytherapyeducation.com.

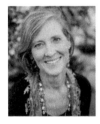

Michele Kolakowski LMT, CD and CPD(DONA), CLC has diverse experience serving childbearing women and babies since 1992. She is an authorized Pre- and Perinatal Massage Therapy workshops instructor and teaches maternity massage at massage schools, spas, destination resorts, hospitals and conferences nationwide. Her experience includes hospital-based maternity massage and attendance at births in homes, birth centers and hospitals. Her private practice is Sanctuary Healing Arts. For more on Michele, visit www.sanctuaryhealingartsllc.com.

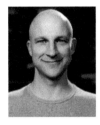

David M Lobenstine BA, LMT, BCTMB has been massaging, teaching, writing and editing for over 15 years in New York City, with a focus on clients at all stages of childbearing. He is an authorized instructor of the Pre- and Perinatal Massage Therapy workshops, and also designs and teaches his own continuing education workshops, both around the USA and online, at Body Brain Breath. For more on David, visit www.bodybrainbreath.com.

SUBJECT MATTER REVIEWERS

Comprehensive Reviewers

Linda Hickey
Registered Massage Therapist
Founder and Director Calgary Maternity Massage
Therapy
Calgary, Alberta, Canada

Yeliz Çakır Koçak, Midwife, Research Assistant,
M.Sc., Ph.D.
Pregnancy Massage Therapist
Ege University Faculty of Health Sciences Midwifery
Department
Izmir/Turkey

Chapter Reviewers

Faith Davis LMT, Certified Yoga Teacher and Certified
Postpartum Doula
Mountain Mama Massage LLC
Boulder, Colorado, USA
(Chapters 1 and 3)

Marjorie Johnson LMT
(Chapters 1 and 3)

Lynn Schulte PT
Birth Healing Expert, Institute for Birth Healing
Founder
(Chapters 1 and 6)

Penny Bussell Stansfield BA(Hons), AdvCD(DONA),
BDT(DONA), LCCE, CLC, BCLMT
Author of *Labors of Love: A Doula's Birth Stories*
(Chapter 5)

Ruth Werner, Board Certified in Therapeutic Massage
and Bodywork
Author of *A Massage Therapist's Guide to Pathology, Disease
Handbook for Massage Therapists* and *Scheumann's The
Balanced Body*
(Chapter 2)

FOREWORD BY PENNY SIMKIN

"It takes a village to have a baby."*

Pregnancy and childbirth represent a permanent transformation to parenthood for the birthing person and to infancy for the fetus. Other new roles are also created: fathers, co-parents, grandparents, siblings and more. In fact, each birth causes a ripple effect that radiates outward from the family of origin to the community and beyond. In every culture, childbearing people are guided and advised through this transformation by a "village" of wise, caring experts. In North America, the "village" includes not only family and friends, but also their medical caregivers or midwives, and some of the following: childbirth educators, nutritionists, yoga teachers, doulas, lactation counselors, mental health specialists, peer group facilitators, chiropractors, physical therapists, acupuncturists, and even numerous books, films, and informative websites about pregnancy, postpartum and childcare.

Another extremely valuable group of maternity professionals are prenatal and perinatal massage therapists, the focal audience for this book. This third edition of *Pre- and Perinatal Massage Therapy* now includes the knowledge and experience of two additional skilled massage therapists and authors – Michele Kolakowski and David M Lobenstine – along with Carole Osborne, the author of all previous editions. The result is a remarkable guide for how to use touch throughout pregnancy, birth and the postpartum period. With this book, you can become part of the village that nurtures the births of mothers and babies.

Many childbearing professionals could benefit from this book's insight and skills as they touch those in their care. Specifically though, massage therapy uses the hands, the head and the heart of the practitioner, organized by the intention and the specific skills to nurture, heal, comfort, soothe and relax the receiver, who places trust in the massage practitioner and then benefits emotionally and physically. Research suggests that the greater sense

of calm and well-being, as well as tension release and pain relief, provided by massage therapy, also benefits the baby.

Let's think for a moment about some of the changes and challenges encountered during the childbearing year – a particularly vulnerable time for all expectant and new parents. Their emotional and physical needs are uniquely altered; their body and mind are affected by the many rapid changes of all kinds: weight gain, bodily discomforts, alterations in posture and balance, emotional lability, feelings of dependency, new perceptions of oneself and their world, reflections on their own childhood and the way they were parented. The fetus within and its safe passage become the birthing parent's major focus. They labor and give birth, undergoing some of the deepest, most intense sensations and emotions they are likely ever to experience – excitement, anticipation, exertion, fatigue, fear, anxiety, vulnerability, pain, uncertainty, nakedness, exposure, unfamiliarity with their surroundings and their healthcare providers, and possible physical injury. The potential for everything from joy and triumph to disappointment and suffering exists. For a positive emotional outcome in childbirth, they need comfort, reassurance and guidance, along with skilled maternity care.

After the birth, one's body returns to a non-pregnant state, but now it feels very strange, and may hold pain or a need to heal in some parts. The "new" body produces breast milk and functions on much less sleep due to the constant need to care for her baby. The new body is physically and emotionally vulnerable, with little time for oneself, possible psychological challenges, or lack of confidence in their mothering abilities.

What keeps them going during this time? How do they deal with these extraordinary challenges? The answer is that some people handle this period better than others. The resilient, emotionally and physically healthy person who has a healthy baby, an adequate support system and self-confidence weathers this time well with pleasing memories, a sense of accomplishment and enhanced self-esteem. As one person said, after giving birth, "After that, I knew I could do anything!" Those who lack some

---

*With acknowledgement of the African proverb, "It Takes a Village to Raise a Child," which inspired my rewording to focus on childbearing.

of these assets may look back on their childbearing experience with sorrow, guilt, shame or anger. They may feel defeated, neglected, incompetent and traumatized.

My own study, "Just Another Day in a Woman's Life?"** found that when birthing persons feel well-cared for by their health care professionals during childbirth, they feel a greater sense of accomplishment, higher self-esteem and greater satisfaction with their birth experiences 20 years later (and probably longer) compared to those who did not feel respected or well-cared for. All had vivid, accurate and poignant memories of their children's births and the professionals who cared for them. Those who reported low satisfaction with their children's births had negative memories of things that were said and done to them by their caregivers, and they felt little or no sense of personal accomplishment.

The massage practitioner, by employing comforting and healing techniques during the childbearing year, is in a perfect position to enhance not only the way the person feels as they go through pregnancy and birth and the postpartum period, but also how they will look back on it in the future. The massage practitioner may not realize it at the time, but they will also be remembered by the birthing person for years to come. I think every massage therapist should ask themselves, while working with childbearing people, how the client will remember each technique, each session, each interaction. This book is a guide to saying and doing what will help to create happy bodies and good memories.

What a privilege it is for skilled, compassionate and sensitive massage practitioners, and other touch professionals, to offer their talents to childbearing people at this pivotal stage in their lives! How fortunate childbearing people are to have this service! Carole, Michele and David are top authorities in the field. They teach and model the skills and compassionate understanding needed for safe and effective work. Let them guide you as you discover the joy and satisfaction of providing massage therapy during this unforgettable time of life.

With best wishes.

Penny Simkin PT, CD(DONA)

Author of *The Birth Partner: A Complete Guide to Childbirth for Dads, Partners, Doulas, and All Other Labor Companions*

Kenmore, WA, USA

November 2020

**Simkin P. (1991) Just Another Day in a Woman's Life? Women's Long-term Perceptions of Their First Birth Experience. Part 1. Birth 18 (4):203-210.

FOREWORD BY LINDA HICKEY

I want you to know how delighted I am to be introducing you to the third edition of *Pre- and Perinatal Massage Therapy*, and to be the one writing these words: *"In your hands …"* I have always loved it when a foreword begins like that, setting the stage for the wonder and excitement to come. Now it is my turn.

You hold in your hands an invitation to step inside the world of maternity massage therapy and to be inspired and enchanted, as I am, with the work, wisdom and words of Carole Osborne, joined in this edition by David M Lobenstine and Michele Kolakowski.

Carole's work over the last four decades has been the respected standard for therapists engaged in evidence-based, women-centred bodywork – work that embodies effective soft tissue treatment and support for clients who may be anticipating pregnancy, growing their babies, labouring them out or mothering, baby in their arms.

Imagine – Carole's wisdom, words and magic joined by David's laser-sharp focus and attention to detail paired with his delight in the work, and Michele's vast experience in the treatment room and beyond, taking the work into hospital settings and massage classrooms around the country.

In the third edition, this dynamic trio revisits the case for massage and bodywork for pregnant and postpartum clients across a broad range of settings. They explore the continuing and growing evidence supporting the importance of the work not just for the mothers-to-be but their babies, their families and the world. They set the stage for why we should and must continue to do this effective, thoughtful and supportive work moving forward in this increasingly complex world.

Together they outline essential concepts when considering the common experiences of pregnant and postpartum alignment and physiology. They introduce you to proven techniques specific to the pregnant pelvis and alignment – all artfully illustrated and effectively described.

Along the way they guide you in caring for yourself in this important work. The foundational body mechanics will help you to grow and stay strong and flexible beside your table in your treatment rooms for many, lovely years to come.

I do speak from experience. I have had the privilege to journey alongside Carole as a student, a mentee, a teaching assistant and instructor, a colleague and dear friend. Carole and I first crossed paths in 1995, me a shiny new massage therapist from Canada enrolled in her early Bodywork for the Childbearing Year program. That meeting pre-dated her first edition of this book (published in 1998), and yes, we did use those romantic words to describe the time frame for the work "back in the day." Just writing those words still makes me smile.

The treatment approaches and techniques I learned from Carole at that time gave me the confidence to approach the changing landscape of the pregnant body thoughtfully, to use my touch to explore and interact with the tissues and joints in ways that honor and support the process underway and the mother's experience of it. Many of those techniques are beautifully illustrated and described in this new edition, and they remain the foundations of my clinical and birthing support work today, more than 20 years later.

The conclusions throughout this edition regarding the intent, effectiveness and safety of the work are well supported through the literature review and updates that are among David's many wordsmithing super powers. We all thank you, David.

The expansion and refinement of the labor, postpartum and special needs chapters reflect Michele's vast experience and infectious passion for the birth process, new mothers and expanding our work to some of the most in need. We all thank you, Michele.

And then, winding their way through the text and illustrations are the stories – thoughtful reflections shared by therapists and clients from around the world. These insights, and the addition of new, beautiful color photographs, give the reader an opportunity to stop, reflect and be inspired as you explore the wealth of information that follows.

All that and more, *"in your hands."*

In Michele's foreword in the second edition, she reflected that her well-worn and loved copy of Carole's earlier work has been beside her like a trusted friend throughout her career. I agree: me too!

So, settle in and get ready to meet a potential new best friend in the words that follow. And with that new friend firmly tucked at your side, welcome to the world of *Pre- and Perinatal Massage Therapy*.

Linda Hickey

Registered Massage Therapist

Pre- and Perinatal Massage Therapist

Calgary, Alberta, Canada

November 2020

PREFACE

Welcome to the third edition of *Pre- and Perinatal Massage Therapy*! We have written this book for you – whether you are a massage therapist or a physical therapist, a birth or postpartum doula, a midwife or a nurse, to name just a few possibilities. You care for pregnant, birthing and postpartum clients, or you aspire to. And touch is an integral part of your work. We are so pleased that you are joining us on this journey to touch more effectively.

Consider this book your comprehensive professional guide – a foundation, both theoretical and practical – to utilizing your skilled touch in order to facilitate well-being in childbearing. We want to empower you to work confidently, safely and effectively with your clients, whether they are pregnant, in the throes of labor, or ensconced in parenting. Our aim throughout is to merge head, heart and hands, as well as science and art, so that you can work with greater understanding, empathy and skill. We highlight relevant research – much of it quite new – and merge this evolving scientific data with what we know about the anatomical, physiological and functional changes of the childbearing years. We also acknowledge that many things about pregnancy and birth remain scientifically unknown; we humbly present these ambiguities when there is not sufficient evidence to make a clear benefit claim or guideline. We also strive for a balance of confident, evidence-based guidelines to inform your work, while recognizing the fundamental uniqueness of every person and every session. As a result of your thorough study of *Pre- and Perinatal Massage Therapy*, you will be prepared to think critically, make informed decisions, and both enrich and be enriched by your childbearing clients. Furthermore, you will be prepared to collaborate with other professionals in perinatal healthcare, as we all work together to improve the lives of mothers, babies and communities.

Who You Are Learning From

Just as relevant research and societal awareness have grown greatly in recent years, so has our understanding of maternity massage therapy – and this book. It was originally conceived, written and published by Carole in 1998.

Carole's 2012 edition grew with a textbook publisher and the nutrition of David's extensive academic research and Michele's meticulous, loving review of the manuscript. How fitting that, for this third edition, we now are a trio of authors! Together we offer you greater depth, unique insights and varied expertise in a specialty that all three of us cherish. Together we have updated, expanded and improved every facet of these pages, making a good book even better. Our new publisher, Handspring, brings a fresh design, full color and other excellent features to this third edition. Just as birth requires a shared, caring collaboration, so did the creative work of the book that you now hold in your hands!

Throughout this book, you will hear our three voices as practitioners, teachers and authors. In addition, we feature the experiences of other seasoned pre- and perinatal massage therapists, and their clients, from multiple continents. These personal stories illuminate the healing potency of pre- and perinatal massage therapy and offer ways to grow and nurture a satisfying career. We also incorporate the data of the scientists and researchers from around the world who enlighten our work, inform our techniques and remind us of what remains to be discovered. We invite you to use all of these informed guides as you find your own voice in this work.

What You Will Learn

Pregnancy, birth and the postpartum period is an endlessly intriguing and complex topic – and so are the mechanisms of massage therapy. This book is our effort to blend the two – childbearing and massage – into a simple, easy-to-read and regularly referenced resource to have by your side. To help manage this complexity, here are the highlights of what you will learn in this expanded third edition.

Techniques

To meet the needs of all your maternity massage clients, we present nearly 70 techniques for prenatal, labor, birth and postpartum work. They range from simple to complex, from superficial to deep, and have a variety of physiological, functional, energetic and emotional intentions.

Each is fully detailed in the Technique Manuals that make up the heart of Chapters 4, 5 and 6, with intentions, a step-by-step procedure, hints and precautions. Each technique is illustrated where possible; additionally, our online resources contain video demonstrations of some. For your ease both before and after your sessions, look for the specially marked, green-bordered pages to find the Technique Manuals.

All of these techniques are the result of countless hours of research, practice and refinement. Many originated through our more than 90 years of combined experience; others are the maternity-modified versions of related modalities that we have studied; and a few "tried and true" labor and birth support techniques are duly credited to their originators as relevant.

You will learn in Chapter 4 how to apply these techniques to clients' most common complaints, as well as to the unique concerns of each trimester of pregnancy. Chapter 5 will teach you how to approach client positioning, and techniques for labor and for both vaginal and Cesarean births. Chapter 6 expands with postpartum applications of earlier prenatal techniques, as well as specific techniques after both vaginal and Cesarean births to effectively address immediate and long-term postpartum issues. Chapter 7 will guide you in how to adapt your pre- and perinatal sessions when special needs arise, including identifying and working with clients with high-risk factors and medical complications.

As we finalized this special needs chapter, a new high-risk factor emerged. The COVID-19 pandemic has profoundly impacted this third edition, along with all our lives. It is clear that this new infection has childbearing impacts which are only beginning to reveal themselves, ones that will continue to evolve long after this book's publication. 🌐

Effective Thinking

Well-worn myths and misconceptions about pre- and perinatal massage therapy are as plentiful as they are counterproductive; these cause worry in potential clients and anxiety in therapists. We identify and explore these myths with our most current synthesis of many deep dives into the available massage therapy research, additional research in various related fields, and the relevant details of maternity anatomy and physiology. Chapters 1 and 2 address these massage myths directly, while every chapter is designed to convey facts, build your confidence, lessen your fears and increase your effectiveness.

Our aim is to help you to recognize your clients' strength and abilities, assess any potential problems, and then alter your own work to best honor her needs. To do this requires not only knowledge but also sound reasoning, often quickly applied on the job. Look to the "What would you do?" features throughout the book for brief, realistic scenarios that you might face. Apply your own clinical reasoning and then check out our sample responses to these questions in our online resources.

In our "Points of view" features, you will find our honest, balanced presentation of ongoing debates, contrasting opinions and areas that require more research – a well-rounded, transparent perspective that is rare in our field. From this abundance of data and honesty, we have formulated our guidelines. You will learn both what we recommend and why, to ensure that you are building a thoughtful, evidence-based practice. You also will be better equipped to add your own curiosity, humility and passion to the future conversations and research that will guide the evolution of pre- and perinatal massage therapy.

Expanded Embrace

If you are like most of the 5,000-plus practitioners who have enjoyed our pre- and perinatal massage therapy continuing education workshops, you are probably reading this book because you are interested in, and perhaps a little scared of, massaging pregnant clients. Our hope is to quell those fears and enhance your prenatal massage skills. We also aim to widen your perspective and possibly your practice, inviting you to embrace a broader continuum of care – through and beyond your clients' pregnancies and into birth and postpartum.

In our "Caring for all" features, we identify various aspects of the diversity of your potential clients. We point you toward more resources about these groups and invite your thoughtful reflections on the ethical, professional and practical aspects of providing all people with quality care.

Practical Details

You will learn how to manage the many practical considerations of growing a satisfying career that includes pre- and perinatal massage therapy. In Chapter 3, we give you equipment options and show you how to use what you choose for positioning based on evidence-informed guidelines. We show you how to gracefully and modestly drape your clients, and reposition them on the table when necessary, all while optimizing your own body mechanics for ease and efficiency.

Business Details

With an eye toward your potential pre- and perinatal clientele, in Chapter 8 you will learn about marketing, recordkeeping, interacting with other perinatal professionals and more. We help you to identify common business challenges and ethical issues, and explore how to overcome these obstacles. We also demonstrate how to apply critical thinking to your clients' varied concerns, both typical and unique.

How You Will Learn

In addition to the features mentioned above, we have provided other aides for your learning:
- "Reminder" boxes punctuate important safety considerations and key concepts.

- Key terms stand out in green boldface when first used, with definitions collected into a glossary at the end of the book.
- Many opportunities for further learning are indicated throughout the book in our references to online resources. Instructions for how to access these materials, made available with your purchase of this book, are located on the inside front cover. The online resources include PDFs of additional content, referrals and recommendations for your clients and you, more profiles in success, lesson plans for teaching clients, samples of forms and templates for various business purposes, suggested session sequences and the progression of treatment for several therapists' clients, and video summaries of selected techniques from the Technique Manuals. These are just a few of the online resource materials available to extend your understanding. You will see this globe icon throughout the book as an indicator of materials accessible with the QR codes on the inside cover and at each chapter's conclusion. ⊕
- We have augmented our own suggestions with the practical experiences of some of the thousands of practitioners whom we have trained since 1988, in our own Pre- and Perinatal Massage Therapy specialization workshops. In addition to the "From the treatment room" stories, you can find examples of how this specialization manifests in Chapter 8's practice profiles from each of us and from other successful pre- and perinatal massage therapists who are also authorized instructors of this work. These discussions illustrate the many possible solutions to the fundamental challenge that all massage therapists face: caring for ourselves as we care for our clients. We believe that the result is a perspective on the what, the how and the why of pre- and perinatal massage therapy that is unparalleled.

Our Goals for Your Learning

We see this book in the hands of advanced students of therapeutic massage and bodywork, as well as seasoned therapists and other pre- and perinatal professionals. We expect that teachers of massage therapy will utilize this new edition of *Pre- and Perinatal Massage Therapy* as a cited, recommended or required professional reference in their courses, as we will continue to do in our own continuing education workshops. We trust that this book will also guide employers, managers and other healthcare providers as they incorporate meaningful pre- and perinatal massage therapy into their work environments.

Our world – thankfully – is forever changing. It is easy to assume that we know who our "typical" maternity clients are. The reality is far more complex. With increasing awareness and acceptance of diverse gender identities and ethnic, cultural, religious and family configurations, we invite you to consider with us the range of clients you might see in your practice. Together in this book, we invite you to recognize all people whom you have the privilege to serve: those of a variety of religions, traditions or countries of origin; heterosexual couples, single-parent families, those with more than two parents, and blended families formed by second marriages; families with gay, lesbian or transgender partners and parents, or non-binary and genderqueer parents who carry and give birth to their babies. In this book, we choose to celebrate diversity and empower support of all families, and we invite you to consider how you can – and to recognize when you cannot – care for all.

After discussion of this diversity with our publisher, we decided to retain gender-specific language, for simplicity, economy of expression and to avoid confusion. Thus, we sometimes refer to the pregnant, birthing or postpartum person as "woman" or "mother." But we also use "people," "persons" and "individuals" to acknowledge that a variety of gender identities impact childbearing, just like every other facet of life. Spouses, partners and significant others are usually referred to as "partner," and often with male singular pronouns, but we mean partner to include people of every gender identification and those with various relationships to your clients. We call all individuals our "clients" when they are in our care. We respect all, strive to care for all, and recognize all individuals and families whose identities transcend the limits of grammar and pronouns!

We also want to be clear about what this book does not detail. We do not meaningfully explore birthwork with transgender and gender non-conforming clients. Nor were we able to adequately present the additional complexities of cancer and its many treatments' effects on childbearing, accommodating pregnant and postpartum clients with physical disabilities, and other applications of this work with special populations. We strongly recommend that interested therapists pursue advanced training in these areas to bring caring intentions into informed practice.

Our Invitation

Wherever you are in your work, and however you use this book, our hope is that it powerfully enriches your educational and business goals. We want you to grow a satisfying career in this pre- and perinatal specialty, and, perhaps even more importantly, we want it to feed your passion for positive change in our world.

We know that skilled, therapeutic touch with childbearing people has the potential to positively influence individuals and their families. Your work can begin to knit an ever-widening fabric of nurturing touch into families and, from there, into communities and throughout the world, helping unite and transform our all-too-often violent, touch-averse societies. Throughout our history, human hands have woven fabrics, shaped vessels, grown food and cared for others. Nurturing, knowledgeable tactile communication has been vital to childbearing in most cultures for thousands of years. No matter our individual origins, over millennia some form of touch has provided loving support and eased childbearing discomforts.

We invite you to continue that tradition through our modern, professional manifestation: the practice of pre- and perinatal massage therapy. Join us, and let your work be another pebble tossed into humanity's pond, creating ripples of healing support for individuals, their families and the coming generations. As you do, be bold and informed, sensitive and effective, and offer your clients the ease, pain relief and growth that they need and deserve.

We want to hear from you about your experience with this expanded third edition. Tell us what you think, and find out more about our continuing education offerings, at www.bodytherapyeducation.com.

Carole Osborne
San Diego, CA, USA

Michele Kolakowski
Longmont, CO, USA

David M Lobenstine
Brooklyn, NY, USA

October 2020

Cover image

This soapstone carving, "Mother and Child," was created in Zimbabwe, and gifted to Carole by her son. It represents for us the continuous, dynamic and fluid connection between mother and baby. Enhancing this connection, from in utero and into early mothering, for each individual and for the family of humanity, is the mission that empowers our work.

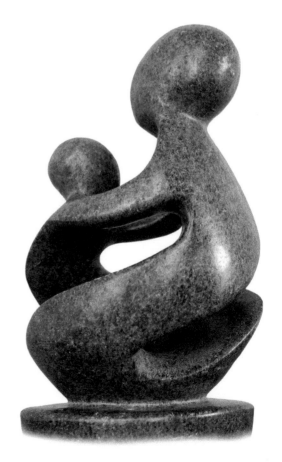

Studying this chapter will prepare you to:

1. describe the societal benefits of maternity massage therapy

2. list six to eight potential beneficial outcomes for individual clients of prenatal, labor and postpartum massage therapy

3. discuss research data that suggest possible positive effects of massage therapy during the childbearing years

4. explain to clients, their families and healthcare providers about the potential benefits of your work with them.

Benefits
Helping Our Clients and Their Babies

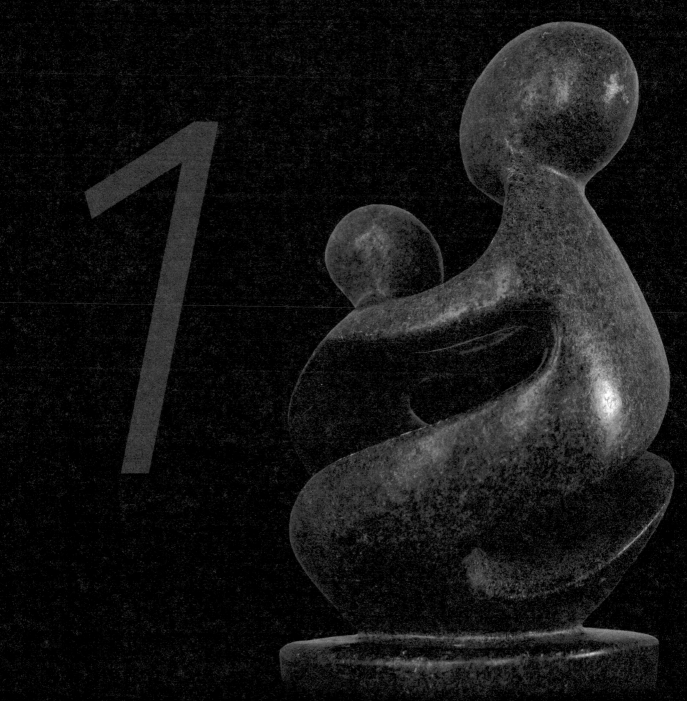

Chapter 1

Chapter Overview

What a gratifying time to be a massage therapist! An ever-growing body of research offers an intellectual expansion of what we have long felt with our hands and hearts. We know more than ever about how and why massage works – and also when and why it is not effective. At the same time, new bits of knowledge prompt additional questions, and remind us of the astounding complexity and wonder of the human body.

It is with this mixture of knowledge and wonder that we approach pregnancy, birth and postpartum – one of the human body's most astonishing transformations. As prepared massage therapists, we have the powerful potential to help facilitate this transformation.

We know that skilled, nurturing touch is good for mothers and their babies. How do we know? We know it by feel, by testimony and by objective data. Every day, another massage therapist feels an expectant client's tension soften and her breath deepen. The therapist's discerning eye sees a client's improving postural integrity, despite that swelling abdomen. Clients regularly leave our therapy tables proclaiming their increased comfort. They report in subsequent sessions their improved mood, sleep and awareness. You will find clients' accounts of these and other positive effects in these pages. You will also find a growing body of data that offers scientific evidence of what many of us have felt anecdotally. Our exploration here will combine personal stories, relevant anatomy and physiology, classic research, and the expanding base of current research in complementary healthcare, to make an emphatic statement: massage therapy, along with other forms of care, improves the outcomes for mothers, babies and their families.

We all need to understand – clients, massage therapists and other healthcare providers alike – that maternity massage therapy does more than just pamper a person (although that, in and of itself, has value!). Massage can improve the well-being of both mother and baby. Your ability to clearly and honestly discuss maternity massage therapy – using precise anatomy and physiology, well-founded theories and substantiated data, as well as acknowledging all that we still do not know – can improve trust, communication and cooperation, both with your potential clients and with other healthcare professionals. With a deeper understanding of the science behind your work, you can reassure all involved that, in almost all circumstances, some form of massage therapy is safe and helpful. With this deeper understanding complementing your technical skills, artistry and intuition, you can offer more effective work.

This chapter highlights the wide range of possible benefits from massage therapy during the **prenatal**, **perinatal** and **postpartum** phases of a woman's normal reproductive life. A comprehensive review of research from varied fields – **obstetrics**, nursing, **midwifery**, physical therapy, **childbirth education**, animal studies and touch therapy – underlies this chapter. These data, augmented with in-depth anatomical and physiological understanding, have led to working theories and guidelines. To these we have added the extensive practical clinical experience of massage therapists, many of whom have worked in maternity massage therapy practices for 30 or more years. We confidently use this ever-evolving body of knowledge as the foundation of our evidence-based specialization in prenatal and perinatal massage therapy. So let us begin to explore the benefits of touch, both holistically and in each of the body systems, for the pregnant client.

Caring for all

In many societies across human history, the ability to conceive, birth and mother has been what defined someone as a woman. Those experiences are a source of great joy and pride for many. But for some, the accompanying expectations are confining. Some people who are pregnant do not identify as women. Others identify as women, but want to avoid the restrictions that gendered language and identities can create. We invite you to consider these enormously complex questions of identity in your own work. A first step is to avoid making assumptions about each client's gender identity or pronoun use. Adopting inclusive language in your **intake** forms, promotional materials and social media facilitates an openness to all. If you want to work with trans or gender non-conforming clients, specialized training in trans health is strongly recommended. How might you adapt your practice so that all people can find safety and comfort in your touch? Our intention in writing this book, as we describe in the Preface, is to provide a similar welcome to all of our readers and the clients we serve.

Touching Humanity, Two Bodies at a Time

Nurturing touch during pregnancy, labor and the post-partum period is not a new concept. Massage and movement during the childbearing experience have long been prominent parts of healthcare in many cultures. India's ancient Ayurvedic medical manuals offer instructions for rubbing specially formulated oils into pregnant patients' stretched abdominal skin. Traditional sculptures depict Eskimo fathers supporting and lovingly stroking their wives' backs during labor (Goldsmith 1984). In contemporary hospitals worldwide, birth doulas or midwives hold and stroke the laboring woman however and whenever she needs (Bohren et al. 2019; Klaus et al. 2012). Midwives, who for centuries have provided most of the world's maternity care, have highly developed hands-on skills. For billions of women, over thousands of years, touch has provided loving support, knowledgeable assistance and much-needed ease.

Anthropological studies indicate that, in the world's more peaceful cultures, touch is prominent during pregnancy and early childhood (Prescott 2005). There is an 80 percent correlation, found across 49 societies, between high levels of infant physical attention – including caressing and carrying the infant on the mother's body – and low levels of crime and violence – including theft, torture, mutilation and slavery (Prescott 2005).

The same researchers studied offspring separated from their mothers – who thus lost the opportunity for bonding – primarily with Harry Harlow's famous research monkeys. These young monkeys spent their formative periods of brain growth apart from their mothers. They were less capable of affection and pleasure and more inclined toward depression, isolation and violence to self and others. The lack of sensory input typically provided by the mother's touching and rocking, it seems, damages the development of the neuronal systems that control affection and mediate violent behaviors (Voltolini et al. 2014; Prescott 2005).

Around the world, we are witness to political, religious and cultural conflicts; so many of these, it seems, are defined by divisiveness rather than dialogue, isolation rather than connection, distance rather than contact.

Though our work is minuscule compared to the scope of the globe's dilemmas, it can make a meaningful difference. Personal stories and an ever-growing body of data suggest that massage therapy has some potential to spread the far-reaching benefits of touch. Massage therapists, we believe, are contributing to a more peaceful world. By nurturing mothers through massage, we aid in the momentous process of pregnancy, birth and parenting; we enable these mothers to better nurture their babies. We now have a variety of studies that suggest massage with pregnant people has multiple positive effects, including a reduction in prenatal and postpartum depression, prematurity and low birth weight; an improvement in sleep patterns; lower cortisol levels; and less pain both during pregnancy and in labor (Field et al. 2010a). The results are convincing: therapeutic touch is global in its benefits, affecting a variety of body systems, and both the mother and the baby. And the results are lasting: when labors have fewer complications, and there are fewer preterm births (Field et al. 1999), that translates directly into less separation of mother and newborn, and more time for and inclination toward the type of bonding that seems so integral to a culture capable of peace, love and happiness.

Given this connection between touch and reduction of violence, massage therapists and others working with childbearing clients should take great pride in their contributions to more loving families, communities and the world, now and across future generations.

Pregnant with Stress

Most people regard motherhood as one of life's most precious opportunities. Often, however, this intense emotional investment is the very thing that can make the many weeks of pregnancy so stressful. Committed to the best for her baby, the mother can pressure herself in so many ways to be perfect. It is hard to eat right, exercise just enough and maintain a job, especially as pregnancy's common discomforts get in the way. For those people who are hesitant about being pregnant, all of these difficulties are heightened. In other words, for nearly all people, in one way or another, pregnancy and stress are inseparable. Where does an expectant person's stress originate? How does it affect pregnancy outcomes? How can relaxation, particularly from massage therapy, reduce the negative effects of stress? These are the questions we address below.

A Time of Transitions and Expectations

Although pregnancy is a welcome blessing for most, it brings many changes for all involved (Figure 1.1). As her body transforms, the woman must adjust to her altered physiological functioning. The shape of her pregnant

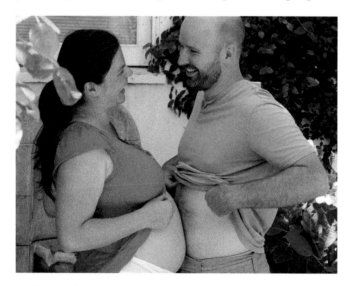

Figure 1.1
Joyful welcoming. Pregnancy may be stressful, but it can bring a family closer as they prepare for the new baby.

body shifts, and her gait and other movement patterns usually alter. As her hair and skin and hormones change, she may feel as though she is no longer her former physical or emotional self.

Pregnancy is often a time of upheaval and anxiety, as well as a time of euphoria and joy. In a single day, a pregnant person's emotions may fluctuate tremendously. Her relationships to her partner, parents, friends and co-workers will all change. Issues that may have been repressed sometimes resurface, including the legacies of physical and emotional abuse. Pregnancy often requires her to be more dependent on others than she is used to and forces a reckoning with what, for some, are uncomfortable societal roles and expectations. A new baby can stretch emotions, finances and careers – often, all at the same time – and can especially strain families with fewer resources.

An alarming number of pregnant people also suffer abuse from their partners (Alhusen et al. 2015). Furthermore, one-quarter of pregnancies are at higher risk of developing serious, sometimes life-threatening, medical complications (see Chapter 7). Pregnant people who are single, or lesbian, or non-binary, or handicapped, or surrogates, often have additional challenges unique to their non-traditional situations. In this period, when every person needs support, many find themselves isolated, without the community and familial support of former times or of kin-based cultures.

Pregnancy is also suffused with expectation. Many women have more apparent control than ever over whether, when and how they become pregnant. They are increasingly likely to delay pregnancy and have fewer children (Mathews and Hamilton 2014; Ely and Hamilton 2018). The result is a growing number of people whose pregnancies are deliberately timed or come after investing years and thousands of dollars in **assisted reproductive technology** treatments. These pregnancies can take on greater significance and emotional investment.

Popular culture can create the expectation of childbearing as a romantic, blissful time; for many people, the reality is more complicated. Some dislike the feeling of being pregnant. Some are overwhelmed by the abundance of childbirth education and other choices available to them, and they worry about all the things that could go wrong. Some plan their "ideal" birth and feel anguish over anything that falls short. Some cling to real or imagined promises of painless, risk-free labor through technology and pharmaceuticals to assuage their fears about the upcoming birth. Health problems, not to mention stresses from the rest of life, increase maternal and fetal risks for some women, adding additional layers of apprehension about the pregnancy's outcome (Ricci 2017).

Reminder

Be prepared to support and care for clients with a wide range of feelings about their pregnancies and those from varying socioeconomic and familial support systems.

Maternal and Fetal Consequences

With all of these concerns, it is no surprise that pregnancy is often a time of increased stress. Stress activates the **sympathetic branch of the autonomic nervous system**. This increases adrenal production of stress hormones, creating a fight, flight or freeze response. Such activation is essential for our survival – think of slamming the car brakes to avoid an accident. However, both acute stressors and chronic sympathetic arousal, provoked by ongoing worries and anxieties, can have negative impacts on mother and baby (Spradley 2019; Reyes et al. 2018).

Today, the topic of stress seems ubiquitous. But amidst our ongoing complaints about how stressed we are, or how stressed out we feel, it is useful to consider the very concrete and far-reaching ways that stress impacts health. In the rapidly growing fetus, and the rapidly changing mother, the manifestations of stress can be many.

In one study, elevated amounts of maternal stress (both psychosocial stress and cortisol levels) early in pregnancy were associated with poorer cognitive performance when the baby was a year old (Davis and Sandman 2010). In addition, prenatal depression – which is both caused by various social and physiological stressors, and

furthers those sources of stress – has been correlated with prematurity and low birth weight (Field 2017).

Multiple systematic reviews reveal a litany of consequences emerging from prenatal stress. During pregnancy and birth, there is an association between prenatal stress and:

- **preterm labor**
- preterm birth
- low birth weight
- restricted fetal growth
- **pre-eclampsia**
- **gestational diabetes** (Field 2017; Coussons-Read 2013).

Those negative consequences can, in turn, continue into the baby's life, manifesting in:

- hyper-responsiveness to stress
- asthma
- allergies
- temperamental difficulties
- affective disorders
- **attachment** difficulties (Coussons-Read 2013).

This growing body of evidence supports the "fetal origins hypothesis," which argues that what the fetus is exposed to *in utero* – not just environmental factors, but also psychosocial ones – "can have sustained effects across the lifespan" of the child (Kinsella and Monk 2009; Monk et al. 2016). Indeed, one review argues that "prenatal stress can have consequences that span generations" (Coussons-Read 2013).

From the treatment room

Massage therapy is so relaxing. I hadn't done much for myself since I became pregnant, and I can really see how it benefits me and my baby by loosening muscles and making me slow down.

– Melissa, client

What We Can Do

The potential burdens of pregnancy are numerous. Yet there is a way to help with all of them: learning how to relax and to focus internally. Relaxation and self-awareness tend to increase well-being for both mother and baby, and the chances for positive birth experiences. Learning relaxation techniques is correlated with a host of benefits: "fewer admissions to the hospital, fewer obstetric complications, longer gestation, reduction of caesarean sections, and fewer postpartum complications" (Fink et al. 2012). Women and their partners who learn relaxation techniques are better able to adapt to stress and pain during pregnancy and labor, and in the days and years of parenting (ACOG 2019; Ricci 2017; Hetherington 2007; Nichols and Humenick 2000).

As a massage therapist, you can offer each pregnant client a unique and potent experience of support and relaxation. Massage therapy supports expectant clients because it generally makes them feel good, function more effectively and feel more optimistic. Massage is often intrinsically relaxing – encouraging a client to turn inward, concentrating on her own body and mind rather than on external events, cultivating the ability to let go (Samuels and Samuels 1996). That is the perfect preparation for coping with the demands of labor and birth.

In fact, in preparation for labor, many perinatal specialists recommend women practice deep and sustained levels of relaxation for 45 to 60 minutes without falling asleep, especially in the last six to eight weeks of pregnancy – the exact length of most massage therapy sessions (Simkin 2018)! A massage therapist can create a nurturing atmosphere, offer a moment of undisturbed quiet and encourage a slow, regular breath – all of which invites deep relaxation to take place.

In contrast to the "fight or flight" effects of stress, support and relaxation activate the parasympathetic branch of the autonomic nervous system. This "rest and digest" branch provides balance and promotes calm. When relaxed, an expectant person will have steadier blood pressure, pulse and respiratory rates; regular blood flow to uterus, placenta and fetus; and healthier immune system functioning, emotional states, and responses to

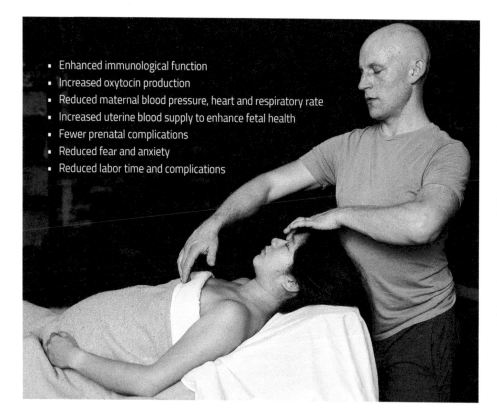

- Enhanced immunological function
- Increased oxytocin production
- Reduced maternal blood pressure, heart and respiratory rate
- Increased uterine blood supply to enhance fetal health
- Fewer prenatal complications
- Reduced fear and anxiety
- Reduced labor time and complications

Figure 1.2
Possible maternal and fetal benefits of prenatal relaxation.

stressful stimuli. Optimal fetal positioning may be more likely too. (Nichols and Humenick 2000; Guan et al. 2014; Lee et al. 2011; Tully 2020).

Reminder

Increased relaxation facilitates healthy circulation to the uterus that improves fetal well-being.

Even a single massage therapy session produces measurable biologic effects, both reducing a client's pain and creating broader changes. Multiple sessions are potentially even more powerful in reducing pain and diminishing anxiety and depression (Rapaport et al. 2010; Moyer et al. 2004). We now have a number of systematic reviews, from the Samueli Institute and Tiffany Field, among others, that make these benefits clear, for people reckoning with injuries, medical conditions and just the inevitable changes of life (Crawford et al. 2016; Boyd et al. 2016a; Boyd et al. 2016b; Field 2016).

The benefits of massage during pregnancy, though infrequently studied, are also becoming increasingly validated. In one study, depressed pregnant women were given 20-minute massages for 12 weeks; compared to the control group that received standard care, the massaged women reported a decrease in depression, anxiety and pain scales, and an improvement in relationships with their significant others (Field 2017).

Massage can create the same positive physiological states and increased alpha brain-wave activity as meditation. Massage strokes provide variations in pressure, rhythm and positioning that flood the sensory nerve pathways with input, increasing body awareness and overriding signals of pain and stress (Benjamin 2016; Juhan 2003).

Massage therapists do not just provide soothing, nurturing touch; they also bring focused attention to their clients' particular concerns. This regular, caring contact can be a vital component of a pregnant client's support system, especially when family and friends are not providing such assistance. All therapists can listen attentively and non-judgmentally; those with complementary skills and training in counseling and emotional processing can offer additional aid as clients reckon with the strong emotions and vast changes of pregnancy. When needed, massage therapists provide referrals to other professionals. They also can educate the pregnant client in ways to use her mind and body that assist in managing and reducing stress. Indeed, how we talk with a client can be as important as the techniques we use (Fogarty et al. 2020).

However extensive the negative effects of stress are, it appears that proper support can counteract these effects (Box 1.1). Many expectant massage therapy clients claim that massage therapy helped them in carrying to full **term**, having fewer complications and feeling more peace (Osborne 2009). One study considered several hundred pregnant women who had many difficult life changes in the two years immediately preceding and/or during their pregnancy. Those who also had strong support systems had significantly fewer complications – both during pregnancy and in the postpartum period – compared to those who experienced similar stresses without a support system (Giesbrecht et al. 2013; Lancaster et al. 2010; Hobel and Colhane 2003; Nuckolls et al. 1972). And during labor, women who had "continuous support" had a host of benefits, from lower rates of **Cesarean births** and **epidurals** to higher levels of satisfaction (Kozhimannil 2013).

Box 1.1
Ways in which prenatal massage therapy reduces stress

- Nurturing, skilled touch
- Attention to individual needs
- Emotional support, especially in the absence of supportive family and friends
- Non-judgmental listening and emotional processing
- Education and encouragement in stress-reducing activities
- Appropriate referrals to other specialists

Researchers are also starting to document what most people know intuitively. Fight, flight and freeze are not the only stress reactions; women also respond with a pattern known as "tend and befriend" (Taylor 2012). In trying times, women instinctively care for others and surround themselves with supportive people. Interestingly enough, the neuroendocrine core of this response seems to be female reproductive hormones, particularly oxytocin – a hormone that is responsible for gestational developments and mothering responses, and that massage therapy seems to increase (Morhenn et al. 2012; Uvnäs-Moberg 2019; Taylor et al. 2000)! How appropriate, then, that so many people seek out the nurturing care of a skilled and supportive massage therapist during this time of stressful and joyous transitions.

What would you do?

A new client spends her entire massage animatedly sharing the details of her pregnancy. She also asks you many questions. You share in her excitement, yet you also know that she is missing out on certain benefits of the session. Why might it be important for her to turn inward and "focus" in her treatments? What can you do to encourage that – with your words, your hands and your environment – while honoring her wish to share?

Physiological Benefits

Long before most people are aware that they are pregnant, the endocrine system has begun to orchestrate a confluence of changes in every system of the body. An intricate sequence of hormonal communications immediately begins preparing the newly pregnant body for the nine months of creative activity ahead (Figure 1.3). Human chorionic gonadotropin (hCG), a hormone detected in home urine pregnancy tests, ensures adequate first-trimester hormonal levels. The fertilized egg itself manages the pregnancy for the first few weeks, and the placenta is fully functioning by 12 weeks, an example of how well the body usually works to ensure a viable pregnancy (Ricci 2017).

The mother's endocrine glands and ovaries enlarge and accelerate production of the hormones that cause the vast physiological adaptations to come. In its functions as an endocrine organ, the placenta produces additional estrogen, progesterone and other pregnancy-specific hormones. These powerful chemicals stimulate positive changes that increase fuel and vitamin and mineral supplies, ensuring sufficient maternal energy levels and robust fetal growth. These changes include increased energy storage in the form of fat in the thighs, buttocks and abdomen.

Progesterone also relaxes smooth muscle linings of the following: (1) the digestive tract, thus maximizing intestinal absorption time and uptake of iron, calcium and other nutrients; (2) the uterine muscles, to prevent excessive, premature contractions; and (3) the vascular walls, to maintain a healthy, low blood pressure. Another of progesterone's effects is increased respiratory efficiency, characterized by greater tidal volume in the lungs and faster respiratory rate to handle increased cardiac output (Ricci 2017).

Meanwhile, estrogen stimulates the following: (1) uterine growth and blood supply; (2) balanced salt, water and insulin levels; and (3) increased metabolic efficiency in sugar and carbohydrate use. Another hormone, relaxin, works together with progesterone and estrogen to soften connective tissue; hormone levels fluctuate as the pregnancy progresses so that joints and soft tissues can accommodate uterine and fetal growth. These vital hormonal adaptations are evidence of the body's "wisdom" in sustaining a healthy pregnancy. They are also responsible, in part, for the mother's initial months of exhaustion, urinary frequency and, often, morning sickness (Ricci 2017).

A small body of scientific evidence, and a large body of anecdotal evidence, tell us that massage therapy may facilitate these essential physiological changes of pregnancy – while, at the same time, helping to minimize many of the attendant discomforts that result. (Note that some of your clients may seek medical, pharmacological and non-pharmacological relief for these secondary symptoms. Although massage therapy

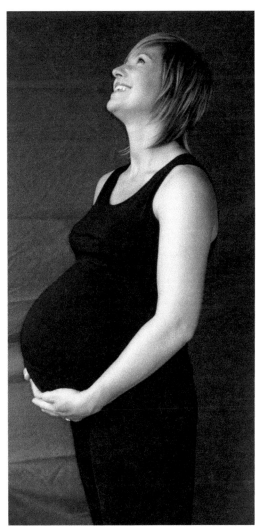

Gland	Hormone produced: function of hormone
Placenta	• estrogen: ensures placental viability, fetal circulation and health; softens ligaments, connective tissue and cervix; relaxes smooth muscles • progesterone: supports endometrium; quiets uterine motility; regulates respiratory changes • four chorionic hormones: support endometrium and breast development and glucose metabolism; increase thyroid production
Ovaries	• estrogen, relaxin: relax ligaments, connective tissue; increase cervical dilation • progesterone: supports endometrium
Trophoblastic cells and fetal adrenals	• two chorionic hormones, estrogen: initiate labor
Pituitary	• prolactin: stimulates milk production • oxytocin: stimulates uterine contractions
Adrenals	• estrogen • progesterone
Thyroid	• triiodothyronine (T3) Together, these hormones regulate the body's • thyroxine (T4) temperature, metabolism and heart rate • calcitonin
Parathyroid	• parathyroid hormone (PTH): regulates calcium and phosphate

Figure 1.3
Prenatal endocrine activity. Many organs produce numerous hormones that have far-ranging effects on mother and fetus.

may help to reduce the intensity or shorten the duration of these symptoms, as well as alleviating them, it is not within our scope of practice to instruct clients to discontinue any medical treatments or medications.)

Below we will discuss these systemic changes in descending order of relevance to us as massage therapists: the circulatory, respiratory, gastrointestinal, integumentary and urinary systems. Our work is so effective for the pervasive changes to the musculoskeletal system that we will explore that in its own separate section.

Circulatory System Benefits

The circulatory system makes brilliant adaptations to provide for the needs of the growing fetus. From as early as weeks 10 to 12, elevated estrogen and progesterone production increases total blood volume. It peaks by weeks 32 to 34, when the body is producing 50 percent more blood than prior to pregnancy. Levels of all blood components – white blood cells, plasma, serum protein and serum enzymes – are elevated. Because red blood cells increase at a lower rate than these other elements, many women develop a physiological anemia. The positive result of all of these changes is more oxygen/carbon dioxide exchange, a higher supply of nutrients and hydration, and better removal of waste for both the mother and the baby (Ricci 2017).

The heart actually enlarges slightly to accommodate this increased load, and by week 32 its output (stroke volume) is 30 to 50 percent higher than before pregnancy. Heart rate increases by 10 to 15 beats per minute, beginning in the second trimester and persisting to term. Progesterone causes peripheral **vasodilation**, to help the vessels accommodate the increased load; one result is that blood pressure actually declines slightly in pregnancy. Blood pressure is at its lowest during mid-pregnancy, but maintains pre-pregnancy levels in the first and third trimesters in normal pregnancies. A significant rise in prenatal blood pressure can be indicative of **gestational hypertensive disorders** (Ricci 2017), a complication that can be a serious risk for both the mother and the baby and needs close monitoring (see Chapter 7).

Most of these normal circulatory system changes go relatively unnoticed by the expectant mother. Far more obvious is the 40 percent increase in interstitial fluid volume over non-pregnant levels. By the third trimester, this increase often results in **edema**, most noticeable in her arms and legs. Both the weighty uterus and myofascial restrictions around the pelvis contribute to this swelling, working much like a cork in a bottle and restricting femoral fluid return (Figure 1.4). As a result, about 75 percent of people experience normal, pregnancy-induced (non-pitting) edema in the lower extremities, usually in the late second or third trimester. Some individuals can develop numbness, tingling and burning sensations in the feet and lower legs as the extra fluid compresses on the tarsal nerve, creating **tarsal tunnel syndrome**. When this fluid increase pervades the pectoral girdle, **carpal tunnel syndrome** can develop, causing moderate to severe pain in the arms and hands, particularly in the middle and index fingers (Zyluk 2013).

These vascular changes can cause **varicose veins** and **spider veins**. Women can feel self-conscious about them, but these are the result of progesterone's wise relaxation of the smooth muscle walls of all blood vessels, which

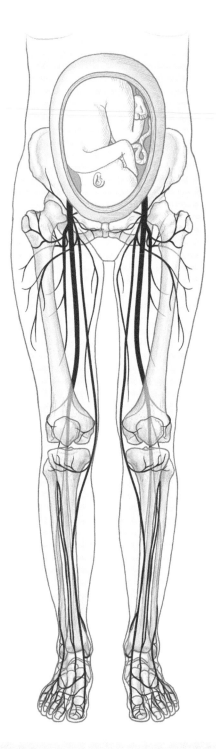

Figure 1.4
Arteries and veins of the leg.

particularly challenges the integrity of the femoral, saphenous and other leg veins. As blood flow from the legs is restricted, due to uterine compression of the iliac veins and inferior vena cava, **femoral venous blood pressure** increases and distends the vessels; varicose veins are the result. A person's heredity and diet, prolonged sitting or standing, and the position and size of her baby help determine the degree of edema and varicosities. Some women also develop varicose veins on the vulva and anus, creating **hemorrhoids**. Spider veins are what result when these dilated peripheral blood vessels burst, creating areas of reddish broken capillaries, typically on the legs, face and upper body (Ricci 2017).

During pregnancy, the blood's ability to clot increases and its clot-dissolving capacity (**fibrinolysis**) decreases dramatically. The change makes her less likely to **hemorrhage** during childbirth, but more likely to develop blood clots called **thrombi**, particularly in the legs and groin. Thrombi are also the result of the growing uterus restricting iliac and femoral circulation and contributing to sluggish blood flow; higher progesterone levels relaxing vascular smooth muscles; and increased metabolic demands elevating blood and interstitial fluid volumes (Devis and Knuttinen 2017; Jefferies and Bochner 1991). Although these changes are mostly unnoticed by pregnant people, we need to be very aware of this increased thrombi risk and take specific precautions during sessions (see Chapter 2).

From the treatment room

Before the massage, I had been holding water in my legs and feet. Afterwards, the swelling lessened, and my whole body felt very relaxed and ready for a peaceful nap.

– Aletha, client

Now let us discuss how massage affects the circulatory system – or does not. It is a long-standing claim that Swedish massage increases circulation – that our work "moves the blood" in one way or another. Though this concept is frequently mentioned, it has never been sufficiently proven or disproven. A few recent, and very small, experiments have demonstrated various shifts in blood flow after massage (Sefton et al. 2010; Munk et al. 2012); other studies have concluded the opposite – that massage has no impact on circulation (Hinds et al. 2004; Shoemaker et al. 1997; Wiltshire et al. 2010).

There is similar uncertainty about whether lymphatic massage techniques (typically taught as either Manual Lymph Drainage or Lymph Drainage Therapy) can be useful for the excess fluid of pregnancy. First, most of the lymph research has been done on postoperative patients, whose lymph nodes have been removed or otherwise impaired. Second, while some research has demonstrated clear benefits (Zimmerman et al. 2012), at least one systematic review found no impact (Huang et al. 2013). Beyond anecdotal evidence that lymph drainage can be helpful both during and after pregnancy (see Chapter 6), there is no scientific consensus or recommendation.

Across the last half-century, several theories have sought to explain how Swedish strokes (as well as lymphatic drainage techniques) might counteract pregnancy's increase in blood and interstitial fluid volumes, and the edema that results. Performed rhythmically, lymphatic strokes might work like a hydraulic pump, shifting excess fluid from the tissues to the blood and lymph vessels (Zanolla et al. 1984). The mechanical effects of compression strokes theoretically increase capillary blood flow and produce local vasodilation through increased histamine release. It is theorized that these effects also may be induced through autonomic vascular reflexes, which promote delivery of oxygen and nutrients and removal of waste materials (Arkko et al. 1983; Linde 1989). But again, these theories are speculative and increasingly dated.

Amidst this uncertainty, it may be helpful to consider one of our profession's other most persistent claims: that massage "releases" or "flushes" toxins from the body. This is little more than a myth, and a good example of how broad, unsubstantiated explanations for why massage feels good does not benefit us or our clients (Walton 2016). Such concerns led some therapists to suggest that breastfeeding moms should "pump and dump" after a massage session – an unfounded precaution that we do *not* endorse.

Instead of insisting on unfounded beliefs, we should educate our clients about what we do know, and be honest about what we do not. If massage does not actually impact the circulation of blood or lymph during pregnancy, is your work any less valuable? No. So instead of this broad, but unverified, claim about "increasing circulation," let us explore two other ways in which our work may benefit the circulatory system.

Though we do not know whether (or how) massage impacts circulation, increasing research suggests that massage does have an effect on the autonomic nervous system, by encouraging parasympathetic activity – the "rest and digest" response (Diego and Field 2009; Field 2016). Massage may, in turn, impact the circulatory system in at least two ways: improving heart-rate variability (HRV) and regulating blood pressure (Guan et al. 2014; Lee et al. 2011). Two small, older studies, in which slow, rhythmic stroking stimulated parasympathetic activity (Longworth 1982; Fakouri and Jones 1987), also suggest that we might be able to normalize heart rate and blood pressure. The Autonomic Sedation Sequence 3–1–1 technique, detailed in Chapter 4, deserves further research, as it potentially could increase relaxation while contributing to the management or prevention of gestational hypertensive disorders. Instead of just "moving" blood, massage's impact on the autonomic realm suggests benefits for the circulatory and just about every other system of the body. This autonomic response also might explain why our pregnant clients proclaim how much better they feel after a prenatal massage.

We also know that the body's circulatory system is inextricably linked to – and can be restricted by – the body's musculature and fascia. And we are aware that both blood and lymph depend on muscular contraction to enable movement. Restrictions in the fascia or soft tissue may reduce local circulation in both upper and lower extremities. **Deep tissue massage** to the pectoralis major and minor and other pectoral girdle structures may help reduce carpal tunnel syndrome symptoms (Zyluk 2013). If pelvic restrictions are found, specific myofascial and/or passive movement techniques that reduce those restrictions may help to relieve edema (Benjamin 2016). Clients derive great benefit from gentle

leg and pelvic work, while we use caution (see Chapter 2) to work safely there.

While new research can seem to minimize our grand claims for the benefits of massage, this evolving understanding should not discourage us. Indeed, new research is often a reminder of the incredible adaptive abilities of the human body, and the fact that our work is most beneficial when we see massage not as changing the body, but as facilitating its own inherent processes.

Respiratory System Benefits

Elevated progesterone production prompts a 30 to 40 percent increase in the exchange of gases with each breath or tidal volume, yet most expectant people still tend to feel short of breath and often hyperventilate. The typical pregnant breathing pattern – rapid, shallow and in the upper chest – is the result of the growing uterus restricting the diaphragm's movement and the chest's expansion (Ricci 2017). Compensating for an enlarged abdomen and breasts, many women also lean back, as though to prevent falling forward. This shifts the upper thoracic area posteriorly while the lower ribcage presses more anteriorly. At the same time, the pectoral girdle tends to rotate anteriorly, further restricting ribcage expansion.

We can help the pregnant client correct counterproductive breathing patterns – whether shallow, or rapid, or **paradoxical breathing** – by guiding them in diaphragmatic (sometimes called abdominal) breathing. Diaphragmatic breathing promotes relaxation, reduces stress, and relieves the musculoskeletal strain of inefficient breathing on the neck, chest and upper back (Xiao, Zi-Qi et al. 2017). Although the inferior ribcage circumference is expanded by the uterus, our clients often benefit from instruction in more lateral and posterior ribcage expansion to foster easier and more effective breathing.

Deep tissue massage, structural realignment guidance, passive and active movement, and **trigger point** therapy may improve breathing by correcting restrictive postural deviations and improving neck, abdomen and chest mobility (Thompson and Brooks 2016). Furthermore, massage seems to increase parasympathetic nervous system activity, which in turn prompts the slow, effortless breathing that is essential as the growing uterus compresses the ribcage and lungs. Myofascial restriction, tender points and habitual holding patterns in the scalenes, sternocleidomastoid, intercostals, pectoralis major and minor, levator scapulae, rhomboids, trapezius and serratus anterior require particular attention (Allen and Pounds 2016).

From the treatment room

I had felt a stitch in my side for weeks. After last session's deeper breathing and those strokes on my ribs, that's gone. Relaxing and breathing to my baby seems to make this all more real to me, too.

– Kim, client

Many women have uncomfortable congestion in the nose and sinuses due to estrogen-induced increased vascularity in the respiratory tract. This worsens when she has a cold, or if she cannot take her typical medication for respiratory allergies or asthma. She will especially appreciate facial massage and use of pressure points that emphasize sinus relief. You also can teach her self-massage that may help ease sinus discomfort (Ferguson 1995; Stillerman 2013).

Gastrointestinal System Benefits

Progesterone seems to have one purpose for the digestive system: to extract every morsel of nutrition to grow a healthy baby. To do so, it relaxes the smooth muscle lining of most of the digestive system. This relaxation decreases peristalsis; the slower movement of food through the gastrointestinal tract allows for maximal absorption. Unfortunately the secondary effects described below are often far more noticeable for pregnant people: constipation, **gastric reflux** and sometimes gall bladder disease.

Twenty-five percent of all expectant mothers are frequently constipated (Ricci 2017). With the decrease in peristalsis, and intestines that are compressed by the growing uterus, food is usually processed more slowly. The resulting higher water absorption, especially in combination with iron supplements, low-fiber foods and

any decreased activity level, creates bloating and strained bowel movements. Often hemorrhoids develop, too.

The enlarged uterus also presses on both the stomach and the gall bladder. Combined with a more relaxed esophageal sphincter, stomach acid is more likely to regurgitate into the upper esophagus, causing burning pain in the mid-chest and throat. Seventy percent of all women have this heartburn, especially in later pregnancy and when lying down (Ricci 2017).

Estrogen, progesterone and hCG are partially responsible for another common gastrointestinal complaint: nausea and vomiting, known as morning sickness. hCG maintains a woman's estrogen levels in early pregnancy, inhibits maternal rejection of the embryo as foreign tissue, and increases basal temperature. Its high level is a suspected cause of morning sickness, particularly common in weeks 6 to 12. But some women continue to feel sick throughout their pregnancies, and some are nauseated all day and night (Ricci 2017).

Many direct massage techniques that therapists use to relieve constipation are potentially unsafe during pregnancy (see Chapter 2). As an alternative, **acupressure** and **reflexive techniques** may assist gastrointestinal functioning. Although data to validate its effectiveness are currently mixed, many therapists and clients report good results from work on specific zones in the feet and hands (see Figures 4.13 and 7.3); along certain acupuncture meridians (Flocco 1993; Enzer 2004; Wang et al. 2008); and using acupressure (Steel et al. 2015). Several studies suggest that nausea and vomiting can often be reduced with daily acupressure to the Pericardium 6 (PC-6) point on the forearms (see Figure 7.3) (Ozgoli and Saei Ghare Naz 2018).

We cannot fix these gastrointestinal discomforts, but it is possible that massage therapy helps counteract the negative nutritional impact of vomiting. Several studies of premature infants documented significant weight gain for infants that were massaged. Researchers have proposed that massage increases vagal nerve activity, which stimulates production of food absorption hormones (Diego et al. 2005; Wheeden et al. 1993). Extrapolating from these infant studies, Swedish massage strokes might improve the pregnant body's ability to use nutrients.

Integumentary System Benefits

Perhaps one of the most significant benefits of prenatal massage therapy is the simple yet profound effect of skin stimulation. Ashley Montagu, anthropologist and "skin scholar," describes the brain as "the inside layer of the skin, and the skin the outside layer of the brain" (Montagu 1978). Not only is our skin the largest organ of the body, but studies show it has an "active interface with the endocrine, immune, and central nervous systems" (Thompson and Brooks 2016).

A number of classic animal studies – comparing rats and mice that were gentled (stroked) with non-gentled control groups – document the widespread importance of skin stimulation through touch. Pups of gentled rats and mice opened their eyes sooner after birth, were more active, developed motor coordination earlier and weighed more at weaning. Stroked animals had stronger immune systems and showed 50 percent more synaptic junctions. They were more sexually active. They were more curious and calmer, made better problem solvers, and had superior mothering skills.

These rats' superior motor, mental and social development lasted their entire lives. The positive results of tactile stimulation increased further when handlers stroked these animals throughout their maturation. The non-gentled control animals in these studies, by contrast, were more excitable, timid and fearful; they tended toward rage reactions in response to frustration, and they often bit each other and their caretakers (Meaney et al. 1989; Pauk et al. 1986; Meaney et al. 1985; Weininger et al. 1954; Rosen 1957; Denenberg and Karas 1960; Tapp and Markowitz 1963; Juraska et al. 1980). Add these studies to the data discussed earlier and, as "professional skin stimulators," the argument for the peace-promoting potential of prenatal massage therapists grows even stronger.

Even more directly relevant to maternity massage therapy, consider the many negative effects observed when pregnant rats could not self-stimulate by licking. An experimental group of expectant rats wore large collars that restricted the characteristic licking of their swelling abdomens and teats. The collared rats' mammary development was 50 percent less than that of the control rats.

These mothers built their nests randomly and ineffectively, and then delivered fewer live offspring than control mothers. They neglected cleaning the afterbirth and licking their young. Fewer pups survived this neglect, and their mothers had difficulties in nursing them. Even their placentas were poorly developed; these trailblazing researchers postulated that the skin stimulation provided by licking promoted the secretion of the hormones vital for healthy pregnancies (see Figure 1.3) (Roth and Rosenblatt 1996).

These studies suggest that:

- Skin stimulation stimulates the brain, creating positive effects in all body systems of both the mother and the baby.

- Touch during pregnancy promotes the production of hormones – especially progesterone, estrogen, oxytocin, **human placental lactogen** and **prolactin** – which seem to improve pregnancy outcomes and encourage appropriate mothering behaviors.

- Massage and other touch therapies inherently provide pregnant, laboring and postpartum people with these broad physiological benefits.

Reminder

Skin stimulation = brain stimulation = improved placental functioning = improved hormonal production.

Pregnancy brings changes in the texture, oiliness and pigmentation of skin. As the abdominal skin stretches over the expanding uterus, it can become dry, itchy and taut. The pregnant client may develop stretch marks called **striae gravidarum** on her abdomen, breasts and other areas where weight and size increases are most dramatic. Darker patches may develop across her cheeks and nose (**chloasma**), and a dark line known as the **linea nigra** may develop from pubic bone to xiphoid process. Oil or other lubricants used during a massage can feel soothing.

As we attend to a pregnant client's aches and pains, it is easy to lose sight of the manifold benefits of our contact with the skin. But we must remember that "touch is the first of our senses to develop, providing us with the sensory scaffold on which we come to perceive our own bodies and our sense of self" (Bremner and Spence 2017). And that perception of self happens via our integumentary system, since "the skin is the site of events and processes crucial to the way we think about, feel about, and interact with one another" (Morrison et al. 2010).

Urinary System Benefits

Pregnancy's effects on the urinary system are the source of many laughs, but it is no joke to expectant people. Urinary frequency is highest in the first trimester and in the final weeks of pregnancy, particularly after the baby's engagement or lightening, when its head (or feet, if in breech presentation) descends lower into the pelvis, further compressing the bladder. The sidelying sleeping common in later pregnancy – and recommended by the American College of Obstetricians and Gynecologists – allows greater blood circulation from the legs, increasing renal perfusion and filtration; most women complain of getting up four or more times a night to use the toilet. Decreased bladder tone and longer emptying time are other bothersome complaints. The swelling uterus compresses both the bladder and its ureters, slowing urination and reducing bladder space. Progesterone simultaneously enlarges the kidneys and ureters, accommodating their increased workload. Urinary output is 40 to 60 percent greater, initially because of hormonal fluctuations, and then, later in pregnancy, because of increased fluid and waste product removal. All of these factors increase the likelihood of bladder and kidney infections during pregnancy (Ricci 2017).

As pregnancy progresses, weight gain also strains the pelvic floor muscles (Figure 1.5). Many women leak small amounts of urine when laughing, sneezing or coughing (urinary stress incontinence). Birth may worsen this condition because of the inevitable stretching – and possible trauma – in the pelvic floor musculature. Both during and after pregnancy, creating a balance of muscle tone and pliability in the pelvic floor is key.

Though outside the scope of practice of massage therapists, partner or self-massage of the pelvic floor muscles may ready the area for birthing, as can numerous, daily repetitions of various pelvic floor (Kegel) exercises. Strengthening these muscles prevents and treats urinary incontinence and improves muscular tone and vascularization (Ko et al. 2011). Additionally, "reverse" Kegels help the pregnant client to practice releasing and softening these vital muscles. Both forms of pelvic floor activity also expand a woman's awareness and control of her pelvic floor, skills especially helpful during labor and birth (Simkin et al. 2018; Franklin 2003). Some therapists report that reflexive techniques on the feet, hands and energy meridians may enhance bladder and kidney function (Enzer 2004).

Reduction of Musculoskeletal Strain and Pain

In one informal survey of prenatal and perinatal massage therapists, relief from musculoskeletal aches and pains was the primary reason why their clients sought therapy. Therapists reported the following areas, in descending order of frequency, as the most problematic: lower back, upper back/neck and shoulder pain, sacral and pelvic pain, sciatica and similar sensations, and abdominal pain (Osborne 2009). Few pregnant people escape the burdens of a growing belly! Back and pelvic pain, as well as other localized musculoskeletal discomforts, is a near-universal experience at some point during pregnancy (see Figure 1.5).

In addition, trigger points are especially common when coping with pregnancy's structural stresses. These hyperirritable spots are quite painful when activated, and they generally create a characteristic referred pain in some other location, sometimes very distant from the trigger point. During pregnancy, trigger points – which can be caused by trauma or strained posture, or by muscle chilling, fatigue, strain or tension – can develop or worsen. Most pregnancy-induced trigger points appear in the musculature of the abdomen, ribcage, upper and lower back, neck and legs (see Figure 1.5). (We are aware of the persistent debate about exactly what trigger points are – or whether they even exist! And if they do, we do not necessarily know exactly what the physiological

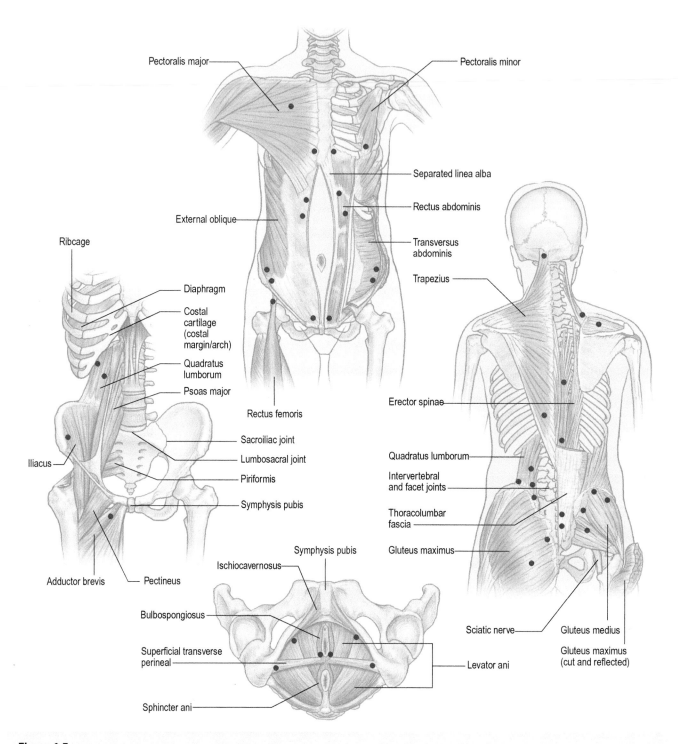

Figure 1.5
Joints and muscles most directly affected by pregnancy. Common trigger points are marked with a *red dot*. (Note that trigger points are marked unilaterally, but often exist bilaterally.)

mechanism is that we are engaging. That said, we find the existing concept useful for many massage therapists, and we witness these points of "exquisite pain" in our clients. Until more convincing evidence emerges, we are continuing to use this terminology where helpful.)

A great pre- and perinatal massage – whether using trigger point therapy or any of our many other modalities – is often just what an expectant person's muscles and fascia and joints need.

Structural Imbalance

The ever-increasing anterior weight generally challenges a pregnant person's structural integrity. As pregnancy progresses, her pelvis tends to rotate anteriorly, spilling the uterus forward against the abdominal walls. The lumbar curvature increases and the abdominal muscles stretch. A double compensation then follows: she leans her upper ribcage more posteriorly, and then her head and neck jut forward anterior of the optimal vertical line. This stretch in the abdomen is most pronounced along the midline, called the linea alba; by the third trimester, the stretch will usually separate the rectus abdominis muscles, a condition known as **diastasis recti**.

These compensations strain the posterior musculature as well, creating fatigue, tightness, trigger points and **fibrosis**. Excessive lumbar **lordosis** correlates with shorter hip flexors, iliopsoas and tensor fasciae latae; it also shortens the thoracolumbar fascia, decreasing spine flexibility. Enlarging breasts pull her pectoral girdle into forward rotation, causing tight pectoral muscles and stretched rhomboids. Increased uterine weight also strains the pelvic floor.

Women commonly respond by broadening their standing foundation, laterally rotating at the hips. Chronic tension then builds in the piriformis and other external hip rotators. Furthermore, with the knee and foot no longer aligned with the hip joint, the iliopsoas cannot efficiently stabilize or flex the pelvis when walking. In compensation, the gluteus medius must first abduct the thigh for the quadriceps to complete a step. This creates the characteristic waddling gait of many pregnant people. To prevent falling forward with the increased anterior weight, the expectant person tends to hyperextend her

knees, and her weight collapses into the medial arches of her weary feet (see Figure 4.6) (Werner 2019).

Back and Pelvic Pain

These postural adjustments, along with weight gain, tend to destabilize, strain and compress the weight-bearing joints and associated myofascial structures (see Figure 1.5); pain and functional limitations often follow. It is estimated that one in five women feel pain in the pelvic region that starts during pregnancy or within the first three months after birth, and that does not have an obvious cause – other than the numerous changes of pregnancy! This is known as **pregnancy-related pelvic girdle pain** (PPGP), sometimes referred to as perinatal pelvic pain syndrome (PPPS) (Katonis et al. 2011). These women feel the greatest discomfort around the sacroiliac joint, lumbosacral joint and pubic symphysis, but other pelvic and leg regions are sometimes painful too

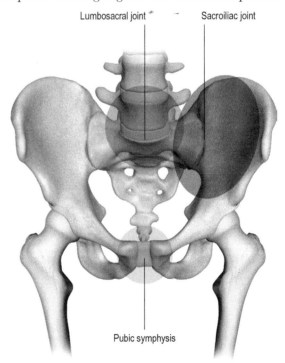

Lumbosacral joint   Sacroiliac joint

Pubic symphysis

Figure 1.6
Joint pain in the pregnant pelvis. *Shaded areas* indicate typical range of pain. Density of shading correlates to the likelihood of pain, with the lightest being the least likely.

(Figures 1.6 and 1.7) (CPWHC 2014; Kanakaris et al. 2011; Verstraete et al. 2013; Howard 2000).

At the sacroiliac joints, the relationship between each ilium and the sacrum shifts dramatically as the enlarged abdomen protrudes anteriorly. When the pelvis anteriorly rotates, the ligaments of these deep pelvic joints are compressed and strained, and can become either hypermobile or hypomobile, and painful, in response. The long dorsal sacroiliac ligament seems to be particularly sensitive; it is the site of pain in as many as 76 percent of women with pelvic pain (CPWHC 2014; Vleeming et al. 2002). Sacroiliac joint strain may refer pain to the lower lumbar region, the buttocks and inner thighs, and as far as the lower extremities (Kanakaris et al. 2011; Slipman et al. 2000).

Distinct from the aforementioned manifestations of pregnancy-related pelvic girdle pain, some people have severe compression at the lumbosacral joint, causing pain from lumbar nerve root impingement. Often this pain is constant, unilateral and movement-sensitive, and it can be felt on any part of the pelvis (Katonis et al. 2011; Vermani et al. 2010; Howard 2000). Besides the aforementioned external rotation of the femur, the hip joints often feel compressed, with little space for free movement. Extra weight gain multiplies all of these strains.

As pregnancy progresses, relaxin and other hormones begin softening the body's connective tissue. This allows more pelvic flexibility and space to accommodate the developing fetus – and, most importantly, its passage through the pelvis during birth; however, as we have seen with other body systems, the pelvis is not the sole target for these hormones' softening effects. Laxity in ligaments, tendons, cartilage and fascia contributes to joint instability and strain on all joints, particularly weight-bearing structures, especially in the lumbar spine and pelvis. Pregnancy makes some people feel like "a loose goose," walking like the scarecrow in *The Wizard of Oz*.

Many people report their first incidence of chronic back pain during a pregnancy. Of them, according to one study, 50 percent suffer pain in the sacroiliac area, 25 percent in the upper back and 25 percent in the lower back. Though buttock and posterior thigh pain may occur, only about 1 percent have true sciatica (rather than pain caused by restrictions other than at the spine) (Riczo 2020; Katonis et al. 2011; Ostgaard et al. 1992). More than two-thirds of pregnant women experience low back pain and almost one-fifth experience pelvic pain (Liddle and Pennick 2015). Onset of pelvic pain is most common in the second trimester, but they are nearly as vulnerable in the first three months postpartum.

As detailed above, back pain is created by posture-induced strain to localized segments of the posterior musculature and ligaments, and/or referred pain from both posterior and anterior trigger points. Poor abdominal tone and diastasis recti can also contribute to back pain. A fetus with a preferred position in the uterus often overburdens that side of the back, making it tired and sore from the unbalanced weight load.

Clients often describe the generalized back pain of pregnancy as fatigue, tightness and achiness. They frequently feel sacroiliac pain as chronic soreness in the upper, medial quadrant of the buttocks, across the iliac crest, or at the posterior iliac spine of the pelvis, which can radiate for several inches in any direction. Prolonged periods of standing or sitting, wearing high heels, and using insufficient back support while seated can all create strain to these joints, which are softened by relaxin and other hormones and stressed by any pelvic rotation. Occasionally, one sacroiliac joint is hypermobile and the other hypomobile. This results in sharp, stabbing posterior pelvic pain when leaving the supine position.

Pain from other pelvic joints varies depending on the source (Figure 1.6). Achiness in the center of the sacral and lumbar areas may indicate strain and compression of the lumbosacral joint. Sharp, stabbing anterior pain in the center of the pelvis indicates instability of the pubic symphysis, known as symphysis pubis dysfunction or pelvic girdle instability. Softened by relaxin and other hormones, this joint is vulnerable to horizontal sheering strains; movements that elevate or depress one side of the pelvis can be excruciating. Trigger points and fatigue of the gluteus medius also contribute to back and pelvic pain (see Figure 1.6) (CPWHC 2014; Jeffcoat 2009; Noble 2003).

The growing uterus itself is also part of the pelvic pain picture. During pregnancy, the pregnant uterus blossoms from a small pear-sized organ to watermelon proportions. There are eight **uterine ligaments** that make this enormous change possible, by suspending and supporting the uterus in the pelvic cavity (Figure 1.7). These ligaments, formed of thickened layers of external uterine peritoneal connective tissue and interwoven with the vast web of intra-abdominal fascia, include the following:

- two broad ligaments that spread laterally from the uterus and attach in the anterior, internal lower iliac region (and that also support the ovaries and fallopian tubes embedded within them)

- two round ligaments extending from the anterior, superior uterine surface near the broad ligament, which continues either through or near the inguinal ligament, and then attaches in the connective tissue of the labia majora

- two sacrouterine ligaments extending from the posterior uterus around the descending colon and attaching to the posterior wall of the pelvis and the anterior surface of the sacrum at S2 and S3

- a small anterior ligament that attaches to the bladder

- a small posterior ligament that attaches to the rectum.

Uterine growth inevitably stretches these ligaments – distortion and pull of their fascial continuations is almost as inevitable (Tully 2020). These changes can result in referred pain (see Figure 1.7):

- broad ligaments: low back, buttock and sciatic-like pain

- round ligaments: diagonal pain from the top of the uterus to groin; usually one-sided, depending on **fetal position**; can extend as far as the vulva and upper thigh

- sacrouterine ligaments: achiness just lateral to or beneath the sacrum and in the lower back.

There are a few other possible pain culprits in the back and pelvis. Severe postural imbalance in the lumbar spine can cause a radiating pain through the buttocks and down the posterior leg. More commonly, chronic tension in the piriformis entraps and compresses the sciatic nerve; this is known as **piriformis syndrome**. From either source, this pain burns, sometimes worsened by tingling, numbness and weakness in the legs. Other nerves, detailed in Chapter 4, may also become compressed with resulting pelvic pain. Some women have coccygeal and other pelvic floor pain, too (see Figure 1.5). The possibilities for back and pelvic pain, in other words, are multiple!

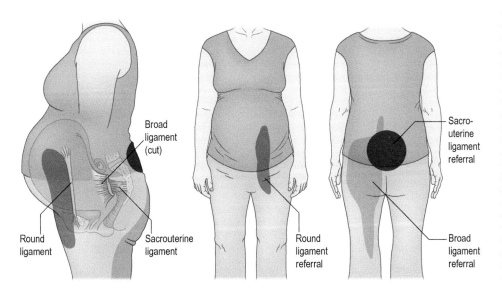

Broad ligament (cut)

Round ligament

Sacrouterine ligament

Round ligament referral

Sacrouterine ligament referral

Round ligament referral

Broad ligament referral

Figure 1.7
Referred pain from uterine ligaments. The sacrouterine ligament (*darkest shade*) is more problematic in the third trimester, whereas round ligament pain (*medium shade*) is more common in the second trimester. Broad ligament pain (*lightest shade*) occurs more from the sixth month on, and can spread into the lateral thigh as well.

Other Musculoskeletal Complaints

Although not as common as back and pelvic pain, pain in the feet, calves, knees, thighs and hips is experienced by many expectant people. Edema produces some of this achy, sore, tense feeling, as does strain to the muscles and joints of the feet and legs. Numbness around the medial malleolus and medial plantar aspect of the foot can occur if edema compresses the tibial nerve; this is known as tarsal tunnel syndrome. Cramping in the gastrocnemius, soleus and the peroneals torments some women's sleep, as do the vibrations and irritations of **restless leg syndrome**. Compression of knee and ankle joints results in soreness and fatigue. Hip joint discomfort and stiffness caused by compression and chronic external femoral rotation often become more severe in later pregnancy, when sleeping positions are restricted to sidelying or **semireclining**. Some women have pain and numbness on the anterolateral side of the thigh, thought to be caused by the inguinal ligament and nearby fascial sheaths compressing the lateral cutaneous femoral nerve (Patijn et al. 2011; Harney and Patijn 2007).

Pregnancy often worsens prior postural imbalances and injuries: anything from lumbar and cervical lordosis, to scoliosis and disc dysfunctions, to **thoracic outlet syndrome**. When strained posture compresses the brachial plexus, there is a characteristic pain, numbness or tingling in the entire hand and along the arm; however, edema-dependent carpal tunnel syndrome pain happens more frequently (Klein 2013; Werner 2019). Ribcage pain may occur in later pregnancy as organ space diminishes. As the lower circumference widens and the ribs spread, they can strain abdominal attachments and intercostal muscles. Trigger points develop, referring pain into the mid- and lower back and sometimes throughout the ribcage. The baby may intensify this discomfort with frequent kicks or stretching (see Figure 1.5).

Headaches are common and often musculoskeletal in origin, the result of tension, strain and trigger points, especially in the neck and upper back. They can be more intense and frequent if the woman hyperventilates, since the overused scalenes will tug on their cervical origins. Other hormonal effects on blood vessel dilation and increased mucus production in the sinuses make sinus headaches more common, too (Ricci 2017; Gibbs et al. 2003).

Our Role in Pain Control

Amidst these seemingly endless structural changes, there is much that we can do. Knowledgeable maternity massage therapists may help their clients to prevent, reduce and manage pain by supporting and encouraging the body's adaptation to these many myofascial and proprioceptive transitions.

The effectiveness of massage therapy for reducing pain has now been validated not just by individual studies (Cherkin 2011), but by a growing number of literature reviews and meta-analyses (Crawford et al. 2016; Boyd et al. 2016a; Boyd et al. 2016b; Field 2016; Miake-Lye et al. 2019).

There is much anecdotal testimony to the effectiveness of massage for pregnancy's pains, but little specific research

(Oswald et al. 2013). In one of the few well-structured studies specifically of massage and pregnancy, massaged clients reported less back pain and a similar reduction in leg pain, among other benefits, compared with those who had an equal amount of relaxation therapy (Field et al. 1999). Depressed second-trimester women had similar reductions in pain when they received massage therapy rather than relaxation sessions or normal prenatal care alone (Field et al. 2004; Field 2017).

Several theories explain this welcomed relief, though with varying levels of validation. A long-standing explanation, the gate theory of pain, holds that massage alleviates painful stimulation and alters the processing of painful input (see Chapter 5). The neuromatrix theory emphasizes that each of us generates outputs of information that create our pain perception. A more elaborate version of that, the biopsychosocial model, posits an interplay of anatomy, physiology, pain experiences, one's judgment or appraisal of the pain, and the behaviors that result, as well as the person's environment (Thompson and Brooks 2016).

Some studies have suggested that massage stimulates the body's pressure receptors and thus enhances vagus nerve activity and reduces cortisol levels (Field 2016). Still other studies have suggested that massage produces a relaxation response; functional magnetic resonance imaging studies have suggested that massage influences regions of the brain responsible for stress and the regulation of emotion (Buckenmaier et al. 2016).

Though we still do not yet fully understand exactly why it works, we do have a variety of techniques that seem to prevent and reduce pain in our prenatal clients (Çakır 2018). Rhythmic passive movements including small-amplitude Trager™ movements, and osteopathic strain–counterstrain and muscle energy techniques are all effective in pain management (Thompson and Brooks 2016). Deep tissue work and other forms of myofascial release may reduce pain by elongating shortened, bunched connective tissue (Ajimsha et al. 2015), and deep cross-fiber friction may reduce pain and the restricted range of movement of fibrosis (Thompson and Brooks 2016; Cyriax and Coldham 1984). Swedish massage, and any other strokes done with mindful attention,

may encourage parasympathetic activation of the client's nervous system (Guan et al. 2014; Lee et al. 2011).

Trigger point therapy, or just focused pressure and appropriate stretching around trigger points, can reduce the pain associated with these points by, scientists speculate, relieving tissue ischemia and allowing restoration of normal tissue blood supply (Liddle and Pennick 2015; Howard 2000). (See Chapters 2 and 4 for abdominal precautions.)

Our pregnant clients welcome the lessening pain these techniques can bring (Steel et al. 2015).

In addition to hands-on techniques, education also helps reduce pain and decrease stress on structures. Correct (and safe) abdominal strengthening activities and body-use guidelines for walking, sitting, sleeping, carrying and other daily activities will further reduce strain in the neck, back and pelvis. These more efficient movement patterns, in turn, reinforce the effectiveness of hands-on therapy (Simkin et al. 2018).

Labor Preparation

Physical flexibility and kinesthetic awareness may equip people to more actively participate in the birth process. Muscle and joint pliability offer more possibilities for movement and positioning, crucial to an active birth (Ricci 2017). Many laboring people want to walk, squat, rock, lunge, kneel or stand during various parts of labor; open hip joints, supple adductors, hamstrings and calf muscles, and resilient postural muscles enable this urge. Any structure connecting to the pelvis needs length and pliability. At the very least, those birthing vaginally must be able to open their thighs to allow the baby's passage.

The same massage therapy methods useful for pain control may be effective in increasing flexibility, especially passive and assisted resisted stretching, deep tissue work and osteopathic soft tissue treatments (Thompson and Brooks 2016). Women can participate in fitness or yoga programs led by instructors with specialized prenatal training. Including strengthening and aerobic exercise helps ready them for the athletic challenges of labor and birth (Simkin et al. 2018; Jorge et al.

2015). Of course, they should consult with their maternity healthcare provider concerning the advisability of prenatal exercise.

Deepening an awareness of their body is one of the many potential benefits of prenatal exercise and bodywork. As a result of the "feedback loop" of the sensory–motor system, increased bodily awareness creates increased sensory awareness and control of muscles (Juhan 2003). Heightened familiarity with her internal landscape means your client may be more likely to make the labor journey with more ease, less pain and a spirit of adventure (Tully 2020).

From the treatment room

I believe that massage therapy helped me so much while I was pregnant. My body would relax, and I'd be so centered within myself and able to focus and go inside, which made a big difference during labor.

– **Ileana**, client

The variety of stimuli introduced by bodywork techniques is one way that this feedback loop becomes activated. Swedish, deep tissue and reflexive modalities, in particular, are built upon modulations in depth, direction and duration of touch. Kinesthetic input varies with changes in the speed, rhythm and intensity of passive and active movements. Some techniques you will learn are passively received by the client; others involve the client's active movement. All of these experiences create a rich influx of information and corresponding responses in the client's body and mind. The result can be heightened perception, new body understandings and more specific awareness.

During prenatal massage sessions, there are numerous opportunities to help your client connect with and express her physical and emotional awareness. As she learns to more fully express her sensations and her needs as a client, she can improve her ability to more effectively communicate with her family and the labor professionals she employs. She is then more likely to be able to access

her feelings and assert her needs during labor. Those with previous traumatic births, or other physical and/or emotionally traumatic histories, often need particularly sensitive assistance to effectively express themselves (see Chapter 7).

If the musculature of the back, abdomen and pelvic floor remains relaxed, the uterus can labor without resistance, the baby can press more firmly against the cervix and birth requires less effort. The laboring person should be able to scan for tension throughout her body. Her labor may be easier if she knows how to release tension – whether through imagery, hypnosis or conscious control (Smith et al. 2018a). Labor also requires the use of specific muscles in a precise, controlled manner. She can develop all of these abilities during prenatal bodywork. Education in diaphragmatic breathing, strengthening the abdominals and pelvic floor, and perineal self-massage are particularly useful in developing awareness and control in these vital birthing muscles (see Chapter 5) (Simkin et al. 2018; Jorge et al. 2015).

Most clients gain self-awareness, relaxation and emotional support from receiving therapeutic bodywork during pregnancy. This contributes to the development of someone who is more able to access those inborn skills and intuitions that have evolved over the millennia of humanity's existence and women's experiences of giving birth (Togher 2017; Samuels and Samuels 1996).

Teaching massage to partners and others who will attend a birth furthers everyone's labor preparedness. Family or friends can accompany the pregnant client to a session to watch and practice simple, yet effective massage movements. Some therapists teach a segment in a childbirth education class or organize a separate class for small groups of women and their loved ones to learn labor massage possibilities. Therapeutic procedures requiring refined palpatory skills and advanced anatomical knowledge are best in the hands of professionals; however, non-professionals can safely rub and knead family members, as long as important safety precautions are included in instruction (see Chapter 5 and online resources). ⊕

Labor Facilitation

Our skilled touch is powerful during labor as well: massage can contribute to shorter, less painful labors with fewer complications, less use of medications and fewer medical interventions. There are no guarantees in labor, of course, but at the least, massage usually helps improve both the mother's and her infant's physical and emotional well-being. What these women inherently and personally know, contemporary research is beginning to verify. Providing the option for such powerful, non-pharmacological pain management is a critical step toward the goal of a more mother-friendly model of maternity care (Budin 2007; Olsen and Clausen 2012). In Chapter 5 we will explore the particulars of labor, and specific techniques that we can use to facilitate it. Here we offer a brief overview of the value of touch during this incredible journey.

Timeless Touch

Skim any history or anthropological study of childbirth (see Cassidy 2006 or Goldsmith 1984 for two of many examples) and the pages overflow with images of laboring people being soothed and reinforced by skilled and loving hands. When pain or stress intensifies, the impulse to reach out and assist someone giving birth comes naturally. Of course, not all laboring people want to be touched, but most appreciate reassuring touch at some point in their labors.

That primal instinct stands in sharp contrast to Western medicine over the last two centuries, which has moved away from "high-touch" and toward "high-tech" birthing. Modern monitoring, pharmacology and surgical procedures have benefited many women and their families. They have also contributed to a birthing milieu that can feel impersonal and disempowering, and statistically is not as safe as many believe (Olsen and Clausen 2012; Budin 2007; Behruzi et al. 2013).

Research on Touch in Labor

A growing number of studies, and several systematic reviews, corroborate what women have long known: that rubbing in general, and massage therapy specifically, can have a variety of benefits during this period of incredible

intensity. As with much massage research, the sample sizes for labor studies are small and the methodologies imperfect. But, as the volume of data grows, we can become more certain of the varied efficacy of massage. Based on numerous studies, involving hundreds of women in multiple settings, we can confidently say that massage has been shown to:

- reduce the perception of labor pain
- increase the ability to cope with the demands of labor
- reduce the length of labor
- provide relaxation
- lower anxiety
- decrease the need for medication
- improve the sense of control
- improve the emotional experience of labor (Smith et al. 2018b; Unalmis Erdogan et al. 2017; Field 2016; Gallo et al. 2013; Simkin and O'Hara 2002).

We should rejoice at such a compelling body of knowledge!

An additional source of reliable data is provided by studies involving professional labor support. Birth doulas provide continuous support – stroking, kneading, holding, and otherwise offering physical, verbal and emotional comfort – throughout labor. In a meta-analysis of six studies conducted worldwide, this consistent physical presence, nurturing touch and emotional support created the following benefits, compared with the control groups:

- 25 percent shorter labors
- 40 percent less use of **pitocin**
- 30 percent decrease in all pain medication use, including 60 percent decrease in requests for epidurals
- 40 percent less need for **forceps**
- 50 percent fewer Cesarean births
- improved infant **Apgar scores**
- enhanced postpartum family adjustment (Klaus et al. 2012).

Numerous more recent studies have demonstrated the abundant benefits of a caring, supportive, well-trained labor companion (Bohren et al. 2019; Gruber et al. 2013). Meanwhile, the practice files of prenatal massage therapists are full of detailed anecdotal evidence of easier, more satisfying and healthier births when we are part of the birthing team (Figure 1.8).

The long-term value of appropriate labor massage therapy is compelling. More people express satisfaction with their childbirth experience and its impact on their lives when they are emotionally supported during labor. In addition, the quality of the woman's relationship with her maternity healthcare provider and the degree of participation she has in decision-making have a long-term impact far beyond the management of labor pain. In fact, receiving nurturing care correlates more significantly than the ease of labor itself – even in long, complicated births – with this overall sense of satisfaction (The Nature and Management of Labor Pain 2003).

Practicing therapists have found many massage therapy techniques as effective during labor as they are prenatally. General massage techniques reduce stress and promote relaxation, both essential for labor. Deep tissue work and stretching may relieve muscle tension, cramping and other soft tissue discomforts. A therapist's focused, calm presence can support the physiological and emotional needs of labor and birth. Stress can significantly reduce blood flow to the uterus, and it may make labor longer, slower and more painful. A massage therapist, in turn, can promote a level of relaxation that facilitates labor and allows a woman to explore the many aspects of the labor process (see Chapter 5).

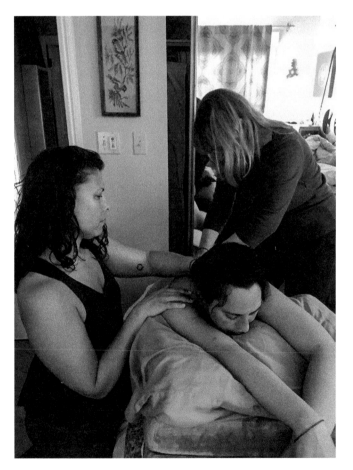

Figure 1.8
Labor massage. The skilled touch of massage therapists and birth doulas may help to ease labor pain.

From the treatment room

We wanted a gentle, unmedicated birth, but 16 hours of intense labor almost ended in a Cesarean. My therapist used every massage technique to keep my hips relaxed, pressed on them, and cradled me on my side to help the baby come out.

– **Pat**, client

Nurturing Maternal Touch

How important is cuddling, stroking and carrying a baby? It is vital. A century ago, American orphanages had infant **mortality** rates of 95 to 100 percent. The orphanages usually provided food and shelter; the little ones there died of tactile and vestibular starvation (Montagu 1978). More recently, we have seen the developmental tragedies of touch-neglected children in the orphanages of communist Romania (Settle 1991).

Research on our mammalian cousins reinforces this message: the need for cutaneous stimulation is so great that monkeys separated from their natural mothers chose a softer, cuddly "mother" substitute with poor milk supply rather than a wire surrogate with abundant milk. Contact is more compelling than nutrients. When mice that were handled during their infancy became moms, they nursed, cleaned and cared for their young better than those in unstroked control groups (Montagu 1978).

Though our instinct to touch runs deep, not all parents hold and care for their children. Nurturing, respectful touch is an experience often lacking in our technological, touch-averse cultures. Some parents, like the research animals described above, have experienced neglect, impersonal contact and physical, sexual or emotional abuse. Lacking a fully embodied sense of appropriate touch (Montagu 1978; Simkin and Klaus 2011), it is hard for them to nurture the next generation.

Massage practitioners have the opportunity to develop their clients' nurturing skills. We can become role models for our pregnant clients; we can help them to embody loving, appropriate touch. Classic nursing studies show that mothers touch their newborns in consistent ways: first with tentative fingertips, then fuller hand contact, and finally complete embraces, leading to a "molding" of the two to each other. This sequence was completed more slowly, or was aborted, by those whose prenatal and perinatal care consisted only of routine, impersonal touch. Researchers concluded that "appropriate, meaningful touch of pregnant and laboring women leads to touching babies in meaningful, effective, and caring ways," thus facilitating the transformation from person to parent (Rubin 1963; Rubin 1975; Rubin 1984).

In addition, massage techniques that you teach for pregnancy and labor can also empower partners and other loved ones to offer meaningful physical nurturing to the mother after the birth. If she feels supported by others, she is more likely to be able to support her new family. The power of touch, in other words, continues to resonate: one study found that from just a few hours of skin-to-skin contact between mother and baby immediately after birth, those babies were less irritable and more self-regulated *a year later* (Bystrova et al. 2009).

From the treatment room

I learned so much in my massages about appropriate levels of touch and so many techniques I can use to get in touch with my baby in the womb and for after she's born.

– Sara, client

To further nurturing touch in the family, many maternity massage therapists teach parents how to massage their infants. Simple sequences of effleurage, kneading and raking can have significant health benefits for all babies, but particularly for those with health challenges. Premature infants who received a 15-minute massage and movement sequence three times daily gained 47 percent more weight and were more active, alert and relaxed than unmassaged premature babies in the control group, and were discharged an average of six days earlier. These babies' superior development continued through the six months of follow-up study, regardless of whether the massage was continued at home (Field et al. 2010b). This study and numerous others (Solkoff et al. 1969; Rice 1979; Rausch 1981; Scafidi et al. 1986; Scafidi et al. 1990; Gunzenhauser 1990; Holst et al. 2002; Feldman et al. 2002; Rad et al. 2016) support the benefits of massage for infants and for their caretakers.

Reminder

Humans need nurturing touch to survive and to thrive.

Facilitating Postpartum Recovery

Even mothers who have experienced massage's many benefits often do not prioritize their self-care during the postpartum period; less than 25 percent of the prenatal clients of surveyed perinatal massage therapists returned for massage after the birth (Osborne 2009). But the emotional, physiological and functional benefits of postpartum bodywork can be just as valuable. Chapter 6 will offer an abundance of techniques to address postpartum's unique demands; here is an overview of the essential adjustments that come after birth and how we can facilitate them.

Emotional Adjustments

After childbirth, many people have an intrinsic need to tell their birth story. Some retell the details repeatedly, oftentimes unsolicited. This storytelling can seem most urgent when the labor decisions were out of the person's control or the outcome was not as anticipated. The psychological integration of her childbearing experience into her sense of self is a critical aspect of postpartum recovery. This is particularly important for women who have been depressed or who are slipping into **perinatal mood and anxiety disorders** (see Chapter 7) (Simkin et al. 2018; O'Connor et al. 2019).

Massage therapists can provide a professional yet caring opportunity for postpartum clients to talk freely. Within a therapeutic session, many clients will celebrate their accomplishments and unburden themselves of the fear, sadness and anger often generated during labor. This may help them to begin to let go of muscular tension, frozen expressions and gestures, and unresolved issues. This is also an opportunity to relate any frustrations and concerns about infant care and their transition into mothering. You can listen compassionately and attentively (and, in the process, identify those who may need the assistance of mental health professionals and refer them appropriately).

Physiological Adjustments

In addition to providing emotional support, postpartum massage therapy facilitates physiological recovery of an exhausted body. Labor is usually an athletic test of a woman's strength and endurance that can result in various muscular aches and pains. As a result, most massage methods may help the mother to recover, as well as giving her a rare moment to focus on herself. This type of physiological assistance is especially helpful for post-Cesarean birth mothers who are recuperating from major abdominal surgery, as well as the strain of pregnancy. Sequential and appropriate therapy to the incision site may speed healing and reduce fibrous buildup in and around the scar (see Chapter 6) (Smith and Ryan 2016; Shin and Bordeaux 2012).

Constipation, difficulty urinating, uterine cramping and perineal soreness are common in the days and weeks postpartum. Swedish techniques, skin rolling and trigger point therapy reduce these pains and aid in rehabilitation of the abdominal skin, muscles and organs. Reflexive techniques to feet, hands, connective tissue and energy meridians may enhance metabolic functioning, both system-wide and in individual organs (Irani et al. 2015; Enzer 2004).

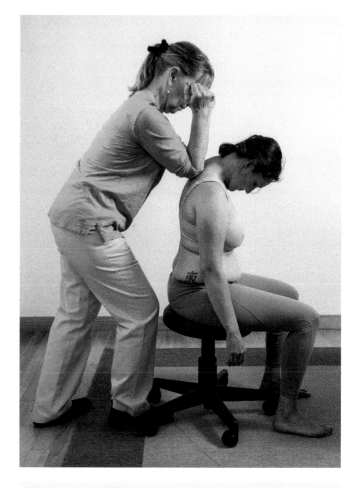

Figure 1.9
Postpartum massage. Newborn care often taxes the lower back, pectoral girdle and neck; postpartum massage therapy can help to relieve these burdens.

Postural Adjustments

Labor sometimes worsens pain originating in prenatal postural imbalances. After pregnancy, women need particular attention to their back, abdomen and pelvic floor. Additional structural stresses emerge during the many hours of nursing, lifting and other childcare tasks (Johnson 2017; Ricci 2017; Pirie and Herman 2003). By reducing tension in postural muscles, re-educating the mother about the use of the iliopsoas muscles for both pelvic alignment and efficient gait, and encouraging proper **body mechanics**, a perinatal massage therapist offers relief from postural and mechanically induced postpartum pain. For optimal postpartum recovery, we recommend that most new mothers receive regular massage therapy for a full year after the birth (Figure 1.9).

From the treatment room

Going for a massage in the first two weeks after my baby was born was the best decision I made for my own health and recovery. I was intimidated by leaving the house so soon with my new baby but I knew Linda's clinic was a safe place for me. A massage was exactly what my sore body and exhausted new mom self needed. I had to breastfeed my baby part way through and Linda helped me get comfortable and massaged my feet while I nursed.

– **Andrea**, client

What would you do?

You are invited to attend a conference for public health nurses in your community as part of their continuing education program. How would you describe the benefits of massage therapy both during and after pregnancy to this group?

From the treatment room

After my Cesarean section, I came in a week later to get a massage. My recovery was quicker this time than it was for my previous two Cesarean sections. Scar tissue was minimized by the massage work that was done to the incision in later sessions. It was also a great support to me to have someone to confide in as far as the nursing.

– **Maria**, client

Chapter Summary

Parents, healthcare providers and massage therapists can feel confident and enthused about the likely positive effects of prenatal and perinatal massage therapy. Skilled, empathetic touch therapy can offer far-reaching, multidimensional benefits to individuals, their loved ones and the human family. Based on research, observation and clients' testimonies, we know that there are numerous ways that touch can be of benefit:

During pregnancy:

- Reduces stress, promotes relaxation and facilitates transitions through emotional support and physical nurturing.

- Reduces negative effects of circulatory system changes, including edema, varicose veins and increased blood pressure.

- Minimizes discomforts of pregnancy's hormonal, respiratory, gastrointestinal, urinary and other physiological adaptations.

- Reduces musculoskeletal strain and pain.

- Develops the flexibility and kinesthetic awareness necessary to actively participate in the birth process.

- Fosters nurturing maternal touch and healthy bonding.

In labor:

- Contributes to shorter, less painful labor.

- Reduces labor complications, medications and interventions.

- Improves infant well-being, mother's satisfaction with the birth and family formation.

In the postpartum period:

- Facilitates postpartum emotional, physiological and family adjustments.

- Reduces musculoskeletal and organ pain.

- Promotes structural realignment of the spine and pelvis, and reorganization of movement.

- Contributes to rehabilitation of abdominal skin, muscles and organs.

- Promotes recovery from Cesarean birth, including healing of the incision.

- Relieves muscle strain and tension caused by childcare activities.

Across society:

- Develops individuals more capable of love and pleasure.

- Builds less violent, more respectful cultures.

Think it through

To deepen your knowledge, go to our online resources, answer the test questions for this chapter and explore further. 🌐

References and Further Reading

ACOG (American College of Obstetricians and Gynecologists) (2019) Approaches to limit intervention during labor and birth. Committee Opinion 766. 133(2), February.

Ajimsha MS, Al-Mudahka NR, Al-Madzhar JA (2015) Effectiveness of MFR: systematic review of randomized controlled trials. J Bodyw Mov Ther. 19(1):102–112.

Alhusen JL, Ray E, Sharps P et al. (2015) Intimate partner violence during pregnancy: maternal and neonatal outcomes. J Womens Health (Larchmt). 24(1):100–106.

Allen L and Pounds D (2016) Clay and Pounds' Basic Clinical Massage Therapy, 3rd edn. Baltimore: Wolters Kluwer.

Andrade C-K, Clifford P (2008) Outcome-Based Massage: From Evidence to Practice, 2nd edn. Baltimore: Lippincott, Williams and Wilkins.

Arkko PJ, Pakarinen AJ, Kari-Koskinen O (1983) Effects of whole-body massage on serum protein, electrolyte and hormone concentrations, enzyme activities, and hematological parameters. Int J Sports Med. 4:265–267.

Behruzi R, Hatern M, Goulet L et al. (2013) Understanding childbirth practices as an organizational cultural phenomenon: a conceptual framework. BMC Pregnancy Childbirth. 13:205.

Benjamin P (2016) Tappan's Handbook of Massage Therapy: Blending Art with Science, 6th edn. Hoboken: Pearson.

Birch E (1986) The experience of touch received during labor. J Nurse-Midwifery. 31:270–275.

Bohren MA, Berger BO, Munthe-Kaas H et al. (2019) Perceptions and experiences of labour companionship: a qualitative evidence synthesis. Cochrane Database Syst Rev. 3(3):CD012449.

Boyd C, Crawford C, Paat CF et al. (2016a) The impact of massage therapy on function in pain populations-a systematic review and meta-analysis of randomized controlled trials: Part II, Cancer pain populations. Pain Med. 17(8): 1553–1568.

Boyd C, Crawford C, Paat CF et al. (2016b) The impact of massage therapy on function in pain populations-a systematic review and meta-analysis of randomized controlled trials: Part III, Surgical pain populations. Pain Med. 17(9):1757–1772.

Bremner AJ, Spence C (2017) The development of tactile perception. Adv Child Dev Behav. 52:227–268.

Buckenmaier C, Cambron J, Werner R et al. (2016) Massage therapy for pain – call to action. Pain Med. 17:1211–1214.

Budin W, ed. (2007) Advancing normal birth. J Perinat Educ. 16:1.

Bystrova K, Ivanova V, Edhborg M et al. (2009) Early contact versus separation: effects on mother–infant interaction one year later. Birth. 36:97–109.

Çakır Koçak Y, Sevil Ü, Ergenoğlu AM (2018) The Effect of Pregnancy Massage on the General Well-Being and Satisfaction Levels of Pregnant Women: A Randomized Controlled Trial, ISS2018 3rd International Science Symposium, "New Horizons in Science," Pristine, Kosova, September 5–8, pp. 97–102 (abstract submission/oral presentation).

Cassidy T (2006) Birth: The Surprising History of How We Are Born. New York: Atlantic Monthly Press.

Chang MY, Wang SY, Chen CH (2002) Effects of massage on pain and anxiety during labour: a randomized controlled trial in Taiwan. J Adv Nurs. 38(1):68–73.

CPWHC (Chartered Physiotherapists in Women's Health and Continence and Directorate of Strategy and Clinical Programmes; Health Service Executive) (2014) Clinical Practice Guideline: Management of Pelvic Girdle Pain in Pregnancy and Post-Partum. Guideline No. 16; revised August.

Cherkin DC, Sherman KJ, Kahn J et al. (2011) A comparison of the effects of 2 types of massage and usual care on chronic low back pain: a randomized, controlled trial. Ann Intern Med. 155(1):1–9.

Chung UL, Hung LC, Kuo SC et al. (2003) Effects of LI4 and BL 67 acupressure on labor pain and uterine contractions in the first stage of labor. J Nurs Res. 11(4):251–260.

Cooper R, Goldenberg R, Das A et al. (1996) The pre-term prediction study: maternal stress is associated with spontaneous preterm birth at less than thirty-five weeks gestation. Am J Obstet Gynecol. 175:1286–1292.

Coussons-Read ME (2013) Effects of prenatal stress on pregnancy and human development: mechanisms and pathways. Obstet Med. 6(2):52–57.

Cranden A (1979) Maternal anxiety and obstetric complications. J Psychos Res. 23:109.

Crawford C, Boyd C, Paat CF et al. (2016) The impact of massage therapy on function in pain populations-a systematic review and meta-analysis of randomized controlled trials: Part I, Patients experiencing pain in the general population. Pain Med. 17(7):1353–1375.

Cyriax J, Coldham M (1984) Indications for and against deep friction, in Textbook of Orthopaedic Medicine. Volume 2 Treatment by Manipulation, Massage, and Injection, 11th edn. Toronto: Bailliere–Tindall.

Davis EP, Sandman CA (2010) The timing of prenatal exposure to maternal cortisol and psychosocial stress is associated with human infant cognitive development. Child Dev. 81(1):131–148.

Denenberg VH, Karas GG. (1960) Interactive effect of age and duration of infantile experience on adult learning. Psychol Rep. 7:313–322.

Devis P, Knuttinen MG (2017) Deep venous thrombosis in pregnancy: incidence, pathogenesis and endovascular management. Cardiovasc Diagn Ther. 7(Suppl 3):S309–S319.

Diego MA, Field T, Hernandez-Reif M (2005) Vagal activity, gastric motility, and weight gain in massaged preterm neonates. J Pediatr. 147(1):50–55.

Diego MA, Field T (2009) Moderate pressure massage elicits a parasympathetic nervous system response. Int J Neurosci. 119(5):630–638.

Ely DM, Hamilton BE (2018) Trends in fertility and mother's age at first birth among rural and metropolitan counties: United States, 2007–2017. NCHS Data Brief, no. 323. Hyattsville, MD: National Center for Health Statistics.

Enzer S (2004) Maternity Reflexology, 2nd edn. UK: Soul to Sole Reflexology.

Fakouri C, Jones P (1987) Relaxation RX: slow stroke back rub. J Gerontol Nurs. 13:32–35.

Feldman R, Eidelman A, Sirota L et al. (2002) Comparison of skin-to-skin (kangaroo) and traditional care: parenting outcomes and preterm infant development. Pediatrics. 110(1):16–26.

Ferguson P (1995) The Self-Shiatsu Handbook. New York: Berkley.

Field T (2016) Massage therapy research review. Complement Ther Clin Pract. 24:19–31.

Field T (2017) Prenatal depression risk factors, developmental effects and interventions: a review. J Pregnancy Child Health. 4(1):301.

Field T, Morrow C, Valdon C et al. (1992) Massage reduces anxiety in child and adolescent psychiatric patients. J Am Acad Child Adolesc Psychiatr. 31:125–131.

Field T, Hernandez-Reif M, Taylor S et al. (1997) Labour pain is reduced by massage therapy. J Psychos Obstet Gynecol. 18(4):286–291.

Field T, Hernandez-Reif M, Hart S et al. (1999) Pregnant women benefit from massage therapy. J Psychos Obstet Gynecol. 20:31–38.

Field T, Diego MA, Hernandez-Reif M et al. (2004) Massage therapy effects on depressed pregnant women. J Psychos Obstet Gynecol. 25:115–122.

Field T, Figueiredo B, Hernandez-Reif M et al. (2008) Massage therapy reduces pain in pregnant women, alleviates prenatal depression in both parents and improves their relationships. J Bodyw Mov Ther. 12(2):146–150.

Field T, Diego MA, Hernandez-Reif MA (2010a) Preterm infant massage therapy research: a review. Infant Behav Dev. 33(2):115–124.

Field T, Diego MA, Hernandez-Reif M (2010b) Prenatal depression effects and interventions: a review. Infant Behav Dev. 33(4):409–418.

Fink NS, Urech C, Cavelti M et al. (2012) Relaxation during pregnancy: what are the benefits for mother, fetus, and the newborn? A systematic review of the literature. J Perinat Neonatal Nurs. 26(4):296–306.

Flocco O (1993) Randomized controlled study of premenstrual symptoms treated with reflexology. Obstet Gynecol. 82:906–911.

Fogarty S, Barnett R, Hay P (2020) Safety and pregnancy massage: a qualitative thematic analysis. Int J Ther Massage Bodywork. 13(1):4–12.

Foldi M (1978) Anatomical and physiological basis for physical therapy of lymphedema. Experientia. 33(Suppl): 15–18.

Franklin E (2003) Pelvic Power: Mind/Body Exercises for Strength, Flexibility, Posture and Balance. Hightstown, NJ: Princeton Book Company.

Gallo R, Santana L, Ferreira C et al. (2013) Massage reduced severity of pain during labour: a randomised trial. J Physiother. 59(2):109–116.

Gibbs RS, Karian BY, Haney AF et al. (2003) Danforth's Obstetrics and Gynecology. Baltimore: Lippincott, Williams & Wilkins.

Giesbrecht G, Poole J, Letourneau N et al. (2013) The buffering effect of social support on hypothalamic-pituitary-adrenal axis function during pregnancy. Psychosom Med. 75(9):856–862.

Glynn L, Schetter C, Wadhwa P et al. (2004) Pregnancy affects appraisal of negative life events. J Psychos Res. 56:47–52.

Goldsmith J (1984) Childbirth Wisdom. New York: Congdon and Weed.

Goldsmith LT, Weiss G (2009) Relaxin in human pregnancy. Ann N Y Acad Sci. 1160:130–135.

Gorsuch R, Key M (1974) Abnormalities of pregnancy as a function of anxiety and life stress. Psychosom Med. 36:353.

Gruber KJ, Cupito SH, Dobson CF (2013) Impact of doulas on healthy birth outcomes. J Perinat Educ. 22(1):49–58.

Guan L, Collet JP, Yuskiv N et al. (2014) The effect of massage therapy on autonomic activity in critically ill children. Evid Based Complement Alternat Med. 2014:656750.

Gunzenhauser N (ed.) (1990) Advances in touch: new implications in human development. Pediatric Roundtable #14.

Harney D, Patijn J (2007) Meralgia paresthetica: diagnosis and management strategies. Pain Med. 8(8):669–677.

Herman H (2004) Pregnancy and Postpartum: Clinical Highlights Seminar. San Diego.

Hetherington S (2007) A controlled study of the effect of prepared childbirth classes on obstetric outcomes. Birth. 17(2):86–90.

Hinds T, McEwan I, Perkes J et al. (2004) Effects of massage on limb and skin blood flow after quadriceps exercise. Med Sci Sports Exerc. 36(8):1308–1313.

Hobel C, Colhane J (2003) Role of psychosocial and nutritional stress on poor pregnancy outcome. J Nutr. 133:1709S–1717S.

Holst S, Uvnäs-Moberg K, Petersson M (2002) Postnatal oxytocin treatment and postnatal stroking of rats reduce blood pressure in adulthood. Auton Neurosci. 99(2):85–90.

Howard F (2000) Pelvic Pain: Diagnosis and Management. Baltimore: Lippincott, Williams & Wilkins.

Huang TW, Tseng SH, Lin CC et al. (2013) Effects of manual lymphatic drainage on breast cancer-related lymphedema: a systematic review and meta-analysis of randomized controlled trials. World J Surg Oncol. 11:15.

Irani M, Kordi M, Tara F et al. (2015) The effect of hand and foot massage on post-cesarean pain and anxiety. J Midwifery Reprod Health. 3(4):465-471.

Jeffcoat H (2009) Help for pubic symphysis pain. Int J Childbirth Educ. Available at: https://feminapt.com/resources/published-articles/help-for-pubic-symphysis-pain [accessed May 27, 2020].

Jefferies W, Bochner F (1991) Thromboembolism and its management in pregnancy. Med J Aus. 155:253.

Johnson KA (2017) The Fourth Trimester: A Postpartum Guide to Healing Your Body, Balancing Your Emotions, and Restoring Your Vitality. Boulder, CO: Shambala.

Jorge C, Santos-Rocha R, Bento R (2015) Can group exercise programs improve health outcomes in pregnant women? A systematic review. Curr Women's Health Rev. 11(1):75–87.

Juhan D (2003) Job's Body: Handbook for Bodyworkers, 3rd edn. Barrytown, NY: Station Hill Press.

Juraska J, Greenough W, Elliott C et al. (1980) Plasticity in adult rat visual cortex: an examination of several cell populations after differential rearing. Behav Neural Biol. 29:157–167.

Kanakaris NK, Roberts CS, Giannoudis PV (2011) Pregnancy-related pelvic girdle pain: an update. BMC Med. 9:15.

Katonis P, Kampouroglou A, Aggelopoulos A et al. (2011) Pregnancy-related low back pain. Hippokratia. 15(3):205–210.

Kinsella MT, Monk C (2009) Impact of maternal stress, depression and anxiety on fetal neurobehavioral development. Clin Obstet Gynecol. 52(3):425–440.

Klaus M, Kennell J, Klaus P (2012) The Doula Book: How a Trained Labor Companion Can Help You Have a Shorter, Easier, and Healthier Birth, 3rd edn. New York: DeCapo Press.

Klein A (2013) Peripheral nerve disease in pregnancy, in Clinical Obstetrics and Gynecology: An Overview. Philadelphia: Lippincott, Williams & Wilkins.

Ko PC, Liang C-C, Chang S-D et al. (2011) A randomized controlled trial of antenatal pelvic floor exercises to prevent and treat urinary incontinence. Int Urogynecol J. 1:17–22.

Kozhimannil KB (2013) Use of non-medical methods of labor induction and pain management among U.S. women. Birth. 40(4):227–236.

Lancaster C, Gold K, Flynn H et al. (2010) Risk factors for depressive symptoms during pregnancy: a systematic review. Am J Obstet Gynecol. 202(1):5–14.

Lee MK, Chang SB, Kang DH (2004) Effects of SP6 acupressure on labor pain and length of delivery time in women during labor. J Altern Complement Med. 10(6):959–965.

Lee YH, Park BN, Kim SH (2011) The effects of heat and massage application on autonomic nervous system. Yonsei Med J. 52(6):982–989.

Liddle SD, Pennick V (2015) Interventions for preventing and treating low-back and pelvic pain during pregnancy. Cochrane Database Syst Rev. 2015(9):CD001130.

Linde B (1989) Dissociation of insulin absorption and blood flow during massage of a subcutaneous injection site. Diabetes Care. 6:570–574.

Longworth J (1982) Psychophysical effects of slow stroke back massage in normotensive females. Adv Nurs Sci. 4:44–61.

Mathews TJ, Hamilton BE (2014) First Births to Older Women Continue to Rise. NCHS Data Brief, no. 152. Hyattsville, MD: National Center for Health Statistics.

Mayo Clinic (n.d.) Domestic Violence Against Women: Recognize Patterns, Seek Help. Available at: http://www.mayoclinic.com/health/domestic-violence/WO00044 [accessed February 14, 2010].

McCormick MC, Siegel J (1999) Prenatal Care: Effectiveness and Implementation. Cambridge: Cambridge University Press.

Meaney, M, Aitken D, Bodnoff S et al. (1985) The effects of postnatal handling on the development of the glucocorticoid receptor systems and stress recovery on the rat. Prog Neuropsychopharmacol Biol Psychiatr. 7:731–734.

Meaney MJ, Aitken DH, Sharma S et al. (1989) Neonatal handling alters adrenocortical negative feedback sensitivity and hippocampal type II glucocorticoid receptor binding in the rat. Neuroendocrinology. 50:597–604.

Miake-Lye IM, Mak S, Lee J et al. (2019) Massage for pain: an evidence map. J Altern Complement Med. 25(5): 475-502.

Monk C, Feng T, Lee S, Krupska I et al. (2016) Distress during pregnancy: epigenetic regulation of placenta glucocorticoid-related genes and fetal neurobehavior. Am J Psychiatry. 173(7):705–713.

Montagu AM (1978) Touching: The Human Significance of the Skin. New York: Harper & Row.

Morhenn V, Beavin LE, Zak PJ (2012) Massage increases oxytocin and reduces adrenocorticotropin hormone in humans. Altern Ther Health Med. 18(6):11–18.

Morrison I, Löken LS, Olausson H (2010) The skin as a social organ. Exp Brain Res. 204:305–314.

Moyer C, Rounds J, Hannum J (2004) A meta-analysis of massage therapy research. Psychol Bull. 130:3–18.

Munk N, Symons B, Shang Y et al. (2012) Noninvasively measuring the hemodynamic effects of massage on skeletal muscle: a novel hybrid near-infrared diffuse optical instrument. J Bodyw Mov Ther. 16(1):22–28.

Nichols F, Humenick S (2000) Childbirth Education: Practice, Research and Theory, 2nd edn. Philadelphia: W.B. Saunders.

Noble E (2003) Essential Exercises for the Childbearing Year, 4th edn. Harwich: New Life Images.

Nuckolls K, Kaplan BH, Cassel J (1972) Psychosocial assets, life crises and the prognosis of pregnancy. Am J Epidemiol. 95:431.

O'Connor E, Senger CA, Henninger ML et al. (2019) Interventions to prevent perinatal depression: evidence report and systematic review for the US Preventive Services Task Force. JAMA. 321(6):588–601.

Olsen O, Clausen JA (2012) Planned hospital birth versus planned home birth. Cochrane Database Syst Rev. 9(9):CD000352.

Osborne C (2009) Pre- and perinatal massage therapy: survey of massage therapists. Available at: www.bodytherapy-education.com [accessed June 1, 2010].

Osborne-Sheets C (2002) Deep Tissue Sculpting, 2nd edn. San Diego: Body Therapy Associates.

Ostgaard HC, Andersson GBS, Karlsson K (1992) Prevalence of back pain in pregnancy. Spine. 17:53–55.

Oswald C, Higgins CC, Assimakopoulos D (2013) Optimizing pain relief during pregnancy using manual therapy. Can Fam Physician. 59(8):841–842.

Ozgoli G, Saei Ghare Naz M (2018) Effects of complementary medicine on nausea and vomiting in pregnancy: a systematic review. Int J Prev Med. 9:75.

Patijn J, Mekhail N, Hayek S et al. (2011) Meralgia paresthetica. Pain Practice. 11(3):302–308.

Pauk J, Kuhn C, Field T et al. (1986) The positive effects of tactile versus kinesthetic or vestibular stimulation on neuroendocrine and ODC activity in maternally deprived rat pups. Life Sci. 39:2081–2087.

Pirie A, Herman H (2003) How to Raise Children Without Breaking Your Back, 2nd edn. Cambridge, MA: IBIS.

Prescott JW (2005) Prevention or therapy and the politics of trust: inspiring a new human agenda. Psychother Polit Int. 3:194–221.

Pryde M (2000) Effectiveness of massage therapy for subacute low-back pain: a randomized controlled trial. Can Med Assoc J. 162(13):1815–1820.

Quebec Task Force on Spinal Disorders (1987) Scientific approach to the assessment and management of activity-related spinal disorders. Spine. 12(Suppl 1):524.

Rad Z, Haghshenas M, Javadian Y et al. (2016) The effect of massage on weight gain in very low birth weight neonates. J Clin Neonatol. 5(2):96–99.

Rapaport MH, Schettler P, Breese C (2010) A preliminary study of the effects of a single session of Swedish massage on hypothalamic-pituitary-adrenal and immune function in normal individuals. J Altern Complement Med. 16(10):1079–1088.

Rausch PB (1981) Effects of tactile and kinesthetic stimulation on premature infants. J Obstet Gynecol Neonatal Nurs. 10:34–37.

Reyes LM, Usselman CW, Davenport MH et al. (2018) Sympathetic nervous system regulation in human normotensive and hypertensive pregnancies. Hypertension. 71(5):793–803.

Ricci SS (2017) Essentials of Maternity, Newborn, and Women's Health Nursing, 4th edn. Philadelphia: Wolters Kluwer.

Rice R (1979) The effects of the Rice sensorimotor stimulation treatment on the development of high-risk infants. Birth Defects Orig Artic Ser. 15:7–26.

Riczo D (2020) Back and Pelvic Girdle Pain in Pregnancy and Postpartum. Minneapolis: OPTP.

Rosen J (1957) Dominance behavior as a function of early gentling experience in the albino rats. MA thesis, University of Toronto.

Roth LL, Rosenblatt JS (1996) Mammary glands of pregnant rats: development stimulated by licking. Science. 264:1403–1404.

Rubin R (1963) Maternal touch. Nurs Outlook. 11:828–831.

Rubin R (1975) Maternal tasks in pregnancy. Matern Child Nurs J. 4:143–153.

Rubin R (1984) Maternal Identity and the Maternal Experience. New York: Springer.

Ruegamer B, Benjamin JD (1954) Growth, food, utilization, and thyroid activity in the albino rat as a function of extra handling. Science. 120:184–185.

Samuels M, Samuels N (1996) The New Well Pregnancy Book. New York: Fireside.

Scafidi FA, Field TM, Schanberg SM et al. (1986) Effects of tactile/kinesthetic stimulation on the clinical course and sleep/wake behavior of preterm neonates. Infant Behav Dev. 9:91–105.

Scafidi FA, Field TM, Schanberg SM et al. (1990) Massage stimulates growth in preterm infants: a replication. Infant Behav Dev. 13:167–188.

Scheumann D (2007) The Balanced Body. Baltimore: Lippincott, Williams & Wilkins.

Schneider ML, Moore CF (2003) Prenatal stress and offspring development in nonhuman primates, in Tremblay RE, Barr RG, Peters RDeV (eds), Encyclopedia on Early Childhood Development. Montreal and Quebec: Centre of Excellence for Early Childhood Development, pp. 1–5. Available at: http://www.child-encyclopedia.com/documents/Schneider-MooreANGxp.pdf [accessed October 27, 2010].

Sefton JM, Yarar C, Berry JW et al. (2010) Therapeutic massage of the neck and shoulders produces changes in peripheral blood flow when assessed with dynamic infrared thermography. J Altern Complement Med. 16(7):723–732.

Settle F (1991) Musica, da? My experience in a Romanian orphanage. Massage Ther J. 64–72.

Shin TM, Bordeaux JS (2012) The role of massage in scar management: a literature review. Dermatol Surg. 38(3):414–423.

Shoemaker JK, Tiidus PM, Mader R (1997) Failure of manual massage to alter limb blood flow: measures by Doppler ultrasound. Med Sci Sports Exerc. 29(5):610–614.

Simkin P (1996) The experience of maternity in a woman's life. J Obstet Gynecol Neonatal Nurs. 25:247–252.

Simkin P, Klaus P (2011) When Survivors Give Birth, 2nd edn. Seattle: Classic Day.

Simkin P, O'Hara M (2002) Nonpharmacologic relief of pain during labor: systematic reviews of five methods. Am J Obstet Gynecol. 5(Supp l186):S131–S159.

Simkin P, Whalley J, Keppler A et al. (2018) Pregnancy, Childbirth and the Newborn, 5th edn. New York: Da Capo Press.

Slipman C, Jackson H, Lipetz J et al. (2000) Sacroiliac joint pain referral zones. Arch Phys Med Rehabil. 81(3):334–338.

Smith CA, Levett KM, Collins CT et al. (2018a) Relaxation techniques for pain management in labour. Cochrane Database Syst Rev. 3(3):CD009514.

Smith CA, Levett KM, Collins CT et al. (2018b) Massage, reflexology and other manual methods for pain management in labour. Cochrane Database Syst Rev. 3:CD009290.

Smith NK, Ryan K (2016) Traumatic Scar Tissue Management: Massage Therapy Principles, Practice and Protocols. Edinburgh: Handspring.

Solkoff N, Yaffe S, Weintraub D et al. (1969) Effects of handling on the subsequent development of premature infants. Develop Psychol. 1:765–768.

Spradley FT (2019) Sympathetic nervous system control of vascular function and blood pressure during pregnancy and preeclampsia. J Hypertens. 37(3):476–487. doi:10.1097/HJH.0000000000001901.

Steel A, Adams J, Sibbritt D et al. (2015) The outcomes of complementary and alternative medicine use among pregnant and birthing women: current trends and future directions. Womens Health. 11(3):309–323.

Stillerman E (2013) Mother Massage: A Handbook for Relieving the Discomforts of Pregnancy. New York: Random House.

Tanaka T, Leisman G, Hidetoshi M et al. (2002) The effect of massage on localized lumbar muscle fatigue. BMC Complem Altern Med. 2:9.

Tapp J, Markowitz H (1963) Infant handling: effects on avoidance learning, brain weight, and cholinesterase. Science. 140:486–487.

Taylor S (2012) Tend and befriend theory, in Handbook of Theories of Social Psychology: Volume 1, pp. 32–49. London: SAGE.

Taylor S, Klein L, Lewis B et al. (2000) Biobehavioral responses to stress in females: tend-and-befriend, not fight-or-flight. Psychol Rev. 107:411–429.

The Nature and Management of Labor Pain (2003) Part 1. Nonpharmacologic Pain Relief. Am Fam Physician. 68(6):1109–1112.

Thompson DL, Brooks M (2016) Integrative pain management: massage, movement, and mindfulness based approaches. Edinburgh: Handspring.

Togher KL, Treacy E, O'Keeffe GW et al. (2017) Maternal distress in late pregnancy alters obstetric outcomes and the expression of genes important for placental glucocorticoid signalling. Psychiatry Res. 255:17–26.

Tully G (2020) Changing Birth on Earth. Bloomington: Maternity House Publishing.

Unalmis Erdogan S, Yanikkerem E, Goker A (2017) Effects of low back massage on perceived birth pain and satisfaction. Complement Ther Clin Pract. 28:169–175.

Uvnäs-Moberg KU (2019) Oxytocin: The Biological Guide to Motherhood. Kindle Edition: Praeclarus Press.

Vermani E, Mittal R, Weeks A (2010) Pelvic girdle pain and low back pain in pregnancy: a review. Pain Practice. 10: 60–71.

Verstraete EH, Vanderstraeten G, Parewijck W (2013) Pelvic girdle pain during or after pregnancy: a review of recent evidence and a clinical care path proposal. Facts Views Vis Obgyn. 5(1):33–43.

Vleeming A, De Vries H, Mens J et al. (2002) Possible role of the long dorsal sacroiliac ligament in women with peripartum pelvic pain. Acta Obstet Gynecol Scand. 81(5):430–436.

Voltolini C, Petraglia F (2014) Neuroendocrinology of pregnancy and parturition. Handb Clin Neurol. 124:17–36. Available at: https://doi.org/10.1016/B978-0-444-59602-4.00002-2 [accessed July 3, 2020].

Wadhwa P, Culhane J, Rauh V (2001) Stress, infection and preterm birth: a biobehavioral perspective. Paediatr Perinat Epidemiol. 15(2):17–29.

Walton T (2016) 5 Myths and Truths about Massage Therapy: Letting Go Without Losing Heart. Massage Therapy Foundation. Available at: www.tracywalton.com [accessed December 12, 2019].

Wang MY, Tsai PS, Lee PH et al. (2008) The efficacy of reflexology: systematic review. J Adv Nurs. 62:512–520.

Weininger O, McClelland W, Arima K (1954) Gentling and weight gain in the albino rat. Can J Psychol. 8:147–151.

Werner R (2019) A Massage Therapist's Guide to Pathology, 7th edn. Boulder: Books of Discovery.

Wheeden A, Scafidi F, Field T et al. (1993) Massage effects on cocaine-exposed preterm neonates. J Develop Behav Pediatr. 14:318–322.

Wiltshire EV, Poitras V, Pak M et al. (2010) Massage impairs postexercise muscle blood flow and "lactic acid" removal. Med Sci Sports Exerc. 42(6):1062–1071.

Witt PL, MacKinnon J (1986) Trager psychophysical integration: a method to improve chest mobility of patients with chronic lung disease. Phys Ther. 66:214–217.

Xiao M, Zi-Qi et al. (2017) The Effect of Diaphragmatic Breathing on Attention, Negative Affect and Stress in Healthy Adults. Front Psychol. 8:874.

Zanolla R, Monzeglio C, Balzarini A et al. (1984) Evaluation of the results of three different methods of post-mastectomy lymphedema treatment. J Surg Oncol. 26:210–213.

Zimmermann A, Wozniewski M, Szklarska A et al. (2012) Efficacy of manual lymphatic drainage in preventing secondary lymphedema after breast cancer surgery. Lymphology. 45(3):103–112.

Zyluk A (2013) Carpal tunnel syndrome in pregnancy: a review. Pol Orthop Traumatol. 78:223–227.

Studying this chapter will prepare you to:

1. list the benefits and safety concerns of different positions during pregnancy

2. adapt your depth of pressure and speed to a beneficial level for prenatal clients

3. explain the safety concerns related to prenatal leg and abdominal massage

4. identify other body areas where you need to make specific prenatal adaptations of massage techniques

5. list adaptations to Swedish, deep tissue, movement, reflexive and other modalities that help ensure safety and effectiveness

6. recognize common signs and symptoms that are not part of normal pregnancy progression

7. list prenatal conditions that are classified as high-risk for creating complications

8. list lifestyle and health history factors that may require additional information and adaptation for prenatal massage therapy.

Guidelines
Massaging Safely and Effectively

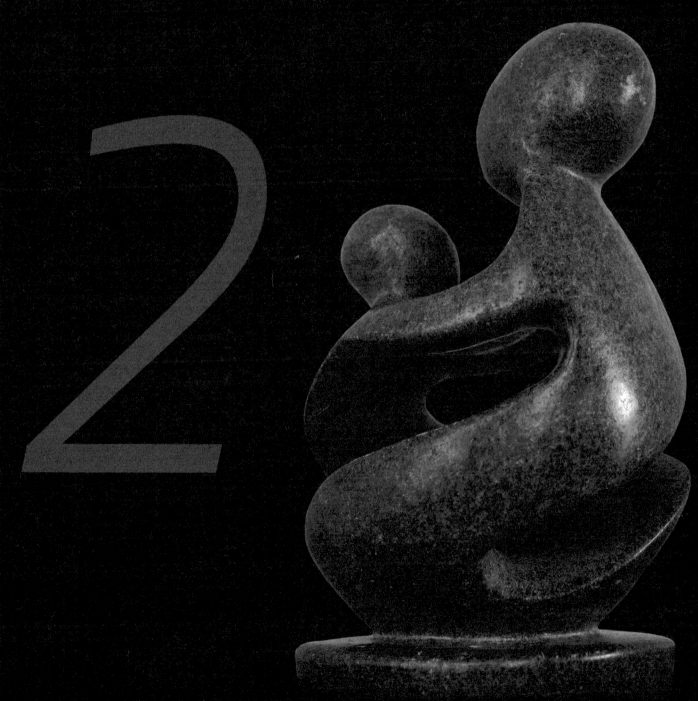

Chapter Overview

With so much potential benefit in receiving massage therapy while pregnant, why would anyone hesitate to receive regular sessions? Other than financial considerations, and the seemingly inevitable difficulty of finding enough time in the day, the ultimate factor in any pregnancy-related decision is: will this be safe for me and my baby? Women, their partners and their healthcare providers need assurance that massage therapy is beneficial and safe. To deliver that assurance, you must assess what is and is not uniquely appropriate for each individual client. You need to understand when the various positions on a therapy table and chair are safe, or not, and how to make every position comfortable. You need to understand and master various appropriate types of therapeutic massage and bodywork. You need to understand prenatal physiology and functioning, and learn how to adapt your touch accordingly. These adaptations include changes in speed, depth of pressure and pain level, an awareness of precautionary areas, and specific modality variations.

To be safe and effective, you must adapt your existing skills to the needs of typical prenatal clients. This chapter will explore how to adapt. That foundation will then be applied to specific prenatal techniques in Chapter 4; massage for labor and birth in Chapter 5; and massage for the postpartum mother in Chapter 6. You also need to be able to recognize when pregnancy and postpartum are not proceeding normally, which is detailed in Chapter 7.

Is Prenatal Massage Safe?

The short answer is: it depends. Nearly every pregnant person can safely benefit from *some* type of therapeutic massage and bodywork. After all, pregnancy itself is not an illness. Pregnant people are not porcelain dolls; they are far from fragile. In fact, many women feel their most sturdy, energetic and fierce when pregnant. As the mother adapts to pregnancy's demands, some form of massage therapy is likely safe in all trimesters (and beyond!).

These factors will determine whether your work is safe: which week/trimester your client is in; how you position and support your client; what body parts you massage; the speed, depth, intensity and intention of your techniques; and the baby's growth and health. In this chapter, you will learn how to create that safety for most pregnant people.

Your safety and effectiveness also will be determined by your ability to understand each client's particular needs and wants, and to adjust your work accordingly. Sometimes a client will prefer to zone out; other times they will want to actively engage. Remember that she may have other conditions unrelated to the pregnancy – infections or injuries, for example – that you need to consider in determining whether and how to work with her.

Of course, pre- and perinatal massage therapy does not replace medical or midwifery care; we work best in collaboration with maternity healthcare providers. In all work environments, remember to seek consultation when you need it – especially if the pregnancy is high-risk, if the client develops or has had prior complications, or if you observe signs of possible complications. With each client, your aim should be to recognize her strength and abilities, assess any potential problems, and then alter your own work to best honor her needs.

From the treatment room

When I started massaging pregnant women for my doctoral study, almost all of the 400 women I invited said that they had never heard of prenatal massage. They and their families were afraid and did not want to have it done. A few in my region of Turkey eventually joined my study. After my research was over, I returned to my clinic. I learned that a pregnant woman had called everyone in the clinic, trying to reach me! I gave her prenatal massages every week. Another participant, after her prenatal massage, said something similar to "That was almost orgasmic." Of course, there was no sexual contact, but she definitely felt the oxytocin effects of this work.

– **Yeliz Çakır Koçak**, therapist

Reminder

When you follow safety guidelines, some form of massage therapy will be safe for virtually every pregnant client.

Points of view: Is massage safe in the first trimester?

But wait! Perhaps in massage school you were taught to never massage in the first trimester; or maybe your employer forbids it. The typical rationale for waiting to start prenatal massage is that pregnancy loss is more common in the first trimester; we do not want a client to associate miscarriage with massage.

Actual accusations of catastrophic results from prenatal massage therapy are rare, but they remain possible (Ernst 2003). Beyond this worst-case scenario, minor injury or just an ineffective massage might occur, especially when a therapist lacks sufficient training. The safety (and effectiveness) of prenatal massage is relative to the therapist's knowledge. The first-trimester prohibition may be a wise legal precaution, especially when the prenatal curricula of many schools are understandably brief and lacking in depth or accuracy (see Chapter 4 for other elements of first-trimester safety).

That said, there is no substantive research that demonstrates that massage is unsafe in the first trimester, when appropriate guidelines are followed. Some erroneous reasons given for the first-trimester contraindication are that it will cause miscarriages or detach the placenta. There is no evidence that either possibility is likely if a therapist works superficially on the abdomen and avoids very specific types of touch on contraindicated points, as discussed later in this chapter. Some teachers claim that first-trimester massage worsens nausea; others say to not massage

at all if a client is nauseated. Again, when performed within the informed guidelines given later in this chapter and in Chapter 4, this should not be a concern; in fact, the parasympathetic stimulation of a good massage may calm a queasy stomach. Of course, if the client is vomiting or extremely nauseated, she is not likely to want a massage anyway.

Increase confidence in the safety of your work by gathering thorough client information, maintaining sufficient communications with their maternity healthcare providers, and following this book's sound guidance.

From the treatment room

When I first met Sharon at the upscale day spa where I worked, she returned a blank health form to me. In fact, she gave the receptionist a hard time, feeling that we were prying into her business; after all, she only wanted a massage!

I explained how massage could certainly address many issues, but that if she had any problems, then I would be better able to serve her by knowing. I could ask more questions that might lead her to see her doctor before her next scheduled monthly visit. She was dumbstruck that so much information went into performing a prenatal massage, and I was grateful that I had the knowledge to care for her.

– **Mia Harper**, therapist

Reminder

You may prefer to delay massage until a client enters her second trimester; however, first-trimester massage therapy is safe if performed according to recommendations.

Safe Positioning

The first practical question most therapists ask when contemplating prenatal massage is how to accommodate that ripe belly. Most of us only work with our non-pregnant clients supine and **prone**, so it is easy for us (and our clients) to feel unsure of any other possibilities. While the pregnant body has unique requirements, the positioning options are abundant. Working in both prone and supine is still fruitful with some clients. But even more advantageous – though initially daunting – is to position your clients on their sides. Safety, comfort and therapeutic effectiveness will determine which positions you use – and when and how (Figure 2.1). We will explore the rationale for all below. Remember that these are not hard and fast rules, particularly regarding their timing. Individual needs change the timing of the recommended positions. But with these guidelines, and a lot of practice, you will be able to efficiently accommodate nearly any pregnant client at any stage of pregnancy.

Prone

Let's face it: many of us are belly sleepers and prefer to not give up that comforting position, even for a massage. And massage therapists are more accustomed to working on a client's back while in prone. But are these reasons enough to use the prone position throughout pregnancy? No. Lying face down may be a safe and comfortable position to rest in (Ricci 2017), but once you apply the pressure needed for an effective massage, it is no longer reliably comfortable or safe for all clients; neither is the three-quarters prone position some of us learned in school. The two potential problems with prone positioning are strain to the uterine ligaments and lower back, and increased pressure inside the uterus, known as **intrauterine pressure** (Figure 2.2). Let us first consider strain to these posterior structures.

Lying prone on a flat therapy table can strain the structures of the lumbar spine, pelvis and uterus. Prone positioning can create a host of negative effects: it shortens posterior musculature; compresses and anteriorly

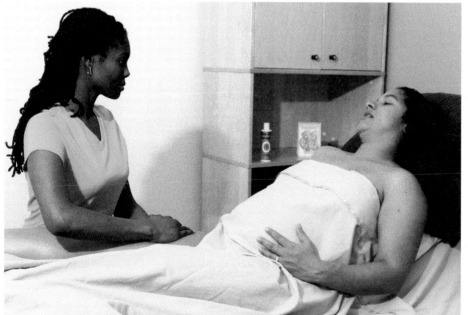

First trimester
- Supine, sidelying, semireclining, prone or in a chair, depending on client comfort.
- Adapt for breast tenderness and other comfort and safety concerns, especially if using prone.

Second trimester
- Prone position is not recommended, even with specialized equipment.
- Supine - use pillow under right lower torso, up to week 22. After 22 weeks, only use semireclining and sidelying positions to prevent supine hypotensive syndrome; chair okay.
- Adapt for breast tenderness, SI joint, and other comfort and safety concerns.

Third trimester
- Sidelying and semireclining positions only; chair okay.
- Adjust for comfort and safety concerns.

Figure 2.1
Overview of prenatal massage positioning. These positions enable comfort, safety and effectiveness throughout the pregnancy.

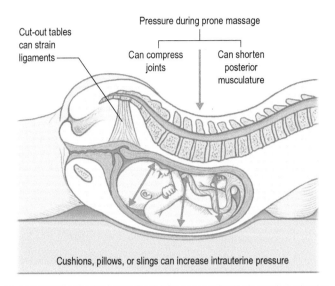

Cut-out tables can strain ligaments

Pressure during prone massage

Can compress joints

Can shorten posterior musculature

Cushions, pillows, or slings can increase intrauterine pressure

Figure 2.2
Potential effects of the prone position. Notice how both safety and comfort can be compromised with improper positioning.

displaces the lumbar vertebrae and lumbosacral junction; rotates and strains the sacroiliac (SI) joints; and increases strain on the sacrouterine ligaments. Because of these effects, lying face down – particularly in later pregnancy – often aggravates the very causes of back discomfort for many. Although some clients feel comfortable in prone, many feel these strains – not to mention the compression of breast tissue and sinuses – which diminishes the effectiveness of their massage.

Pillows, or specialized equipment marketed for pregnant clients, may mitigate these problems to some extent. However, one-size cut-out tables or prone cushions do not fit all bodies, especially with multiples and various breech fetal positions. Nothing – not pillow props; cushions; pregnancy pillows; tables with cut-out ovals, with or without a sling or net designed to support the belly; or most massage chairs – can alone solve all of the problematic aspects of prone positioning completely. If the client is cushioned sufficiently high to keep pressure off the uterus, then further strain to posterior structures and the taxed sacrouterine ligaments is likely. To prevent that posterior strain, the belly must rest against the table, and that increases intrauterine

pressure, especially as you apply sufficient pressure to address the posterior structures. It is the proverbial "catch-22."

Lumbar and pelvic pain is among the top reasons why women come for massage (Osborne 2009). No matter how well intended, even the best effort to maintain pelvic and lumbar alignment while in prone does not relieve strain from all painful structures. The **bodyCushion**™ – when used appropriately, as described in Chapter 3 – can be useful for prenatal and postpartum work. When used under a prone client, it supports the pelvis at the anterior superior iliac spine (ASIS), often normalizing the lumbar curve and helping to prevent lumbar and SI joint strain. However, it does not protect the vulnerable sacrouterine ligaments from strain. When this or any similar support lifts the prone pelvis sufficiently to prevent pressing the **gravid** uterus against the therapy table, the (weighty) uterus is left dangling from these ligaments. The fascial attachments of these ligaments on the anterior sacrum, and the associated connective tissue that wraps around the pelvis, are already strained by any anterior pelvic misalignment during daily activities. The area can become even achier during a session, especially for the length of time and with the amount of pressure needed to work effectively on the posterior body. In short: for your client's sake, you must be aware of prone position's significant problems, and be wary of any prone props or tables, however well intentioned, that claim to solve those problems.

Now let us consider the increase in intrauterine pressure. Because of gravity, the weight of the torso presses the prone client's abdomen into the table, or into any additional supportive device. This increases the amount of pressure already exerted against the inner walls of the uterus by the fetus(es), **amniotic fluid** and placenta(s). The amount of increase depends on the firmness of the table or props and on the client's weight and abdominal size. As you press on her back with any but the lightest touch, your body weight further increases this intrauterine pressure. If you use deeper pressure, especially in the problematic lumbar and pelvic areas – in other words, just posterior of the uterus – that could create even more, albeit unintentional, intrauterine pressure.

Considering all that, how safe is the prone position? We do not have enough direct data to supply a confident answer. Here are some considerations, though.

- The only recommendation that the American College of Obstetricians and Gynecologists (ACOG) currently makes regarding positioning is that pregnant women should sleep on their sides after 13 weeks.

- Pregnancy itself enhances the contractibility of the uterine muscles. Increase in intrauterine pressure (due to tight clothing, excessive amniotic fluid and other causes) irritates the uterine muscles (Ricci 2017). These smooth muscles contract when irritated. Because the uterine muscles are already in a hypercontractile state, those contractions may be mistaken for preterm labor or may potentially contribute to preterm labor or miscarriage.

- Avoiding increased intrauterine pressure is of particular relevance with multiples, placental dysfunction, amniotic fluid imbalances and other high-risk factors and complications (see Chapter 7).

- Extra caution is also needed if there is heightened concern about fetal blood supply, uterine competence and/or a history of miscarriages. People diagnosed with these conditions are often uninformed about how they can be impacted by bodywork. Some of these problems go undetected until someone is specifically screened for them, or until bleeding, cramping or other overt signs of problems have occurred to warrant further diagnosis.

- There is a small amount of recent research that finds little harm for brief periods in the prone position, but also does not offer any conclusive findings about the added pressure that comes with massage (Ray and Trikha 2018; Dennis et al. 2018; Oliveira et al. 2017).

This much is clear: in most uncomplicated, low-risk pregnancies, a mild, temporary increase in intrauterine pressure – such as occurs while resting briefly in prone – is acceptable. During the first 13 weeks, the anterior iliac spines usually protect the uterus from significant increased pressure. Use the prone position in the first trimester if you or your client prefer, but remember that, even in the first trimester, prone can be problematic with the conditions mentioned above, or when the embryo is larger than normal or your client is obese. Because of the fragmented nature of what we do know about prone positioning, and the enormous amount that we do not know, our recommendation is this: to avoid any potential risk of excessive intrauterine pressure, use the sidelying and semireclining positions with all pregnant clients needing posterior work.

Reminder

Prone positioning – especially in second and third trimesters – can increase intrauterine pressure and/or strain posterior ligaments and muscles.

In addition to these safety concerns, there are very compelling comfort reasons to avoid prone positioning. Even in the first trimester, when the abdomen is not significantly larger, prone positioning exerts pressure on enlarged breasts. In fact, first-trimester women often have extremely sensitive breasts. One way to minimize this pain when prone is to use a cushion that has breast recesses carved into the foam foundation. Another alternative is to use a pillow or rolled towels at the clavicles and at the lower ribs so the breasts lie between.

Pregnant people may have more congestion due to a hormonally induced increase in mucus. Those with colds, allergies and other sinus conditions are particularly uncomfortable because their maternity healthcare providers may advise them to discontinue medications that alleviate congestion.

On the emotional side, some clients are uneasy with the idea of "lying on my baby." Similarly, the confines of face cradles and other prone positioning devices can hamper verbal and emotional sharing, important for stress reduction and, for many, a crucial part of a nurturing massage experience. We also lose the ability to gauge the client's experience by observing her facial expressions.

Often the prone position is also the least therapeutically effective position in which to receive a massage session. Stomach sleeping often creates or contributes to back pain, hip and neck dysfunction and other musculoskeletal misalignments (Pirie and Herman 2003). Do we want to contribute to our clients' problems by using this position when there are beneficial alternatives? And as you will see, working from the sidelying and semireclining positions, rather than from prone, offers more ability to engage and move the most problematic parts of the pregnant client: the posterior body, the hip and the shoulder.

In summary, to ensure the safety and comfort of every pregnant client, and to improve session outcomes, we recommend that you eliminate the prone position after the first 13 weeks – regardless of your or the client's preferences. Even in the first trimester, use caution and make reasonable adaptations.

Supine and Semireclining

The other presumed massage position, of course, is lying face up. For prenatal massage, the safety of the supine position is determined mostly by maternal and fetal circulation. The inferior vena cava is the body's major vessel returning blood to the heart from the lower body through the iliac veins. It runs up the right side of the vertebral bodies along the posterior abdominal wall. The inferior vena cava is unaffected by supine positioning in the first trimester: the uterus has not grown beyond the pelvic cavity, and it is not very wide or heavy. Once past 13 or so weeks, when an expectant person lies on her back the weighty uterus and its contents rest against the common and internal iliac veins and the inferior vena cava. Extended compression of these vessels will result in low maternal blood pressure and decreased maternal and fetal circulation, called **supine hypotensive syndrome** (Figure 2.3). Some women report uneasiness, dizziness, weakness, nausea, shortness of breath or other discomforts when lying flat on their back, although others seem entirely content. However, with or without notable negative maternal effects, decreased fetal circulation can occur, particularly if the placenta is embedded posteriorly, its most likely location (Ricci 2017).

Some authorities advise pregnant women to never lie supine, even when resting or sleeping (Stone et al. 2017;

Heazell et al. 2018; Callahan and Caughey 2007), primarily when there is increased concern about fetal oxygenation because of complications. Others caution pregnant women only to avoid supine exercising for long periods (ACOG 2015). From these parameters, it appears safe throughout pregnancy for most of our clients to lie on their backs briefly: say, for up to five minutes. Of course, if she becomes uncomfortable, or if her maternity healthcare provider places greater restrictions on supine positioning, you should adjust accordingly.

There are some options for longer supine work: in the early second trimester of a single-gestation pregnancy, you can use a pillow support under the right side of the lower torso, thus shifting uterine weight toward the left and reducing compression of the vessels. After 22 weeks, the rapidly expanding uterus will compress a sizeable section of the vena cava, even with the pillow under the right pelvis. Instead, you need to utilize what is ultimately the optimal position for face-up prenatal work: semireclining, which we will discuss below.

Comfort is another reason to avoid prolonged supine positioning. More than a few minutes on her back can aggravate the expectant client's SI joints and cause back pain. This is more likely if the back is poorly supported, if she is on an inadequately padded table, or if she is in the last trimester. These conditions can create an immediate,

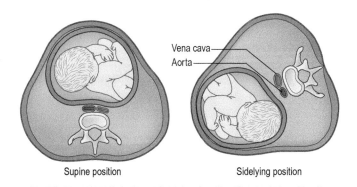

Supine position   Sidelying position

Figure 2.3
Supine hypotensive syndrome. In supine position (left), the enlarged uterus compresses the inferior vena cava. In sidelying position (right), torso vessels are free of the weight of the uterus.

painful, locking sensation in the upper buttock and iliac crest, usually on one side, particularly if one SI joint is hypomobile and the other is hypermobile (Riczo 2020; Noble 2003). Consider a minimum of 3 inches (7.6 cm) of triple-density foam padding for massage therapy tables used prenatally.

No matter how briefly you place the client in supine position, be aware of supporting and reducing lumbar lordosis, when needed. You can best accomplish this with sufficiently high knee bolsters to help mechanically relax the lumbar area against the table. To help relieve lower-extremity edema, place another pillow under her calves and feet level with the knees.

The solution to nearly all of the potential problems of supine prenatal work is to use the semireclining position (also called semirecumbent), either in addition to or instead of supine. Chapter 3 offers detailed instructions for creating this and all recommended positioning adaptations, but the basics are simple: you support the client's torso, assuring an angle of 45 to 75 degrees from her hip to her head. With a few modifications to your own body position as well, what you normally do in supine can be performed in semireclining, without any of the difficulties.

If a client has multiples or is overweight, you should switch to a semireclining position after the first trimester, and not use the pillow under the right pelvis at all. Other clients will be fine using a combination of supine in first trimester, then the pillow under the right pelvis for part of the second trimester, and then semireclining for the remainder. But remember that some clients will prefer the semireclining position throughout their pregnancy, particularly those who are obese or short of breath, or have heartburn. (As discussed in Chapter 6, semireclining can be valuable in postpartum as well.)

Reminder

When the client is supine, use a pillow under the right lower abdomen (weeks 13 to 22), or prop her in a semireclining position, to prevent supine hypotensive syndrome.

Sidelying

The position that offers the greatest combination of safety and comfort, for nearly all clients, and throughout the pregnancy, is the sidelying or **lateral recumbent** position (Figure 2.4). When sufficiently supported by pillows, bolsters and/or positioning systems, most clients find great relief and are happy in this position (see Chapter 3). Properly aligned sidelying position minimizes musculoskeletal and uterine ligament strain. It avoids pressure on the uterus, sinuses and breasts, and enables emotionally helpful conversation. This position offers the psychological comfort that comes from being in (or similar to) the fetal position. Nestled comfortably on her side, the client may feel more able to talk about her excitement, and her concerns, without the obstruction of a face cradle (as when prone) or the confrontational effect of talking face to face (as when supine or semireclining).

Physicians and midwives recommend the sidelying position for sleeping and resting. In sidelying, the vena cava is not compressed, and with proper abdominal support, the strain on uterine ligaments is reduced (see Figure 2.3). In many high-risk pregnancies, or when complications occur, women are told to sleep only in the left sidelying position, which allows for maximum maternal cardiac functioning and fetal oxygenation (Ricci 2017).

Unfortunately, this requirement is often exaggerated to an overly cautious and ultimately uncomfortable conclusion: that all pregnant people should lie exclusively on their left sides. Not only is it perfectly safe for most to lie on either side, but sleeping on both sides may even improve sleep and digestion (Silver et al. 2019). Unless their physician or midwife requires otherwise, feel confident to position your clients on whichever side they prefer or that offers you best access to problematic areas; or divide your session time between left and right sidelying positions. (Also, note that clients who sleep mostly on their left side often need the left side worked more extensively.)

Reminder

Sidelying is the safest (and usually most comfortable) position for prenatal massage therapy when the client is properly supported.

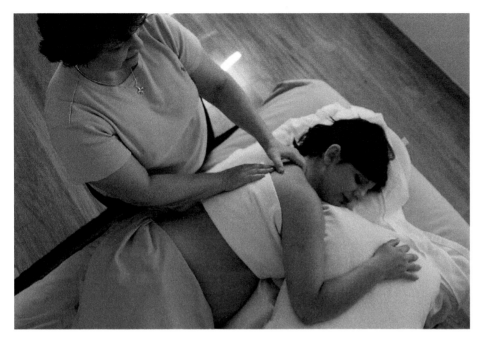

- Improves access to pectoral and pelvic girdle for therapist
- Avoids increased uterine pressure and supine hypotension
- Decreases edema
- Maximizes maternal cardiac function and fetal oxygenation
- Avoids sinus congestion, breast compression
- Psychologically comforts and soothes
- Facilitates sharing

Figure 2.4
Advantages of the sidelying position. When properly supported, the sidelying position benefits mother, fetus and therapist.

Points of view: Positioning

Positioning a pregnant client is one of the most confusing, and contentious, aspects of prenatal massage therapy. So it is important to clarify both the places of overlap and the places of disagreement. With little to no direct research on positioning for prenatal massage therapy, other evidence – anatomy, physiology, and nursing and obstetrical best practices – can provide some objective guidance.

All maternity massage instructors agree on one aspect of prone positioning: after the first trimester, a woman should not lie prone directly on a massage table without some type of accommodating equipment. The area where differing opinions arise is regarding whether any supports sufficiently reduce the problems of second-and third-trimester prone positioning: increased intrauterine pressure and strain to the posterior structures. Some claim that specially contoured cushions will prevent these problems while the client is in prone. Such cushions may be effective for those massage therapists and other providers, such as chiropractors and physical therapists, who do very brief prone treatments (Stillerman 2008) or whose pressure is superficial. Unfortunately, there is no published evidence to confirm or negate this safety concern for the length of most massage therapy sessions or with deeper pressure.

Recommendations for supine positioning have more variance. Some instructors advise to never use supine without modifications to prevent supine hypotensive syndrome, even in the first trimester. Given the small weight of the fetus (1 ounce/0.03 kg) and the size of the gravid uterus (4 inches/10 cm high and barely wider than the pubic bone) at the end of the first trimester, significant compression of the vena cava is highly unlikely before 14 to 20 weeks, except when there are multiples.

Among instructors who advise use of supports under the right side, as described above, there are small variances in placement and timing. Some suggest a wedge or blanket all the way from the shoulder to the iliac crest. Because the inferior vena cava bifurcates deep in the abdomen, into the common and then internal and external iliac veins (which then descend into the pelvis), having the support underneath both the abdomen and the right hip seems more accurate. There is also disagreement as to when to move the client from this modified supine position to semireclining: at 14 weeks (Stager 2010), 18 to 20 weeks (Stillerman 2008), or as late as the last couple of months (Yates 2010). In a singleton pregnancy with average fetal growth, the uterus reaches maternal umbilicus level at 20 to 22 weeks, and is wide enough to press on the iliac veins and the inferior vena cava. Thus, positioning her in semireclining has the desired effect: directing uterine weight more toward the pelvic floor. But in semireclining, using additional supports under the right side is a redundancy, and makes stability in this semi-recumbent position more tenuous.

In summary – and until more direct research on the issue is available – we wholeheartedly recommend the sidelying position for prenatal massage therapy, regardless of possible inconvenience to, or the preference of, the massage therapist. It offers the most advantages and avoids some potential discomforts and risks, especially of prone positioning (see Figures 2.2–2.4). Another safe option, although generally not as comfortable for the expectant client, is seated massage therapy on either a household chair or a stool. Note that most massage chairs are a safe alternative only when the pregnant client rests her back against the pad normally used for chest support, for the same reasons as described in the prone positioning discussion above (and see Chapter 3).

Effective Modalities for Prenatal and Perinatal Massage

Most basic massage therapy training programs teach at least one therapeutic method that is readily adaptable for maternity care. Simple Swedish massage routines and introductory deep tissue or neuromuscular techniques can reduce stress, help relieve achy joints and muscles, and help the client feel nurtured. In other words, you already have some techniques that will help pregnant clients. Chances are, in whatever modalities you currently practice – from myofascial release to Reiki, from Shiatsu to Swedish – you have much to offer a pregnant client.

There is no single method or sequence that is *the* ideal prenatal or postpartum session. To limit yourself in that way would deprive your clients of the extensive benefits of the many somatic practices available to the professional massage therapist. Assess the methods you know to determine which can best help your pregnant clients. During the childbearing year, you will likely need to significantly modify some of those techniques and eliminate others. Use the guidelines and precautions here to carefully evaluate the physiological, structural and psychological impact of every technique from any method you contemplate using. Box 2.4 later lists critical guidelines for making technique choices and modifications.

In later chapters, you will learn many specific pre- and perinatal techniques from a variety of modalities. Let these details spark your creativity and personalize your approach to your clients. As with all hands-on skills, your education will be more complete if you also participate in a comprehensive continuing education program that includes demonstrations of specifically adapted, clinically tested techniques, and then hands-on practice and feedback. ⊕

Moderating Pressure, Speed and Pain

If *whether* and *how* are our first concerns when working with pregnant clients, usually the next is finding the appropriate level of pressure, speed and pain. To some therapists, pregnant clients seem so vulnerable, yet certain methods seem to require deep work to be effective. As mentioned, prenatal clients are far from fragile, but their preferences do vary widely. Determine each client's needs, and recognize that they can be very different in different parts of her body and on different days. Furthermore, cultivating your palpatory sensitivity will make you even more effective; the more aware you are of her tissues, the more you will be able to modify your work to her needs (Chaitow 2017).

Certain techniques in certain areas, such as abdominal effleurage, need to be superficial, reaching only into the skin and superficial fascia. Others, such as deep tissue and trigger point work, need therapeutic depth, but no deeper than what the client experiences as pleasure at the borderline of pain. And in certain parts of the body, especially the medial leg and abdomen, deep work may be dangerous (as detailed below). Just as with non-pregnant clients, you will be able to work as deep as clients want and need in most areas, while still calming them, if you work more slowly, especially when entering and exiting from the tissue.

Always learn the client's pressure preferences, perception of pain, tension level, and needs in a given body area. Her general health, injuries or other safety considerations (discussed later in this chapter) may dictate lighter pressures than those used with non-pregnant clients. Explore with her what qualities of your touch and what techniques best help her to relax, to experience less pain and to expand her enjoyment of her childbearing experience.

Provide her with a reliable means to communicate her experience of your pressure; generic responses like "that feels fine" do not really tell you anything. One option is a number scale (Box 2.1).

Alternatively, try imagery rather than numbers. Pregnant people often relate better to right-brain metaphors than left-brain linear concepts, as pregnancy expands right-brain functioning (Naperstek 2007). You could introduce a color scheme for pleasure and pain feedback that follows the common correlation of a traffic light (Box 2.2). Soliciting your client's feedback can deepen her own engagement with, and control over, your work together.

Regardless of modality, remember that a client's pain level is greatly influenced by the depth and speed of your pressure. Gradually adding your body weight to your working tool makes the client more receptive; their tissues yield rather than guard, and invite greater depth. Instead of forcing or "fixing" your client's tight areas, think of facilitating or encouraging your client towards a position of greater ease. That shift will usually enable you to work more easily and with greater depth, and often makes your client more engaged. As you develop their awareness, their sessions will likely feel more pleasurable and informative. An actively participating client also means that your work will be often less effortful for you, physically and emotionally.

Mechanical considerations, such as table height, positioning and your own body use, also contribute to a client's pain perception. Chapter 3 will give you many tips

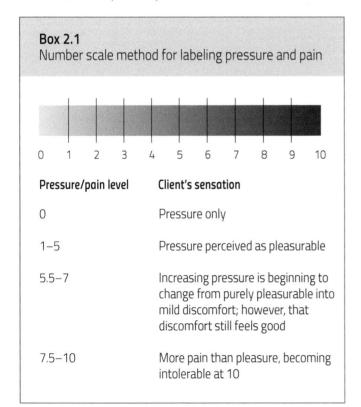

Box 2.1
Number scale method for labeling pressure and pain

Pressure/pain level	Client's sensation
0	Pressure only
1–5	Pressure perceived as pleasurable
5.5–7	Increasing pressure is beginning to change from purely pleasurable into mild discomfort; however, that discomfort still feels good
7.5–10	More pain than pleasure, becoming intolerable at 10

Box 2.2
Color method for labeling pressure and pain

Color	Client's sensation	Therapist's response
Green	Completely pleasurable	Keep on going
Yellow	Pleasure tinged with mild discomfort but still feels good	Proceed with caution
Red	More pain than pleasure	Decrease pressure

and directions to make your work deep, effective and comfortable for your client and for you.

From the treatment room

I loved my first experience with massage therapy. I definitely feared it would be too harsh; it was nothing like that. It was warm, attentive and wonderful. I wished it would go on forever. I felt more balanced, and the specific tight areas I came in with just melted as my therapist worked gradually deeper.

– **Roselle**, client

Maintaining an awareness of your client's experience of pleasure and pain ensures that you will cultivate the intended relaxation response during your session. By contrast, ignoring your client's perception of your work risks the opposite: a counterproductive sympathetic arousal in the mother and her baby. Remember that pain activates adrenal production of the hormones that elevate blood pressure, heart rate and respiratory rate, and lower immune function and blood flow to the uterus. Because these hormonal signals diffuse into fetal circulation through the placenta, the fetus is also negatively impacted (Ricci 2017; Togher et al. 2017; Monk et al. 2016).

Furthermore, forceful and abrupt movements activate the client's defensive withdrawal reflexes, which trigger increased muscular tension rather than relaxation. When pain becomes too intense, the entire body instinctively pushes away from the source of pain. Remember, it is only in a receptive state that clients can readily explore and learn new behaviors, such as more effective breathing, relaxation and postural alignment (Juhan 2003). For your client to relax and to learn as much as possible from your work, you must perform even the deepest work gently.

Reminder

Avoid extremely painful techniques to better achieve the goals of prenatal massage therapy: reduce stress, relieve pain, educate.

Navigating Extreme Emotions

Most expectant people inevitably will feel intense emotions during their pregnancy – everything from anger to fear to sadness to joy – and on your table, they may feel supported enough to explore and express these feelings. Enabling this emotional expression can be as powerful as any soft tissue technique in reducing production of stress hormones and in making your client feel more grounded in her pregnant body. But you also must create a balance – based on intuition and physiology – between those benefits and the potential negative effects of diving into strong emotions. Also, remember to stay within your professional boundaries. Aim to support as complete an expression as your client pursues. Allow for her emotional outbursts, but always follow her lead, and never encourage or push her to the point of emotional overwhelm. (See Chapters 4 to 7 and online resources for more guidance in supporting your clients emotionally.) ⊕

Throughout, remember that treating psychological dynamics is outside of the massage therapist's scope of practice and expertise. You can (and should) be a supportive resource, but you should not treat her psychologically or tell her what to do. As a part of your development as a maternity massage therapist, you should establish a reliable network of professionals who are knowledgeable and experienced in working with maternity mental health.

Areas Requiring Caution

The need for a solid grounding in anatomy, physiology, research and other evidence is particularly important when working with prenatal clients. Pregnancy's changes run the gamut from cellular to full body, in both their magnitude and their complexity. Our approach to working with pregnant clients must be equally comprehensive. Our guidelines must rest on a solid foundation of evidence, not myths or hearsay. The precautions and recommendations in the following section reflect our in-depth understanding of the current evidence available – and a respect for all that we do not currently know. Maximize your understanding of this evidence and of normal and abnormal prenatal developments. That understanding, combined with your good intentions and skillful techniques, will ensure that each client's care is thoughtful and individualized, safe and effective.

Abdominal Massage

When we first started massaging in the 1970s, the existing texts considered pregnancy a total contraindication to massage – often with little or no rationale. So a handful of curious, passionate pioneers, including us, began collecting evidence. Since then, we have been boosted tremendously by a still small, but growing, body of research. That "total contraindication" myth has been debunked. Nevertheless, several controversies relating to maternity massage therapy persist (see "Points of view" boxes throughout this book). The pregnant abdomen is at the top of that list.

Some teachers warn students to never massage the belly for fear of provoking miscarriage. That fear is supported by only one study, described below – a study that was small and flawed, and about deep abdominal massage. That said, caution seems reasonable for students lacking a comprehensive education in prenatal massage. Then, as we deepen our prenatal training, it is critical that we all follow certain guidelines when massaging the abdomen to ensure the safety of client and baby.

When and How to Massage the Abdomen

With a client's permission, superficial abdominal massage is generally beneficial. Some clients report that it soothes nausea. When performed within certain parameters, it may help, through parasympathetic stimulation, to counter the negative effects of stress. It may help women to connect emotionally with their unborn child, reinforcing prenatal bonding (Figure 2.5) (Nichols and Humenick 2000; Fink et al. 2012; Wang et al. 2015; Field 2016).

We touch the abdomen only with the client's permission, and our general safety guidelines are simple:

- Effectively position and support her, as detailed earlier in this chapter and in Chapter 3.
- When applying these guidelines, consider the borders of the pregnant abdomen to be the pubic bone, inguinal ligaments, xiphoid process, distal ribcage

and the lateral borders of the quadratus lumborum, and observe all precautions within those boundaries.

- Touch the pregnant abdomen no deeper than the skin and superficial fascia level.
- Use the entire flat, relaxed palm of your hand for broad, superficial effleurage strokes. For smaller strokes, such as superficial fanning, use only the broad edges of your thumbs, and avoid pointed pressure.
- Completely "mold" your hand to the belly's contours so that there is no space between your hand and the belly. This molding creates full, relaxed contact that is soothing, without being ticklish or too deep. (See Chapter 4's Technique Manual for specific techniques.)
- Modify stretches and other mobilizations to avoid creating deep pressure to the abdomen, such as during hip flexion, internal rotation during deep flexion, or sidebending and flexion of spine/ribcage.

To reinforce the importance of the above guidelines, let us consider what could happen if we ignored these guidelines. To be clear, the points below are all hypothetical, but they are important to consider in order to move beyond the unhelpful and fear-inducing contraindication against any and all abdominal massage. Without proper caution, abdominal massage could cause:

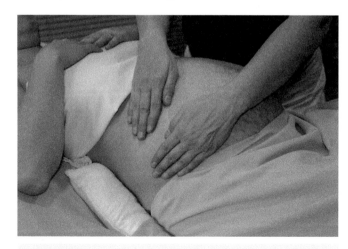

Figure 2.5
Abdominal massage. Gentle but connected strokes can both soothe the mom and connect her and her baby.

- hyperirritability of the smooth muscles of the uterine walls, causing premature contractions

- detachment or damage to the placenta (of particular concern if the attachment is already tenuous and/or not in its ideal location on the posterior uterine wall)

- damage to the blood vessels supplying the uterus that are embedded and supported in the uterine ligaments, particularly the broad ligament (through sustained, deep and pointed pressure into the anterior iliac region)

- dislodging of any thrombi in the iliac veins (see detailed discussion of thrombi later in this chapter).

Again, all of these are theoretical. No reputable studies have found evidence of trauma with abdominal massage using the guidelines above. However, there is one study that has caused a lot of fear. That study examined traditional abdominal massage practices in southern Nigeria, which consisted of stroking and kneading of the anterior abdominal muscles and gentle lifting of the soft tissue over the abdomen. (It also may have involved kneading of the thighs – the study details are vague. That, separate from the abdominal work, could be problematic as well, due to risks of thrombi.) Of the 284 pregnant women in this study, 15 percent had this type of abdominal massage. The mortality rate of the massaged women was almost 5 percent, and that of the infants was 14.3 percent. These numbers seem terribly high, but it is hard to decipher their meaning: the sample size of the study and of massaged women in the study was small, and the researchers included no control group comparison to women who had not received massage. Nevertheless, the researchers recommended that women stop receiving this type of abdominal massage (Ugboma and Akani 2004).

We believe that caution is useful, but fearful avoidance is not. The precautions here can be applied to any and all somatic practices, including deep tissue, trigger point and acupressure, to ensure safe and comforting abdominal work. For added safety, also find alternatives to deep abdominal work aimed to improve peristalsis. In the second or third trimester, the uterus is between your touch and the intestines that you seek to affect with these techniques anyway, rendering them mostly ineffective. You will have more success using reflexive techniques, such as zones on the feet and hands. When you are addressing iliopsoas tension and inactivity, avoid mechanical pressure anywhere along these muscles and their attachments. Try stretching, passive movement and other awareness and educational techniques. (See online resources for more on deep abdominal work. See Chapter 4 for safe and effective abdominal techniques.) ⊕

When deciding if and how to massage a client's abdomen, it seems reasonable to adopt the level of precaution of many obstetricians and midwives. Not knowing the therapist's education and/or adherence to conservative practice, they commonly qualify their approval of massage therapy for a patient by contraindicating abdominal massage, especially if there is some increased concern about miscarriage, complications or high-risk conditions. Of course, you will follow those directions when issued specifically for your client.

It bears repeating that touching her abdomen requires the client's permission. For many reasons, some clients prefer to skip abdominal techniques entirely. Others might be eager to learn how she and her partner can massage her belly, enjoying that intimate, bonding time with their baby on their own. You should explain why abdominal massage might be useful, answer any questions and honor her preferences either way.

Reminder

Superficial strokes on the pregnant abdomen are usually soothing and safe.

When and Why Not to Massage the Abdomen

Although gentle abdominal massage following the guidelines above is safe for most pregnant clients, some therapists prefer to avoid touching a client's abdomen entirely until after the first trimester, to ensure that neither they nor their clients ever question the safety of their work. In addition, in cases in which clients are at high risk for miscarriage, preterm labor or other complications, you may prefer, for liability reasons, to avoid the abdomen throughout the pregnancy (Box 2.3). If a client shows signs of these complications (see Box 2.5 and Box 7.2), you should consult with her maternity healthcare provider before proceeding with abdominal massage.

Miscarriage (also known as **spontaneous abortion**) is a natural termination of pregnancy before the fetus has reached viability, occurring in the first trimester in approximately 80 percent of cases. It is the most common complication of pregnancy, occurring in at least 10 percent of

clinically identified pregnancies (ACOG 2018b). Preterm birth – when labor begins between 20 and 37 weeks – jeopardizes the health and lives of the mother and the fetus in 12 percent of American pregnancies (Ricci 2017).

Here's how to recognize potential problems. One of the most common symptoms of both preterm labor and miscarriage is low back, thigh and/or pelvic pain, referred from the contracting uterus. However, there are usually other identifying symptoms as well, such as bleeding, amniotic fluid leakage, abdominal cramping or regular uterine contractions (see Box 7.2).

Ask the client's physician or midwife to rule out miscarriage, labor or other possible causes of back pain, such as urinary tract infection, other organ or neurological dysfunction, or prior, unresolved injuries before beginning or continuing massage therapy. If that consultation is not possible, remember that musculoskeletal back pain is usually relieved with a change in position or activity, whereas referred organ pain is not. Take full prenatal and medical histories, and evaluate your client's progress thoroughly at *each* massage therapy session (see Chapter 8).

Certain maternal conditions, high-risk factors and complications of pregnancy may increase the occurrence of miscarriage or preterm labor. Some of the most common are: a history of previous miscarriage or preterm labor, fetal genetic or developmental abnormalities, and acute and chronic stress. Consult Boxes 7.1 and 7.2 for the full list of high-risk factors and signs and symptoms to be alert for.

To be clear, the above issues do not rule out massage. Indeed, a client enduring one or more of these issues likely needs massage all the more. These lists are intended to help you become appropriately cautious, to seek consultation, and to figure out how and where else you can use your massage skills for their benefit.

Box 2.3
Liability considerations

A sobering reality of American maternity care is particularly relevant to massage and other somatic therapists: nearly 90 percent of obstetricians and gynecologists are sued (Riley et al. 2016), and nurses and other maternity healthcare providers are more and more frequently being included in these lawsuits (Gilbert 2011). We must be aware of this litigious atmosphere in childbearing; but at the same time, there is no need for alarm. Even amidst this increase in lawsuits, our best estimate is that less than 1 percent of suits against massage therapists are brought by pregnant clients, and no therapists have been found liable in a pregnancy loss (Higdon 2019). The chances of legal repercussions are especially small if you do the following:

- Encourage parasympathetic stimulation.
- Follow the safety recommendations of this text and of clients' healthcare providers.
- Ask each client to complete a written health history form at the first appointment and make thorough progress notes that document each appointment. (See Chapter 8 for more guidance.)
- Practice conservatively, ethically and conscientiously, staying within the scope of your profession.
- Pursue a comprehensive, hands-on education in pre- and perinatal massage therapy.

Reminder

Determine whether high-risk factors or complications make it more prudent to eliminate abdominal massage with some clients.

From the treatment room

Even with my uterine abnormalities, my doctor encouraged massage therapy. He felt it was safe. With my risk of delivering early or miscarrying, it was a tremendous physical and emotional support. I was able to stay relaxed and calm, for the baby and for me.

– Jennifer, client

Leg Massage

Many of us are unnecessarily apprehensive about abdominal massage. But at the same time we are often unaware of the potentially more critical implications of leg massage. Remember all those changes to the circulatory system detailed in Chapter 1? Those effects are nowhere more apparent than in the legs. A variety of aches and pains – calf cramps and leg tension, achy feet and edema, just to name a few – prompt pregnant clients to seek your help. As a caring, responsive therapist, you want to meet their needs, but you also must respect necessary modifications for the legs.

Blood Clots

As we have discussed in Chapter 1, normal circulatory system adaptations create several potentially problematic changes during pregnancy. Increased blood and interstitial fluid volume, combined with uterine restriction of the iliac vessels, results in an expected increase in femoral venous pressure. Since elevated progesterone levels relax the smooth muscular walls of the perforator and deeper leg veins, they are more prone to developing varicose veins and accumulating stagnant blood. Those areas, in turn, are more likely to generate blood clots – which, due to the decrease in clot-dissolving factors, are not readily dissolved.

Clots can form in any vein during pregnancy; however, **thrombophlebitis** and **deep vein thrombosis (DVT)** are most likely, and most dangerous, in the veins where blood is most stagnant. Thus, the leg veins most likely to harbor clots during pregnancy are the deep iliac, femoral, and both superficial and deep saphenous veins, and, to a lesser extent, the more superficial **perforator veins** such as the popliteal and posterior tibial veins (Figure 2.6) (Walton 2011). When clots accumulate in these vessels, they may create some discomfort, but they pose no major threat, unless inflammation is severe and/or infection develops. DVTs in the larger, deeper veins are more serious: if they dislodge, they begin to move through the bloodstream, and eventually could become stuck in the smaller vessels in the lungs (causing a pulmonary embolism). This blockage is one type of the larger category of **thromboembolisms**, which occur four to five times more frequently in pregnant than in non-pregnant women, and can be fatal (ACOG 2018a).

Because a major contributing factor to DVT is high levels of estrogen and progesterone, most pregnant people will likely develop clots. In addition, the more sedentary a person is, the higher the likelihood of thrombi. Those who are on **bed rest** are especially prone to clot production, as are smokers, those over 35, those who have recently used birth control pills, are obese, have lupus, have been pregnant multiple times before or are carrying multiples (Devis and Knuttinen 2017). (DVT is even more common postpartum, so consult Chapter 6 on this topic too.) Again, a clot is not usually a problem by itself; the problem is the potential for it to become dislodged and occlude a blood vessel.

The characteristic symptoms of leg thrombi include increased edema in the foot and/or leg (often unilaterally), localized swelling, heat, redness, and painful, achy legs that can be tender with palpable, ropy veins. These symptoms are particularly worrisome if they increase when the pregnant person walks. But to be clear, legs that are painful or achy are a hallmark of pregnancy, so these symptoms alone do not guarantee a blood clot. A clear determination of the presence of clots is also difficult because thrombi are often asymptomatic (Callahan and Caughey 2007).

Given the increased likelihood that blood will coagulate in pregnancy, the difficulty in determining the presence of clots, and the potential harm of freely circulating clots, it seems prudent to treat all pregnant clients as though they have leg clots. With that assumption, our

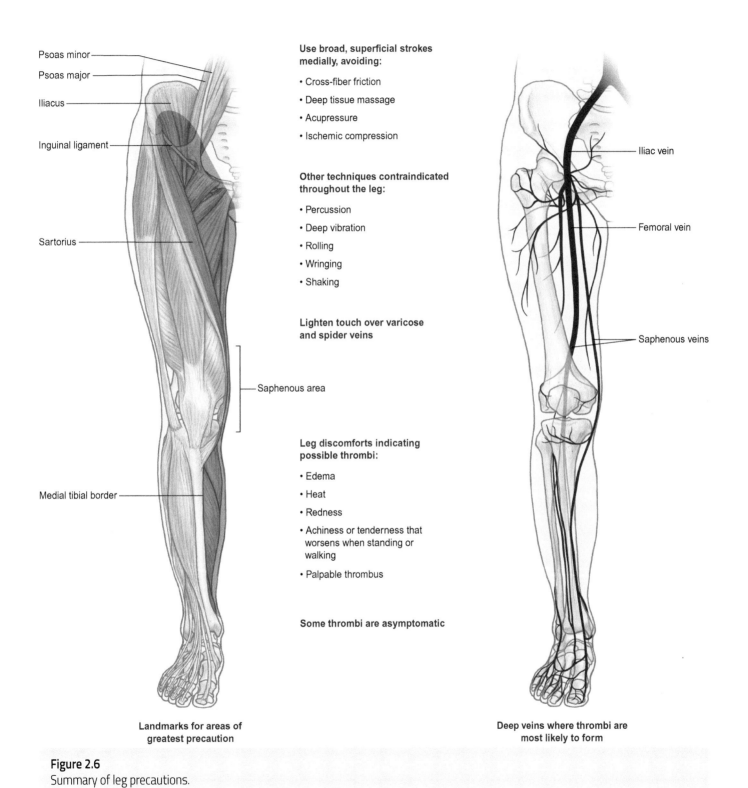

Psoas minor

Psoas major

Iliacus

Inguinal ligament

Sartorius

Saphenous area

Medial tibial border

Use broad, superficial strokes medially, avoiding:

- Cross-fiber friction
- Deep tissue massage
- Acupressure
- Ischemic compression

Other techniques contraindicated throughout the leg:

- Percussion
- Deep vibration
- Rolling
- Wringing
- Shaking

Lighten touch over varicose and spider veins

Leg discomforts indicating possible thrombi:

- Edema
- Heat
- Redness
- Achiness or tenderness that worsens when standing or walking
- Palpable thrombus

Some thrombi are asymptomatic

Iliac vein

Femoral vein

Saphenous veins

Landmarks for areas of greatest precaution

Deep veins where thrombi are most likely to form

Figure 2.6
Summary of leg precautions.

response is obvious: to be totally safe you should eliminate massage procedures that have the potential to move thrombi from their likely harbors in the leg veins (Sutham et al. 2020). The data are not conclusive about the types of touch listed below, and whether they create such localized or systemic circulatory effects. Nevertheless, we think it wisest to still observe the following precautions:

- Do not press deeply or for a sustained length of time into the lower pelvis or inguinal area, where the iliac vein crosses the pelvis.

- Use only superficial, whole-hand pressure in the places where problematic veins traverse: throughout the medial surface of the legs, specifically for several inches along and posterior to the sartorius muscles, distal to the medial knees, and along the medial tibial borders.

- Avoid deep, pointed or stationary pressure that may restrict localized blood flow (ischemic pressure) in these areas – regardless of the type of technique and its otherwise potential benefits. The movement of blood that seems to be propelled when

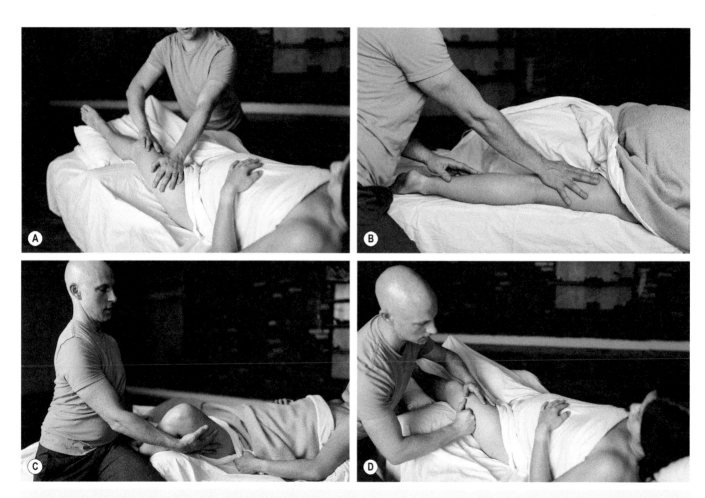

Figure 2.7A–D
Possibilities for working the medial leg. A few of the many ways that you can be cautious and still do effective work. **(A)** Alternating strokes; **(B)** gentle effleurage in sidelying; **(C)** passive relaxation of the adductors; **(D)** light strokes on medial leg combined with deep strokes on lateral leg.

you release your pressure can potentially move clots more proximally. Only use deep pressure – including cross-fiber friction, trigger point therapy, deep tissue and acupressure – on the lateral leg, or the anterior and posterior leg if pressure vector is *not* medially directed, and in the absence of varicose and spider veins.

- With less active clients, avoid tapotement (percussion), as well as any technique that creates a jiggling of leg tissues, such as rolling or wringing. Be gentle and slow with all of your leg strokes and movements of the hips, knees and ankles, to avoid shaking clots loose from leg vessels.

- When a client is on bed rest or has other conditions increasing clot risk, eliminate leg work altogether, except for stationary, energy work or the most superficial strokes (just to spread lubricant on the skin). If you work under direct medical supervision, you may be able to safely do more with these clients' legs. Seek and follow any physician guidelines given. (See Chapter 7 for more on bed rest.)

- Massage therapists without hands-on verification by an instructor of appropriate leg techniques would be wise not to work with the legs of clients with high-risk or complicated pregnancies in which thrombosis formation is higher.

While these precautions are essential, we also want to be clear that there is still lots of valuable work that you can do on the legs, from light alternating effleurage strokes in both semireclining (Figure 2.7A) and sidelying (Figure 2.7B), to passive lengthening of the adductors (Figure 2.7C), to lighter medial strokes combined with deeper lateral strokes (Figure 2.7D). (See Chapter 4 for an abundance of other specific leg techniques.) Remember, caution should not equal avoidance!

Varicose and Spider Veins

Following the guidelines above will also protect vascular areas commonly weakened by progesterone, which usually manifest as spider veins and varicose veins. These reddish, broken superficial capillaries – that look like multilegged spiders – indicate capillary fragility. Squiggly, bulging varicose veins often develop in the

same blood vessels as blood clots. These varicosities are more noticeable in the more superficial veins, but varicosities in deep veins will not necessarily be visible. In any areas of varicose or spider veins, additionally modify massage therapy techniques according to the severity of the condition. With extreme varicosities – palpable, raised and convoluted, often with discolored surrounding tissue – use only featherlight touch and energetic (that is, non-contact) modalities (Werner 2015).

Regardless of varicose vein severity, use procedures to help relieve pelvic congestion (described in Chapter 4); these may help reduce pressure on weakened vessels and encourage movement of blood and edema proximally. However, if thrombi have been confirmed in any vein, do not massage that leg without direct medical supervision, and consult with the client's physician or midwife regarding the advisability of massage on the other, unaffected leg. If there are lesions, ulcerations, inflammation (phlebitis) or infection, do not massage directly over these areas. Gentle techniques proximal of the area can be effective and safe.

Points of view: What adaptations to leg massage are critical during pregnancy?

Most contemporary authors and instructors think that totally contraindicating leg massage during a normal pregnancy is unnecessarily conservative and outdated. However, there is considerable discrepancy on how to determine normalcy and how to safely massage the legs (see, for example, Jordan 2009; Stager 2010; Stillerman 2008; Yates 2010).

Several experts suggest a straight-leg lifting test – where pain is taken for presence of thrombi – to determine the safety of proceeding (Stillerman 2008). The problem with this test, known as Homan's sign, is that there are many other reasons for leg pain with this maneuver, making a solid assessment difficult. For this reason, it is no longer a test recommended by nursing experts (Ricci 2017).

Regarding safe strokes for leg massage, deep, long strokes on the legs often are not recommended. This is unnecessarily restrictive, particularly on the lateral leg, where the long bones offer considerable protection from the possible vein-stripping effects of such work. As your hands work more medially, lightening up and shortening your strokes make good sense. Similarly, your caution should increase as clot risk factors increase or systemic edema occurs; as needed, you can decrease your pressure for any technique on the medial legs to the point of extreme superficiality (see Figure 2.7 for examples).

Reflex and Acupuncture Points

Reflexologists and zone therapists claim that deep pressure to specific areas of the feet and hands stimulates relaxation, facilitates metabolic functions that support pregnancy, and helps to reduce common prenatal discomforts. Amidst these broad claims of positive results, however, there are several reflexive cautions during pregnancy (Enzer 2004).

Feet, Legs and Hands

In reflexive zone therapy, the center of the medial and lateral calcaneus is linked, respectively, to the uterus and ovary. Common anecdotes suggest that deep, bone-to-bone pressure to these zones can potentially initiate labor or strengthen weak labor contractions. There are little to no data to either confirm or dismiss these claims for foot zone therapy. But to be safe, we recommend that you avoid ischemic compression or deep pressure to the center of the medial or lateral calcaneus during pregnancy. Be particularly cautious with these areas in the first trimester and with clients more prone to miscarriage or preterm labor (Enzer 2004). Other types of touch – effleurage, fanning, mobilizations of the foot or ankle – in these areas will not stimulate a reflex response in the respective organs.

Some practitioners caution those without comprehensive training in reflexive zone therapy to avoid extensive reflexive touch (bone-to-bone, rhythmic compressions) on the feet of clients with high-risk factors or serious complications (such as threatened miscarriage, preterm labor, or pre-eclampsia, and when DVT is more likely).

Asian bodywork therapies, rooted in Chinese medicine and the philosophy of Qi, contain many protocols to enhance women's pregnancies (Citkovitz 2019; Jin 1998). Practitioners, whether of Shiatsu, acupressure or many other forms, also learn where to withhold their energy-focused pressure. There are varying opinions on whether these points can actually impact a pregnancy or prompt early labor (Simkin et al. 2018; Schlaeger et al. 2017), but it is wisest to avoid deep, pointed pressure to the acupuncture points traditionally needled to promote uterine contractions (Figures 2.8 and 2.9) (Smith et al. 2017; Jin 1998). These include:

- Spleen 6 (SP-6), four client-fingerwidths proximal to the malleolus, along the medial tibial border

- Kidney 3 (KI-3), on the superior border of, and just posterior to, the medial malleolus

- Urinary Bladder 60 (BL-60), behind the ankle joint, in the depression between the prominence of the lateral malleolus and the Achilles tendon

- Urinary Bladder 67 (BL-67), on the dorsal aspect of the little toe, at the junction of lines drawn along the lateral border of the nail and the base of the nail, just beside the corner of the nail

- Liver 3 (LV-3), at the proximal border of the first and second metatarsal bones

- Large Intestine 4 (LI-4), the complementary Hoku hand point at the junction of the thumb and index finger.

If you observe the precautions concerning blood clots listed in the previous section, you will never activate most of these leg points.

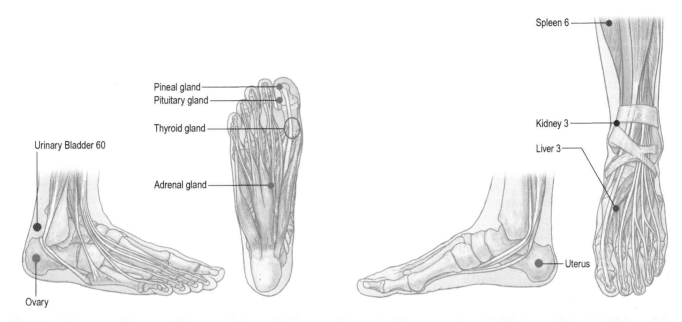

Figure 2.8
Contraindicated points and precautionary zones of lower body. Avoid deep, bone-to-bone pressure on reflex zones *(labeled with an orange dot)* and acupuncture points *(labeled with a red dot).*

Torso

Though reflexive points in the torso are generally regarded as less potent, address soft tissue needs in the following areas with pressure that is broad and general rather than specific and pointed (see Figure 2.9):

- Urinary Bladder 31–34 (BL-31 to BL-34), on the sacrum, at each sacral sulcus

- Gall Bladder 21 (GB-21) halfway between the nape of the neck and the acromion at the trapezius apex (Deadman et al. 2016).

Be precise in your application of deep, pointed pressure anywhere nearby, so that you avoid inadvertently activating these points.

But precision should not mean avoidance! Some clients will inevitably be worried that any massage to their ankles or feet will cause miscarriage or labor.

This misconception has unfortunately been spread by authors who are not trained in acupressure or reflexive zone therapy. Their desire to protect the pregnancy is understandable, of course, but the level of warning is excessive. Indeed, one recent review suggests that no caution is necessary! It found that needling the acupuncture points typically "forbidden" during pregnancy did not cause miscarriage or preterm labor, or otherwise alter birth outcomes (Carr 2015). This finding is a reminder of the paucity of clear data on the effects of alternative medicine; it is a reminder of the need to continue to follow the research, and to ensure our work is guided by caution but not fear. A safe guideline to follow is that only bone-to-bone, energy-focused pressure to these exact reflex areas – usually repeated in prescribed sequences – has the potential to *possibly* create these stimulating effects. Misconstruing this precaution as a total contraindication to touching the heels or the feet of pregnant women deprives them of the soothing relief and grounding possible from other ways of massaging in these areas.

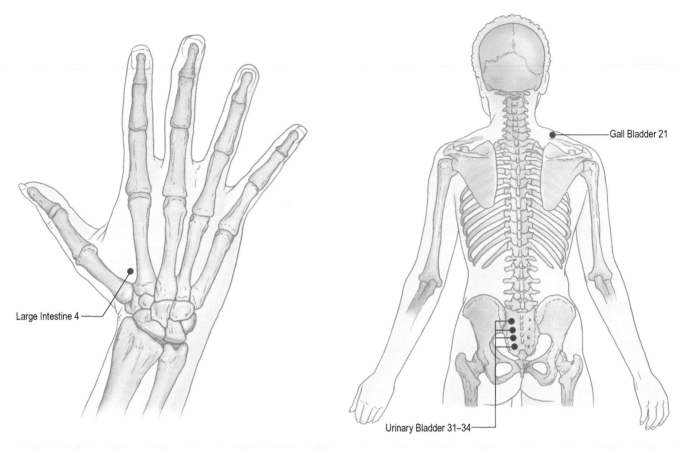

Figure 2.9
Contraindicated points of upper body. Use broadly applied techniques over these acupuncture points on the hand and back.

What would you do?

As you spread oil on the feet of a new pregnant client, her eyes suddenly pop open in alarm and she exclaims, "I heard that having my feet massaged could cause a miscarriage." How will you respond to her concerns, ease her worry and proceed with an appropriate session?

Although these areas do – at least according to anecdotal evidence – have labor-stimulating potential, they reach their full potency only when a woman is in labor

or on the verge of it, and when all points are methodically and repeatedly stimulated by a person trained in interacting with energetic pathways (see Chapter 5 for a discussion of **labor induction** and **labor augmentation**). If you compress with a broad contact or sweep over these points, you will not create unwanted reflexive responses.

Reminder

Modify work on the legs for risks related to blood clots, varicose veins and reflexive points.

Joint Precautions and Passive Movements

Because relaxin and other hormones soften connective tissue, keep all joints within the normal range of motion and avoid overstretching. Lengthened ligaments can result in joint instability and can mean more pain, both prenatally and long-term. Modify all techniques that focus on lengthening: assisted–resisted stretches, positional release, Swedish gymnastic movements, range of motion, and other passive and active movements, such as those in sports and Thai massage.

Symphysis pubis dysfunction (Figure 2.10) is perhaps the most debilitating manifestation of pregnancy-induced joint instability. There are several ways, all detailed in Chapter 4, that you can help your client avoid that sharp, midline pain in the front of the pelvis.

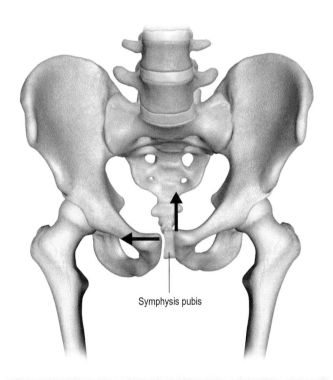

Symphysis pubis

Figure 2.10
Symphysis pubis dysfunction. This anterior pelvic joint, softened by hormones, can spread horizontally, or shear vertically, or both.

Both the gastrocnemius and the peroneals are more likely to spasm and cramp, especially as the pregnancy progresses. When working on a client's feet, maintain them in a neutral or dorsiflexed position to reduce the chance of inducing a cramp.

Clients suffering nausea may not appreciate any rhythmic, rocking movements that can worsen morning sickness. Be sure to use gentle, slow techniques, even on the extremities, and avoid rocking the torso. Once nausea has passed, perform all passive movements with small amplitude and slow, rhythmic frequency.

Take care that any passive or active movements do not increase intrauterine pressure. Those most likely to do so would be knee-to-chest leg and lumbar stretches, hip circumduction, ribcage mobilizations, torso flexion and similar maneuvers. Many Thai massage techniques and range of motion maneuvers, for example, need considerable modification to avoid pressing into the enlarged abdomen.

Smells, Skin and Spa Treatments

During pregnancy, one's sense of smell can be heightened and triggered without warning. When techniques require lubrication, use only unscented oils, or those with fragrances that your client finds appealing.

We recommend pure nut or seed oils such as almond, apricot kernel or grapeseed; fractionated coconut oil is a good lighter option. You may want to use a single ingredient to minimize the risk of allergic reaction; in the rare case where there is an allergic reaction, you will know exactly what it is – the one ingredient! Most lotions or creams, even those touted as "natural," contain preservatives and a large number of potentially skin-irritating ingredients. Natural vitamin E oil, as well as cocoa butter and shea butter in their pure form, are helpful in relieving itchy, stretched skin. Shea butter, cocoa butter and extra-virgin coconut oil – as well as some minimally studied products – contain hyaluronic acid, theorized to hydrate the skin and stimulate new skin cell regeneration below the top layer of the epidermis (Narurkar et al. 2016; Pilkington et al. 2015). There is minimal research evidence of such lubricants reducing stretch mark formation, but many clients choose to give them a try.

There are many varying opinions as to which **essential oils** are safe and effective for the mother and the baby. Unless you are a highly trained **aromatherapist** or work with one to create specific oils for your practice, you should avoid using these powerful plant essences. ⊕

If you are doing more complicated spa treatments, be sure that all products you use are safe for pregnant clients. Here are a few suggestions:

- Consult the master or originator of the spa treatment, and the manufacturers of the products used, to confirm their safe use.

- Research the actions and precautions of essential oils during pregnancy with a reliable source.

- Before applying any product, as mentioned above, check the aroma to determine whether it is pleasing to clients, especially those with sensitive noses or queasy stomachs.

- Or, keep the structure of the spa treatment but replace all products with a simple, pure unscented oil.

Spa treatments are customarily performed with the client prone or supine on a table. Remember the safety and comfort positioning guidelines detailed above, and adapt your wraps, facials and other treatments accordingly.

With spa treatments or other modalities involving heat, modify the duration and extent of applications, particularly in the first trimester. Prolonged heat exposure over large body areas can increase maternal core temperatures. In early pregnancy, this can interfere with fetal development or even cause fetal death. Saunas, steam cabinets, hot tubs and other heat immersion treatments are generally contraindicated in the first trimester. If women do use these at any time, they should carefully monitor their body temperature and keep exposure to around ten minutes (Simkin et al. 2018).

No studies have yet confirmed the appropriate amount of time for local heat application. Common-sense application of the data concerning core body temperature suggests that you limit your local use of heat – whether hot

wraps, hot packs, heat lamps or hot stones – to less than 20 minutes. If a pregnant client becomes uncomfortably hot or if her oral temperature rises 1 degree or more (Fahrenheit), discontinue heat treatment. No modifications in use of cold are required prenatally or perinatally.

Other Precautions

The variety of ways that we can work with pregnant clients are as numerous, and as varied, as pregnancy itself! It should be clear that you can adapt many somatic modalities for pre- and perinatal use. Some particular

---

Box 2.4
Is this a safe technique during pregnancy?

Once you understand the rationale for the guidelines and precautions included in this chapter, you can safely expand your repertoire of prenatal techniques. Answer these questions before using any technique with a pregnant client.

Do I need to adapt:

1. the customary client position for this technique to meet prenatal positioning requirements?
2. the customary speed or pressure of this technique to avoid sympathetic arousal?
3. the emotional intensity of this technique to avoid sympathetic arousal?
4. to avoid ischemic compression on the iliac vein and other medial leg veins, or to avoid dislodging blood clots in the legs?
5. to avoid pressure over weakened veins and capillaries?
6. to avoid increased intrauterine pressure or other irritants to the uterine muscles?
7. to avoid bone-to-bone contact on the reflexive points contraindicated before a client's due date?
8. to protect vulnerable joint structures?
9. due to an existing prenatal complication or a higher risk of complications?
10. to avoid increasing core body temperature?

considerations for adaptations you should contemplate are included in Box 2.4. That said, detailed maternity applications for every possible somatic practice cannot be adequately explored in this text. When you want to use polarity therapy, Thai massage, Watsu or any other method not covered in these pages, study with a master practitioner and/or instructor of those systems prior to working with expectant clients. Always observe pertinent, general contraindications, as well as any restrictions issued by a client's maternity healthcare provider. Furthermore, even when you are using the methods discussed in these pages, certain techniques sometimes require specific safety and comfort adaptations. You will find these specific adaptations included in the detailed instructions for techniques in the coming chapters. And last but not least, just to be clear: the precautions, guidelines and contraindications covered so far in this chapter apply to those with healthy, low-risk pregnancies. See the section below and Chapter 7 for pregnancies with complications and high-risk factors. And remember that the best thing you can do for your own career, and your own clients, is to take advanced training in your areas of specialization.

When Challenges Arise

Pregnancy induces extensive – but normal – changes throughout the body, and extensive – but normal – aches and pains, as described in Chapters 1 and 4. However, roughly one in four pregnancies deviates from these expected physiological adaptations or is at higher risk of certain complications (Ricci 2017). Most of this one-quarter of pregnant people can still benefit from maternity massage therapy, but their needs can be more complex, and require more specific adaptations to your work. Here, you will learn to recognize when a pregnancy is not proceeding normally. When her doctor or midwife identifies that a client's pregnancy has medical complications requiring additional considerations, you can refer to Chapter 7, where you will find guidance for how to make appropriate adaptations. Your sessions with clients undergoing complicated and high-risk pregnancies have the potential to improve their chances for a positive outcome, provide some stress reduction, and offer support if her or her baby's condition deteriorates. Work with such clients can be intimidating, but it is often highly rewarding (Figure 2.11).

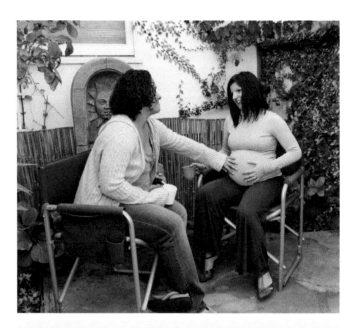

Figure 2.11
Supporting high-risk pregnancies. When a pregnancy is not proceeding as anticipated, add your support to that of the client's family and friends.

Reminder

Collect information about your client at each session to alert you to any developing prenatal complications or high-risk factors.

Recognizing High-Risk Factors and Complications

The obstetrical profession has identified a number of what are called "high-risk factors" – conditions, traits or circumstances that increase the likelihood of medical complications. For some of these high-risk factors, the chances that they will lead to complications are low; however, others can lead to complications more than 50 percent of the time. Just because a client has a high-risk factor does not mean that anything is wrong; there is just a higher probability that problems *may* develop. (And remember that complications can arise spontaneously – during pregnancy or birth or postpartum – even in healthy childbearing people without high-risk factors.)

Below is a list of common risk factors and complications:

- age (younger than 15 or older than 35)

- autoimmune diseases

- cardiovascular disease

- **chronic hypertension**

- diabetes and gestational diabetes

- inadequate support system and abuse (physical and emotional)

- infections (COVID-19, sexually transmitted and other viral and bacterial diseases)

- lack of prenatal, birth and postpartum care

- **multiple gestations** pregnancy

- **parity** – first pregnancies and **grand multiparity**

- perinatal mood and anxiety disorders, or a history of depression and mental health conditions

- placental dysfunctions

- smoking and substance abuse (Ricci 2017).

See Box 7.1 for a more detailed list, and see Chapter 7 for massage guidelines for clients with high-risk factors and complications.

Members of all ethnic and socioeconomic groups experience these risks and complications. However, American research indicates that many of these issues are more common in clients of a non-white ethnicity and/or in poverty. Such disparities in maternal health are painful evidence of continued structural inequalities and socioeconomic injustices. As we treat each client as a unique individual, we also must remain aware of the larger forces that shape their health and well-being.

Remember that while the danger of higher **morbidity** and mortality is real, most people who are dealing with high risks and complications can have healthy pregnancies. Despite – and maybe because of – these stress-provoking concerns, there is much that we can do to help these clients; we just need to do so with knowledge and caution.

Recognizing Signs and Symptoms

At each session, and especially your first time seeing a client, thoroughly assess her general state of health. Inquire about recent appointments with her physician or midwife. Observe and assess and palpate. Pay particular attention if she mentions anything that concerns her or her healthcare provider. Refer to Box 7.2 as often as you need to for a detailed list of signs and symptoms of complications. A few of the most common signs and symptoms you should be alert to are: vaginal bleeding; pre-term abdominal cramping; pitting or systemic edema; excessive thirst; and painful leg cramps with redness, heat, swelling and/or **cyanosis** (Ricci 2017). When a client has any of these or any other of the signs and symptoms in Box 7.2, you need to carefully and appropriately respond, following the guidance detailed in Chapter 7.

Some massage settings do not require health history intake forms. Owners and staff should carefully consider the possible safety, quality of care and legal consequences of these practices with their prenatal clientele. At the very least, the following basic screening questions are necessary: How far along are you? Do you have any conditions that your doctor/midwife is concerned about? What are you hoping to gain from your prenatal massage session today? (See Chapter 8 for more on intake questions.)

What would you do?

A prospective client calls you for an appointment. She is 33 weeks into her first pregnancy and has been having back pain this past week, primarily in her lumbar and sacral areas. Her prenatal exercise teacher has referred her to you for this and for help with her very tense thigh muscles, especially her inner thigh muscles. She is also beginning to notice that her shoes are very tight and her ankles swell in the afternoon and evenings. What additional information would you need to make knowledgeable decisions about her care? Is it likely that she has any complications? What precautions should you take in addressing her edema and medial thigh tension?

Chapter Summary

Following this chapter's precautions and recommendations (summarized in Box 2.5), you and your clients can know that prenatal massage therapy is safe in most pregnancies. Be thorough in acquiring sufficient client information and make conservative decisions on when and when not to massage and what positions to use. As

---

Box 2.5
Summary of general methodological precautions and contraindications by trimester

Abdominal Massage (Any Method)

First trimester:

- Consider eliminating as a liability precaution.

Second and third trimesters

- Superficial effleurage and gentle rocking only.

First through third trimesters

- Liability precaution with hypertensive disorders, and with symptoms or risks of preterm labor, miscarriage or placental dysfunction, and some other risk factors.

Swedish Massage (All Trimesters)

General directions

- Direct strokes toward heart. Work proximal areas first. Work superficially, then more deeply.
- Use procedures that help relieve pelvic congestion.

Precautions for varicose veins

- *Mild (visible/ropy) and spider veins:* Use only appropriate Swedish and lymphatic drainage strokes at moderate pressure.
- *Moderate (palpable/raised, ropy):* Use only appropriate Swedish and lymphatic drainage strokes with a light touch.
- *Extreme (palpable/raised, convoluted, often with discolored surrounding tissue):* Use only featherlight touch and energetic work.

Precautions for clot (thrombi) endangerment sites

- Use soft, whole-hand pressure on the medial thigh.
- Do not use deep or pointed pressure on the medial border of the tibia, on the saphenous area of the knee, along or posterior to the sartorius muscle, and at the inguinal and iliac area.
- Avoid percussion (tapotement), wringing, brisk rocking or other movements, and vibration, either on the legs or that travels to them.

Leg Massage of Any Modality (All Trimesters)

- See Swedish precautions above for legs.
- Avoid acupressure, cross-fiber friction, deep tissue, trigger points, or other deep ischemic pressure into the medial leg.
- Leg massage is contraindicated for clients on bed rest and those with increased clot risks, except with direct medical supervision.

Reflexive Modalities (All Trimesters)

- *Reflexology:* Uterus and ovary points are contraindicated; use caution with endocrine gland points; use caution with substance abusers, those with unhealthy lifestyles and those with high-risk factors or complications.
- *Acupressure:* Avoid pointed stimulation of Spleen 6, Kidney 3, Urinary Bladder 60 and 67 and 31 to 34, Liver 3, Large Intestine 4, Gall Bladder 21.

Deep Tissue (All Trimesters)

- Avoid in abdomen; use only on structures chronically stressed by pregnancy.
- On legs, observe precautions for varicose veins and clots as above for Swedish and leg massage.

Passive and Active Movements

First trimester

- Rocking movements are contraindicated with nausea.

Second and third trimesters

- Rocking movements are contraindicated with nausea.
- Use extra caution on hips and legs with symphysis pubis dysfunction.

All trimesters

- Avoid hyperextension of joints.

Consult master teachers of other somatic practices prior to applying techniques prenatally and perinatally. Modify for complications and high-risk factors as described in Chapter 7. Observe any restrictions issued by maternity healthcare providers.

you use a variety of modalities to create sessions, modify the depth, speed and intensity of techniques, paying particular attention to your work in the abdomen and the legs, with joints and on reflexive points. Throughout your clients' pregnancies, be alert for deviations from normal physiology and any risk factors that could lead to a complication. Within these safety parameters, you can expect your work to benefit prenatal clients greatly and to promote healthy outcomes for both them and their babies.

Think it through

To deepen your knowledge, go to our online resources, answer the test questions for this chapter and explore further. 🌐

References and Further Reading

ACOG (American College of Obstetricians and Gynecologists) (2015) Physical Activity and Exercise During Pregnancy and the Postpartum Period. Committee Opinion 650. December.

ACOG (American College of Obstetricians and Gynecologists) (2018a) ACOG Practice Bulletin No. 196: Thromboembolism in Pregnancy. Obstet Gynecol. 132(1):1–17.

ACOG (American College of Obstetricians and Gynecologists) (2018b) ACOG Practice Bulletin No. 200: Early Pregnancy Loss. Obstet Gynecol. 132(5):e197–e207.

Callahan T, Caughey A (2007) Obstetrics and Gynecology. Baltimore: Lippincott, Williams & Wilkins.

Carr DJ (2015) The safety of obstetric acupuncture: forbidden points revisited. Acupunct Med. 33(5):413–419.

Chaitow L (2017) Palpation and Assessment in Manual Therapy: Learning the Art and Refining Your Skills. Edinburgh: Handspring.

Citkovitz C (2019) Acupressure and Acupuncture During Birth: An Integrative Guide for Acupuncturists and Birth Professionals. London: Jessica Kingsley.

Deadman P, Al-Khafaji M, Baker K (2016) A Manual of Acupuncture. East Sussex: Journal of Chinese Medicine Publications.

Dennis AT, Hardy L, Leeton L (2018) The prone position in healthy pregnant women and in women with preeclampsia – a pilot study. BMC Pregnancy Childbirth. 18:445.

Devis P, Knuttinen M (2017) Deep venous thrombosis in pregnancy: incidence, pathogenesis and endovascular management. Cardiovasc Diagn Ther. 7(Suppl 3): S309–S319.

Enzer S (2004) Maternity Reflexology, 2nd edn. UK: Soul to Sole Reflexology.

Ernst E (2003) The safety of massage therapy. Rheumatology. 42(9):1101–1106.

Field T (2016) Massage therapy research review. Complement Ther Clin Pract. 24:19–31.

Fink NS, Urech C, Cavelti M et al. (2012) Relaxation during pregnancy: what are the benefits for mother, fetus, and the newborn? A systematic review of the literature. J Perinat Neonatal Nurs. 26(4):296–306.

Gibbs R, Karlan B, Haney A et al. (2008) Danforth's Obstetrics and Gynecology, 10th edn. Baltimore: Lippincott, Williams & Wilkins.

Gilbert E (2011) Manual of High-risk Pregnancy and Delivery, 5th edn. St. Louis: Mosby.

Heazell AEP, Li M, Budd J et al. (2018) Association between maternal sleep practices and late stillbirth – findings from a stillbirth case-control study. BJOG. 125:254–262.

Higdon D (2019) Risk Management/Special Services, Associated Bodywork & Massage Professionals, email correspondence with authors, November 13.

Jin Y (1998) Handbook of Obstetrics and Gynecology in Chinese Medicine. Seattle: Eastland Press.

Jordan K (2009) What about varicose veins? Massage Today. May. Available at: https://www.massagetoday.com/articles/10245/What-about-Varicose-Veins [accessed May 6, 2020].

Juhan D (2003) Job's Body: Handbook for Bodyworkers, 3rd edn. Barrytown, NJ: Station Hill Press.

Lett A (2000) Reflex Zone Therapy for Health Professionals. London: Churchill Livingstone.

Monk C, Feng T, Lee S et al. (2016) Distress during pregnancy: epigenetic regulation of placenta glucocorticoid-related genes and fetal neurobehavior. Am J Psychiatry. 173(7):705–713.

Naperstek B (2007) Guided imagery: a best practice for pregnancy and childbirth. Int J Childbirth Educ. 22(3): 4–8.

Narurkar VA, Fabi SG, Bucay VW et al. (2016) Rejuvenating hydrator: restoring epidermal hyaluronic acid homeostasis with instant benefits. J Drugs Dermatol. 15(1 Suppl 2):s24–37.

Nichols R, Humenick S (2000) Childbirth Education: Practice, Research and Theory, 2nd edn. Philadelphia: WB Saunders.

Noble E (2003) Essential Exercises for the Childbearing Year, 4th edn. Harwich: New Life Images.

Oliveira C, Lopes M, Rodrigues AS et al. (2017) Influence of the prone position on a stretcher for pregnant women on maternal and fetal hemodynamic parameters and comfort in pregnancy. Clinics (Sao Paulo, Brazil). 72(6):325–332.

Osborne C (2009) Pre-and Perinatal Massage Therapy: Survey of Massage Therapists. Available at: www.bodytherapyeducation.com [accessed May 1, 2010].

Pilkington SJ, Belden S, Miller RA (2015) The tricky tear trough: a review of topical cosmeceuticals for periorbital skin rejuvenation. J Clin Aesthet Dermatol. 8(9): 39–47.

Pirie A, Herman H (2003) How to Raise Children Without Breaking your Back. Cambridge, MA: IBIS.

Ray BR, Trikha A (2018) Prone position ventilation in pregnancy: concerns and evidence. J Obstet Anaesth Crit Care. 8:7–9.

Ricci S (2017) Essentials of Maternity, Newborn, and Women's Health Nursing. Baltimore: Lippincott, Williams & Wilkins.

Riczo D (2020) Back and Pelvic Girdle Pain in Pregnancy and Postpartum. Minneapolis: OPTP.

Riley W, Meredith LW, Price R et al. (2016) Decreasing malpractice claims by reducing preventable perinatal harm. Health Serv Res. 51 Suppl 3(Suppl 3):2453–2471.

Schlaeger JM, Gabzdyl EM, Bussell JL et al. (2017) Acupuncture and acupressure in labor. J Midwifery Women's Health. 62(1):12–28.

Silver R, Hunter S, Reddy U et al. (2019) Prospective evaluation of maternal sleep position through 30 weeks of gestation and adverse pregnancy outcomes. Obstet Gynecol. 134(4):667–676.

Simkin P, Whalley J, Keppler A (2018) Pregnancy, Childbirth, and the Newborn, 5th edn. New York: Da Capo Lifelong.

Smith CA, Armour M, Dahlen HG (2017) Acupuncture or acupressure for induction of labour. Cochrane Database Syst Rev. 10(10):CD002962.

Stager L (2010) Nurturing Massage for Pregnancy. Baltimore: Lippincott, Williams & Wilkins.

Stillerman E (2008) Prenatal Massage. St. Louis: Mosby/Elsevier.

Stone P, Burgess W, McIntyre J et al. (2017) Effect of maternal position on fetal behavioural state and heart rate variability in healthy late gestation pregnancy. J Physiol. 595(4):1213–1221.

Sutham K, Na-Nan S, Paiboonsithiwong S et al. (2020) Leg massage during pregnancy with unrecognized deep vein thrombosis could be life threatening: a case report. BMC Pregnancy Childbirth. 20:237.

Togher KL, Treacy E, O'Keeffe GW et al. (2017) Maternal distress in late pregnancy alters obstetric outcomes and the expression of genes important for placental glucocorticoid signalling. Psychiatry Res [Internet]. 255:17–26.

Ugboma H, Akani C (2004) Abdominal massage: another cause of maternal mortality. Niger J Med. 13(3):249–262.

Walton T (2011) Medical Conditions and Massage Therapy. Baltimore: Lippincott, Williams & Wilkins.

Wang ZW, Hua J, Xu YH (2015) The relationship between gentle tactile stimulation on the fetus and its temperament 3 months after birth. Behav Neurol. 2015:371906.

Werner R (2015) A Massage Therapist's Guide to Pathology, 6th edn. Baltimore: Lippincott, Williams & Wilkins.

Yates S (2010) Pregnancy and Childbirth. Edinburgh: Churchill Livingstone/Elsevier.

Studying this chapter will prepare you to:

1. establish and maintain an appropriate environment for maternity massage therapy

2. choose and adjust your massage table to ensure effectiveness and comfort, for both client and therapist, in a variety of positions

3. arrange and maintain pillows and other supports on your table to safely and comfortably work with your prenatal clients in a variety of positions

4. modestly and smoothly drape and undrape each client as you massage

5. provide assistance for pregnant clients to get on your table, shift positions and get off your table

6. practice proper body mechanics to enhance the ease and effectiveness of your work.

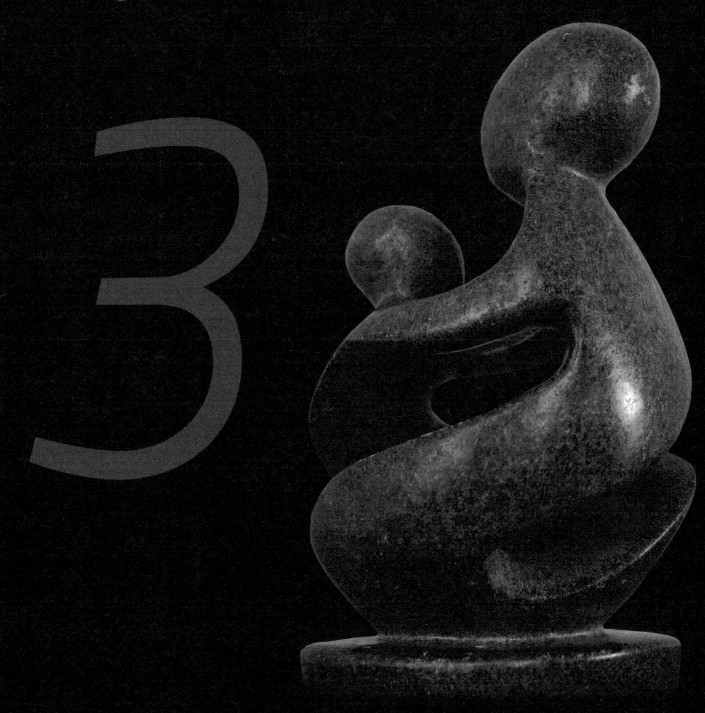

Practical Considerations:
Caring for Your Clients and Yourself

3

Chapter Overview

You have learned why prenatal and perinatal massage therapy is beneficial. You know when to and when not to massage, and generally how to modify your work for prenatal clients with normal pregnancies. In this chapter, we move into the massage therapy room to explore the physical practicalities of your work. The chapter shows you the many ways to make this work effective for your client and comfortable for you both.

As your client is nurturing her baby, you are nurturing her birth as a mother. In that profound process, everything matters, starting with your environment and the equipment you choose. You will learn how everything you use – from table to products, from linens to pillows – can enhance or detract from your session.

Some therapists, especially those who are accustomed only to prone and supine work, are daunted by the positioning needs of pregnant clients. With clear, step-by-step instructions, you will overcome these doubts and embrace the nuances of comfortable, safe and secure client positioning, as well as draping and helping the client move around the table.

The sidelying position quickly becomes a favorite for perinatal massage therapists, even for their non-pregnant clients; however, this happens only when you embody the principles of body mechanics adapted for this position. You will need to adjust your stance and alignment and your use of body weight; then you will need to modify again when your client is semireclining. We will explore tai chi principles as the foundation of those adaptations – decreasing your strain, and increasing your efficiency, fluidity and adaptability as a result.

General Considerations

If you work in a spa or another healthcare provider's office, your employer likely assigns you a room, perhaps not considering its readiness for prenatal massage clients. By knowing the key priorities for a prenatal client, you can work satisfactorily even in the most difficult therapy room. At the other extreme, you might be asked to help set up the rooms in that facility. Or you might be in private practice, where all decisions are yours, like it or not. In any case, here's what to think about and plan for, wherever you work – even in your clients' homes.

Environment

Our most basic goal is simple: we want to safely help our clients feel good. Thus, your therapy room should encourage parasympathetic stimulation whenever possible. You can make a small room feel cozy and womb-like, but if it feels cramped or confined that will detract from relaxation. Pregnant clients are often larger, sometimes feel clumsy, and often in the last few months cannot see their feet as they walk. They need room to maneuver. Postpartum clients might need to bring their little one, so you should also allow space for the inevitable accessories. A room with at least 10 feet × 16 feet of usable space is ideal (Box 3.1).

Box 3.1
Environmental qualities conducive to maternity massage therapy

- Encourages parasympathetic stimulation
- Adequate size for you and the client
- No distracting noise or odors
- Decorative and educational décor
- Sturdy and easy-to-use furniture, adapted for maternity needs
- Restroom adjacent or nearby

Limit outside noise and voices so as not to disturb your ambiance; ensure that people outside your room cannot readily hear your clients. Eliminate the use of strong odors or scents, and, when possible, minimize those smells outside your room, too. Use soothing color combinations on walls, furniture, equipment and accessories.

Some therapists use decoration to convey pregnancy's fluidity, or the power and grace of the pregnant and laboring woman, or the joy of cuddly, happy babies. Like many midwives and obstetricians, some therapists affectionately display photographs of "their babies."

That said, be sensitive that photos of healthy babies may emotionally trigger those clients with unexpected outcomes. Also, you may not want to overwhelm your non-pregnant clients with too much "baby stuff," particularly if you have a diverse clientele.

Educational items, from charts to models to books, are also useful in your décor. The ability to refer to images of joints and muscles, or models of the uterus or pelvis, will reinforce everything that you teach your client and her partner. ⊕

Beyond the room itself, consider how easy it is to access. Is parking close enough for a third-trimester client to arrive at your room without being out of breath and overheated? Even a few stairs can be challenging for some expectant clients, and a full flight or two impossible; an elevator is ideal when you are not at ground level. Be sure that your chairs and tables are sturdy, not too low and adaptable for those coping with larger bellies, ligamental laxity, round ligament strain and other physical discomforts.

Consider where the nearest restroom is. Remember that your client will likely need to use the toilet immediately before and after a session, and sometimes in the middle of it. Ideally, access to the restroom should be private so that she does not have to be fully dressed to reach it. Changing and cleaning her baby is easier with a convenient and equipped restroom, too.

Equipment Requirements

Below are essential items that are specific to an effective prenatal and perinatal massage therapy office setup:

- high-quality massage therapy table (see details below on features to prioritize)

- sturdy, wide, step stool, ideally with a hand support, to help clients move on and off the table

- wedge pillow for under the abdomen and right hip ⊕

- six to eight pillows (including one very firm king-sized pillow, several of standard size and firmness, and one or two thin, pliable ones) plus a foam wedge or other foundation for semireclining support (see positioning instructions below for various options)

- or, preferably, a **Side Lying Positioning System** or a bodyCushion™, plus four firm pillows of various sizes and densities, will for many clients feel even more stable and comfortable ⊕

- twin-sized sheets, including fitted bottom sheets

- breast drapes (king-sized pillowcases are ideal)

- enough pillowcases to be able to launder after each use

- cleaning supplies, as well as vinyl coverings that can be sanitized, to prevent viral and bacterial spread

- unscented oil or lotion (see Chapter 2 for precautions on lubricants)

- at least one prenatal and one anatomical reference book, chart or model.

Equipment Recommendations

While the previous list is essential for effective work with prenatal and perinatal clients, the list below contains items that are recommended, though not required. That said, having most of these can take your maternity work to a higher level.

- lightweight blanket for those extra-chilly days

- one or two double- or queen-sized cover sheets, so that you can modestly drape clients of all sizes

- two or three hospital gowns (or large button-down shirts, worn backwards) to easily drape a client when assisting them on or off the table or for seated massage

- robe for when a client needs to use the bathroom during your session

- 4- to 6-foot-long strip of non-slip shelf liner to secure your pillows

- height-adjustable rolling stool for you

- library of books, DVDs and other educational materials for reference or lending ⊕

- models of the pelvis and uterus

- comfortable chair for resting and nursing, ideally in a secluded area for more privacy

- ottomans or other structures in your waiting area for elevating clients' legs

- full-length mirror to use in coaching alignment

- childcare provider so that moms can more readily schedule sessions

- retail products that you use in your practice and which clients might find useful at home, such as oils or abdominal wedge pillows.

Reminder

Create an environment that promotes parasympathetic stimulation and increased self-awareness, and reinforces the educational benefits of maternity massage therapy.

Massage Table Particulars

When choosing a massage table with maternity work in mind, you will need to consider the model type, width, height adjustability, padding and covering.

Width, Height and Model

Your massage table should be about 30 inches (76 cm) wide to accommodate the sidelying belly and supports; 27 inches (69 cm) is the absolute narrowest width to consider. Sidelying, the position most commonly used with pregnant clients, usually requires working with your table at a higher height than that needed for prone and supine positions. An adjustable-height table is essential. To measure your ideal working height, stand up straight with your arms at your sides; the top of the table should be between your wrist and your knuckles. Be sure that any table you consider safely adjusts up to this height.

With the body mechanics suggested later in this chapter, this height will facilitate the more horizontal weight transfer that sidelying clients require. When your client is semireclining, you may want the table a couple of inches (5 cm) lower than this. This will give you leverage when working on her upper body and more gravitational lean toward the table when working the legs.

In addition to width and height, choose the appropriate table model for your needs. Of course, a hydraulic or electric **lift table** is ideal since it allows you to adjust the table height during a session. Moreover, you can lower the table at the beginning and end of the session, which makes it easier for clients to get on and off. A lift table may seem financially out of reach for you, but remember that it will also accommodate other clients with special needs; it may also be eligible for considerable tax credits under the Americans with Disabilities Act (ADA) or equivalent elsewhere.

Another table model to consider is one with the **tilt-top table** feature. Because you can lift one end to a variety of angles, these tables make sturdy and secure semireclining positioning very easy to achieve with fewer supports. Of course, a lift table with this tilt-top feature would be even better!

However, with the right supports and a willingness to adjust, any table (of the right width and height) can be used. But one note of caution: beware of those marketed as "prenatal massage tables." These may have a cut-out section for the abdomen to hang into while prone, a supportive sling under that hole, and two additional cutouts for the breasts. Despite their well-intended features, these tables are problematic for all of the reasons detailed in Chapter 2 on prone positioning.

From the treatment room

I like my table higher for my prenatal clients so that my alignment is better, and I can use my stool more. I use 4 × 4 blocks (custom-made to my height by a friend), and I simply move the table off the blocks to lower it. That saves time and wear and tear on the table knobs and my back. I often have prenatal clients as well as regular clients scheduled during a single day, and it has been helpful.

– Nanci Newton, therapist

Padding and Covering

Manufacturers usually do not design their standard massage tables with the sidelying or semireclining client in mind. The sidelying position can be uncomfortable at the client's shoulder joint – especially for those with broader shoulders, edema, carpal tunnel syndrome or thoracic outlet syndrome – and the hip joint, especially for those who already have hip pain; in the semireclining position, the sit bones can be uncomfortable (especially for those with sciatic-like sensations). If the foam padding is inadequate, these areas will press against the wooden foundation beneath the table's padding. Look for a table with at least 3 inches (7.6 cm) of triple-density, high-quality foam. Another option is to add a thick padded cover to your table. A primary benefit of some positioning systems is they are designed to reduce pressure at these achy spots.

Most table coverings (whether vinyl or another material) are satisfactory for perinatal needs. Although we joke about "waters breaking" at the most inopportune times, rarely does that happen, so you need not be concerned about excessive fluids soiling your table. You will want your table to have a covering that you can sanitize, to prevent spread of infectious diseases or odor buildup. Most covering materials are odorless after an initial break-in period, but be sure that the vinyl is not emitting smells that could bother your sensitive prenatal clients.

Helping the Client onto the Table

Most pregnant people move about without undue difficulty. These clients can get onto your massage table unassisted. Clearly explain or demonstrate how you want the client to lie on the table (and make sure you clarify where she should be, relative to the supports you already have in place). Provide a sturdy step stool, particularly if you are taller than she is. Give her a little more time than usual for undressing and settling on the table.

If your client appears particularly uncomfortable with normal movements, or if she has signs of pelvic instability, symphysis pubis dysfunction or diastasis recti, ask if she would like your help. Place your footstool at the side of the table that you want her back to face (if moving into the sidelying position), and approximately where her pelvis will be when she lies down. Stand next to the stool with your feet grounded and at least shoulder-width apart. A hand, or your forearm under hers, will give her secure support to step onto the stool. Next, have her sit on the table. Ask her to keep her thighs mostly parallel and to bring her legs onto the table along the edge where you want her to lie. Then she should use her arms to gradually bring her torso down.

If you must be in the room with her as she gets on the table, it can be useful to have a garment that opens in the back for her to wear. After she is settled, you can open the gown and have her slip it off each arm as you work on that side. She will be able to reposition it to modestly get off the table.

Reminder

Assess and ask your client whether she needs your assistance getting on or off the table.

Client Positioning

Follow these essential guidelines for positioning your client in the prone, supine, semireclining, sidelying and seated positions. Box 3.2 summarizes the main points for each position.

Box 3.2
Positioning checklists

Prone (first trimester only)

- Support for pelvis at anterior superior iliac spines
- Support under chest or breast recesses, if breasts are tender
- High bolster under ankles

Supine

- Additional supports for weeks 14 to 22: small wedge pillow, 2 to 4 inches (5 to 10 cm) thick, under right side from lower ribcage to hip joint
- High bolster under knees, adding a pillow under calves and feet
- Pillow under head, if desired
- Soft surface to prevent sacroiliac pain

Semireclining

- Head-to-hip elevation to between 45 and 75 degrees
- Sufficient lumbar and cervical support
- High bolster or pillow under knees
- Additional pillow under calves and feet

Sidelying

- Firm supports to prevent rolling onto abdomen
- Small wedge pillow, 2 to 4 inches (5 to 10 cm) thick, under abdomen
- Entire ceiling-side leg supported anterior of other leg with firm bolster and pillows; maintain horizontal line between hip, knee and ankle; hip flexed at 55- to 80-degree angle to torso and knee flexed
- Table-side leg on table, slightly flexed
- Horizontal and slightly flexed spinal alignment
- Appropriate-height head pillows to avoid cervical hyperextension or sidebending and acromioclavicular compression
- Possible additional supports: under both arms, lumbar spine, ribcage and/or greater trochanter
- Side Lying Positioning System or bodyCushion™ highly recommended

Prone

If you or your clients prefer the prone position for first-trimester sessions, you must decide if you think that the position is preferable to sidelying for each unique individual (see Chapter 2 for more on positioning considerations). Use the suggestions below to minimize compression of her abdomen into the table when you are working on her back, and to reduce other negative aspects of prone positioning. After the first trimester, we recommend avoiding prone positioning, especially for working on the back and pelvis.

Suggested Supports

To help prevent increasing intrauterine pressure, use two pillows (which should provide 3 to 5 inches/7.6 to 12.7 cm of lift), one placed under each anterior superior iliac spine, or a four-part bodyCushion. You will also need a high ankle bolster or other such support, in order to avoid deep plantarflexion of her ankle joints, which can induce calf cramps.

Additional Safety and Comfort

Some clients also like a third pillow or rolled towel or blanket under their clavicles and anterior shoulders to reduce the pressure on their sensitive breasts. Be sure to adjust the face cradle to a comfortable height. Use this position for the shortest possible time to reduce the possibility of undesired effects. Minimize your pressure on her back to avoid excessive compression of her abdomen.

Supine

You may find that you can reach the head, neck and anterior surface of your client's body most easily when she is supine. Although many clients may be happy to stay on their backs, follow the guidelines of the American College of Obstetricians and Gynecologists and avoid the supine position for "long periods" (ACOG 2015). Check in frequently for any sign of supine hypotensive syndrome. We recommend three to five minutes as a conservative target for supine work, and 20 minutes as the longest time without any adaptations. If your client is supine for longer, be sure to shift her uterine weight off the vena cava during weeks 14 to 22 (see Chapter 2 for rationale, and for when to use semireclining instead).

Suggested Supports

This position requires no extra equipment in the first trimester; just use a knee bolster high enough to help flatten her lumbar spine to the table. Offer her a head pillow if she prefers one. At 14 weeks, begin using an 8- to 10-inch (20 to 25 cm) square wedge, or a pillow that is 2 to 4 inches (5 to 10 cm) thick, covered with a clean pillowcase. Place it directly on top of the bottom sheet. Position it under her right side, with the narrowest side of the wedge tucked at her spine and sloping laterally to her right side (Figure 3.1). Elevating her right side from the lower ribcage to the hip joint in this manner usually will prevent supine hypotensive syndrome, as discussed in Chapter 2.

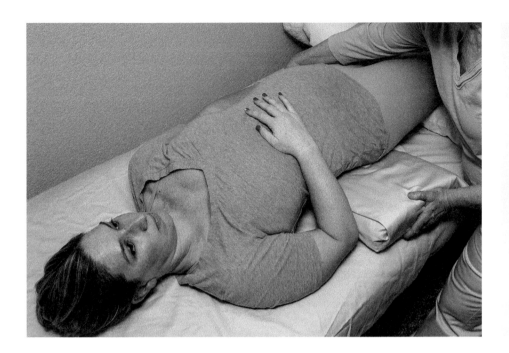

Figure 3.1
Supine positioning: weeks 14 to 22. Use a small wedge-shaped pillow under the right pelvis to shift weight off the vena cava.

Additional Safety and Comfort

Occasionally, a woman will feel that the wedge under her lower torso creates an uncomfortable spinal or pelvic twist. If so, you can add additional pillows under the rest of her right side so that her entire body is canted slightly off to her left but still aligned. Some therapists use the bodyCushion with the wedge placed under the right side for improved supine comfort. Regardless of your other equipment, add a pillow under her calves and feet so that they are level with her knees. Use additional padding on your table if your supine client experiences sacroiliac pain (see Chapter 2).

Semireclining

You should shift from the supine to the semireclining position after week 22 in most pregnancies or if the client has heartburn or is short of breath. Use semireclining when your client has multiple gestations or feels dizzy, light-headed or uncomfortable when supine, regardless of week of pregnancy (Figure 3.2).

Suggested Supports

The goal of the semireclining position is to shift the abdominal weight toward your client's pelvic floor rather

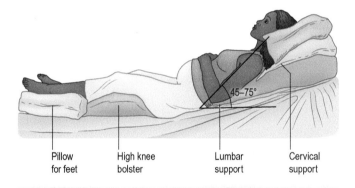

Figure 3.2
Semireclining positioning: week 23 to term. Use props to elevate the client's torso from the hip to head between 45 and 75 degrees; add an additional knee bolster and foot pillow.

than posteriorly onto her vena cava. Do this by elevating her entire upper body – from hip joint to head – 45 to 75 degrees above the level of the table. You will need sufficient equipment to create a firm, steady and secure foundation for propping your client to this height (Figure 3.3). If you only have pillows available, use three of your firmest, biggest ones for this foundation

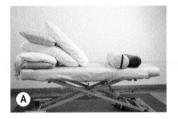
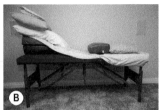
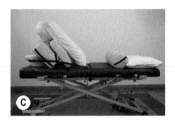
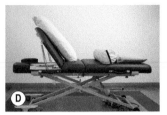

Figure 3.3A–D
Prop options for semireclining positioning. **(A)** Pillows; **(B)** bodyCushion™; **(C)** Side Lying Positioning System reconfigured for semireclining; **(D)** tilt-top table.

(Figure 3.3A). Other foundation options are to choose a dense, foot-high foam wedge or to fold the two sections of a bodyCushion to form that wedge (Figure 3.3B). If using the Side Lying Positioning System, weave and secure its strap around the sections, according to the manufacturer's instructions, to assemble a foundation (Figure 3.3C).

After creating your foundation at the head end of the table, cover it with a sheet. Next, begin stacking any additional pillows you need onto the covered foundation. They will be more secure if you alternate them – lengthwise and then widthwise – on the stack. If you have accurately estimated the height of pillows needed for her torso length and width, you may only need to make small adjustments after she settles onto the table.

She might need, for example, an additional small pillow or rolled towel against her lumbar spine to accommodate her increasing lordotic curve. Similarly, adjust her head and neck until in a neutral position, neither hyperflexed nor extended. Use a high, firm knee bolster to help keep her body from sliding down the table. For added comfort and edema relief, elevate her lower legs with a pillow under her calves and feet. If you have angled her back sufficiently, you will not need the pillow under her right pelvis.

If you use a tilt-top table (Figure 3.3D), adjust the movable section to at least 45 degrees. With all but the tallest of clients, you may only need additional bolsters or small pillows to provide both the lumbar spine and the cervical spine with essential support – plus knee and calf bolsters, of course.

Additional Safety and Comfort

Here are a few ideas for helping to secure your semireclining foundation, which sometimes shifts when the client leans back.

- If you have an adjustable-tilt face cradle, position it so that the cradle faces the foot end of the table, at a 90-degree angle from the table top. (Do be judicious in using your face cradle in this way, as manufacturers only test them to support a client's head, not the torso.)

- Some therapists prefer to back their table up against a wall for the ultimate in solidity behind their supports. (You will then need to reach her upper body from each side of the table rather than from behind her.)

- Check that you are locking the strap of the Side Lying Positioning System firmly into the table hinge, using it to better secure the system sections together.

If your table's covering is smooth or slippery, you may want to place a 4- to 6-foot-long strip of non-slip shelf liner between it and your foundation supports. Even with a non-slip covering, weaving this strip between your pillows as you add them will help to hold them together, too. For added safety, test the security of your foundation by leaning back against it yourself before your client does.

When you direct her into the semireclining position, have her bring her buttocks completely against the supports before she lies back, so that she does not have to scoot further back once she is lying down. If she slumps, so that her lower back is actually flat on the table, help her to reposition, adding other supports as needed so that she can truly be upright from hip to head. Monitor her position as you work to be sure that she does not slide down, thus risking supine hypotension.

As described above, your supports need to be secure enough that, when she leans back, she does not feel as though she is pushing them off the table. They also must have enough side-to-side stability for her not to feel tilted to the left or right. "Weaving" a few larger pillows, rather than piling up oodles of smaller ones, will assist with this.

You can also help to stabilize her with one hand as you work with the other, particularly on her arms and torso. Use some traction with one hand on her arm or shoulder to counter any pressure that could move her to the opposite side.

Fine-tune the position of her head and neck. Try a small wedge, your face cradle cushion or a cervical roll, until you find the perfect support for her cervical spine. If your table is wide enough, you can also place matching bolsters or pillows or towels under each forearm and hand, and she will feel like the "queen mom."

Remember: taking extra time to arrange the supports precisely will not distract from your session. If she is slumping, tilting or just not as comfortable as she could be, pausing to adjust the supports will increase her relaxation because she will feel more secure.

Reminder

Monitor your semireclining client's position and maintain it so that her entire torso, from hip to head, stays elevated somewhere between 45 and 75 degrees.

Sidelying

You may be surprised at how quickly you become both proficient in and enthusiastic about the sidelying position. With the proper equipment, an understanding of your

goals and some practice in the efficient maneuvering of your supports, you will make the sidelying position both efficient and effective. In explaining this position, ceiling side will refer to the side of your client's body that is available to work with; the side she is lying on will be called table side.

A sidelying position that is secure and comfortable requires the following:

- enough supports to help her stay directly lateral on the table side of her torso and thigh, without her feeling she needs to hold herself in position

- enough supports to keep her spine horizontally aligned

- attention to preventing strain to joint or uterine ligaments or pressure on the abdomen

- stabilizing her pelvis and legs with supports sufficient to align her ceiling-side hip, knee and ankle on the same horizontal plane

- minimizing painful pressure on her table-side hip and shoulder and both breasts.

Suggested Supports

We recommend three different sets of equipment, each of which can be used to achieve the ideal sidelying positioning: the Side Lying Positioning System, the bodyCushion and a variety of pillows (Figure 3.4). Each has advantages and disadvantages. Experiment to find what works best for you and your clients. Whichever setup you choose, start by creating a foundation: head support, torso cushioning and one or two leg supports. Place that foundation on top of your fitted bottom sheet, which makes it easier to shift these components when your client turns over. Position the head and torso supports off the table's midline – you want your client to lie as close to the back edge of the table as possible. Cover the head and torso elements not enclosed in pillowcases with another flat sheet, folded in half lengthwise.

Most therapists arrange their foundation, show or tell the client where to lie, and then leave the room so she can get undressed and on the table. They then come back to fine-tune her positioning and pillow placement.

(If she needs your assistance, remain in the room to help as above.) Below are a series of general instructions to optimize the various support options.

Once she settles onto the table, help her to center her entire torso into the torso cushion so that her back is parallel with the table edge, and her entire pectoral girdle is between the torso and head cushions. If you are using only pillows, help her to align herself an inch or two (2.5 to 5 cm) from the back edge of the table. Then you will need to fine-tune your supports (refer to Figure 3.4 as you read the directions below).

With her permission, gently check that her belly is fully supported, especially at pelvic level. If there is space between the supports and her belly, slide a small wedge or towel into that space so that her belly is sufficiently cradled. This extra support will reduce painful strain to the ceiling-side uterine broad and round ligaments. (Use a small enough belly pillow, though, to avoid her feeling as though she is rolling backwards off the table.)

Her legs and pelvis will feel more stable if she extends the table-side leg, positioning it posterior of the ceiling-side leg (which should be flexed somewhere between 55 and 80 degrees). Then you need to place bolsters and/or pillows beneath the ceiling-side leg, high enough to create a horizontal line between this hip, knee and ankle. Some clients will want to keep both legs together and flexed, and to have a pillow between the knees. That arrangement is usually not as stable, forcing clients to tense to maintain their position. (However, this might be more comfortable if she has signs of symphysis pubis dysfunction.)

Visually assess the alignment of her ceiling-side leg. If her knee medially rotates so that it is lower than her hip, check to see if the pillows need to be further under her thigh and knee. One corner should be near the groin with 2 to 3 inches (5 to 7.6 cm) of pillow forward of her anterior thigh. Align the pillows lengthwise with the table rather than skewed at an angle. If her knee still slumps down, you may need additional pillows. Getting the knee and ankle level may require yet another pillow or two placed under her foot, particularly with taller clients. Placing smaller pillows or wedges between larger ones, rather than on top, usually is more stable.

After supporting the belly, leveling the ceiling-side leg is usually the most important part of sidelying propping, and is worth whatever time it takes. Optimal height and support will usually:

- prevent strain on the sacroiliac joints and the lumbar spine

- stabilize the client so she does not roll anteriorly onto her belly

- provide stable, easy access to many problematic areas of the lower torso and extremities

- mechanically assist in the reduction of leg edema

- provide some relief from painful varicose veins.

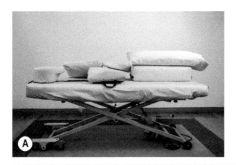
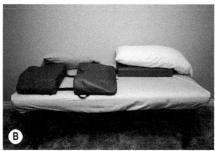
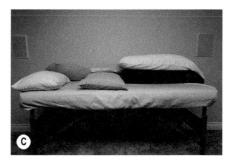

Figure 3.4A–C
Prop options for sidelying positioning. **(A)** Side Lying Positioning System; **(B)** bodyCushion™; **(C)** pillows.

Let's look at her torso now. When used correctly, both the systems in Figure 3.4A and B have a great advantage over the use of pillows only: they take some of the torso weight off the table-side shoulder and hip. Just be sure that the entire scapula area is between the head and torso cushions, thus lying directly on the table. In that position, these systems better accommodate the space between the acromioclavicular joint and the head. Check that her cervical spine aligns with her torso, without hyperextending or sidebending her neck and head. If you are using pillows instead, a full pillow placed under the neck, and a relatively flat one placed under the ribs (with a sufficient gap for the shoulder girdle to rest between), can provide a workable alternative. If her lumbar spine sags toward the table, then put a very small pillow or rolled towel or sheet between her lower ribs and iliac crest, to lift her lumbar spine so it is horizontal with the thoracic spine.

Finally, no matter what setup you use, give her a pillow to place under her ceiling-side arm. That pillow should be of sufficient height and firmness to lift the arm off her breast, help to prevent anterior rotation of her body, and open the anterior pectoral region for circulation. If her hands are swollen, you may want to use an additional pillow to level her hand with her shoulder. If you place these arm pillows on top of her cover sheet, they also will help to hold that drape in place over her breasts. In addition, if her table-side forearm and hand are not fully resting on the table, prop with a small wedge or rolled hand towel underneath.

The Oakworks Side Lying Positioning System (Figure 3.4A) was specially designed to help you achieve the parameters described above, and supports most clients comfortably and securely. The bodyCushion (Figure 3.4B) was not designed specifically for sidelying work, but some therapists use its head, torso and leg pieces to good effect. Other therapists prefer to use pillows: one or two head pillows, a thinner torso pillow, the abdominal wedge pillow, and dense king-sized ones for under her ceiling-side leg (Figure 3.4C). Note that a long body pillow, folded in half, can form a good foundation – both for the ceiling-side leg in sidelying, and for the semireclining position – but you will still need to add other pillows to achieve the appropriate alignment. (See online resources for additional pointers on refining sidelying and semireclining supports.) ⊕

From the treatment room

Good positioning is not only important for your techniques to be effective – good positioning does half your work for you! Almost all of my clients, upon being effectively supported in the sidelying position I have mastered, say, "I haven't felt this comfortable in weeks!" Before I have kneaded, or rocked, or gently stretched any of their areas of discomfort, my clients already feel significantly better.

– **Anne Gilbert**, therapist

Additional Safety and Comfort

As mentioned previously, uncomfortable pressure at the shoulder and hip joints can occur if your table padding is inadequate. Either of the two positioning systems will help prevent this. If just using pillows, you could lay down a thin pillow or two under the shoulder and hip for more cushioning. Another alternative is a specialized cushion for under the hip joint. ⊕

If her table-side shoulder is uncomfortable, the client's instinct might be to move her arm behind her back. That position is counterproductive, as it shifts her upper torso posteriorly and rolls more of her weight onto her belly. Instead, help her to reach her table-side arm further in front of her. And if needed, adjust the thin pillow along the ribcage until it is just below the armpit, which might reduce pressure on the shoulder. For all these situations, choosing your pillows for the needs of each individual client is essential.

As the pillows compress and the client relaxes under your touch, you may find that you periodically need to adjust your supports or add more. Depending on her relaxin levels and resulting ligamental laxity, you may find her skeleton loose and hard to keep stabilized. Monitor her alignment, adding and subtracting supports so that she stays comfortable and stable throughout your session. If you make these adjustments gracefully and calmly, they will not detract from your session.

Instead, she will feel attended to and cared for by your detailed attention to her comfort.

Often clients remark that this setup is what they need to sleep more comfortably. Point out the essential elements of your setup that she can provide for herself: a belly pillow, level hip, knee and foot alignment, and adequate head pillows.

> ## Reminder
>
> Fully supporting the abdomen and leveling the ceiling-side leg are the most important parts of a safe and comfortable sidelying position.

Seated

If there is no table available or the client does not feel comfortable in any other position, you can still do a partial session with her seated. Clients who might be more comfortable seated include the extremely obese, those carrying twins or triplets, or those with severe symphysis pubis pain (all of whom might have trouble getting onto a table even using a step stool and your help); clients with severe gastric reflux; and clients who are fearful about lying down and feel more control when seated.

You can use a typical dining room or kitchen chair, or even a folding chair – one that is very sturdy, relatively firm and that will not compress excessively under your pressure. The lower the back support, the easier your access to her neck and shoulders. Prop her legs up on an ottoman or another chair to help reduce edema, and encourage her to scoot her gluteal muscles as far back in the chair as is comfortable, to avoid her feeling as if she is sliding forward as you sink into her shoulders. If she can comfortably externally rotate her hips to straddle the seat, you can have her turn around and sit backwards, which allows you to work on her back. Use a firm pillow or cushions between her body and the chair back. You will need to be superficial in your posterior work so as to avoid increasing intrauterine pressure, but this is a viable alternative. If you place the chair back against the

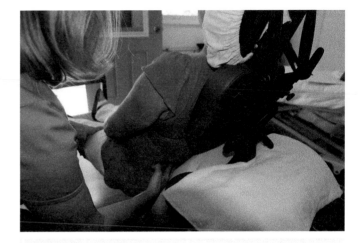

Figure 3.5
On-site massage chair adapted for prenatal sessions.

edge of a table, you might also stack enough pillows or cushions on the table so that she can rest her forearms and head, too.

Alternatively, use an **on-site massage chair** in an unorthodox manner to achieve a semireclining position (Figure 3.5). If the client sits in the massage chair as it was designed, you will risk straining the uterine ligaments or increasing intrauterine pressure. Instead, adjust the angle of the chair to between 45 and 75 degrees, fill in the space between the seat and chest support (if possible), and then have her sit backward on it. Offer a stool for her feet, and encourage her to place her forearms in her lap or on her belly; then she can lean back against the chair in an approximated semireclining position. You will need to adapt your own body mechanics to this unusual setup, but you will be able to work on most of the body, including the lower back.

Draping

Draping has the same purpose in prenatal massage as in all therapeutic massage: keeping the client modestly and comfortably covered and warm, while allowing you maximum access to structures. There are, not surprisingly, a few unique considerations in prenatal draping.

Some clients will feel more modest, perhaps shameful, about their increased size. Others are comfortable, even proud and flamboyant, about their "baby bump" and their rounder body shape. You need skill in professionally draping clients along all points of the modesty spectrum. Due to increased vaginal secretions, many clients will leave their underpants on for massage; use these garments to anchor your linens so they never feel exposed. Increased breast size and tenderness can mean some will leave their bras on, too. If you need further access to the client's back, remember to ask permission to unhook her bra, never assuming permission or coercing her to do so.

The increased basal body temperature means pregnant clients often prefer more lightweight sheets. It is best to have a selection of varying weights, and your heavy flannel sheets can work as lightweight blankets, if needed. Any sheet sets you purchase should include a cover sheet that is at least twin-sized. For breast drapes, king-sized pillowcases are ideal.

As a professional massage therapist, you are already comfortable with draping prone and supine clients. With practice, your semireclining and sidelying draping will be just as graceful. There are some significant differences, though. For instance, in the semireclining position, it is easier for drapes to slip down and expose the breast area. In the sidelying position, the buttocks and even the genital area can feel more exposed, even when completely covered. For these reasons, it is important not only to adequately position your drapes, but also to securely tuck them in rather than leaving them loose. Your client usually needs to be able to feel that these intimate areas are covered so that she can more completely relax. Remember to redrape each body segment after completing your work before uncovering another. Now we will look at how to efficiently drape for these two positions.

Semireclining

In many ways, semireclining draping is very similar to supine draping, particularly for the legs. Your biggest, unique challenge will be in anchoring the cover sheet and/or breast drape over her chest and swollen abdomen. A twin-sized cover sheet will be wide enough for you to center it on your client and cover her completely, with a foot or more on each side left over to tuck under her if necessary. Tuck from her torso to her upper thigh, or just tuck at chest level. Of course, you should only secure the drapes, not make them constrictive, especially over her abdomen.

We recommend discussing abdominal and ribcage work before your client is on your table, including how you will keep her modestly covered. If agreed upon, then at that point in the session, first tell your client about the draping changes about to occur. Add a breast drape and ask her to hold the top of it, so she feels a sense of control over what is happening. Maneuver the cover sheet as you do with a supine client by gently sliding the sheet inferior of her abdomen, and then anchor it under her buttocks on each side, positioning your palms against the table – not her buttocks – as you tuck.

If her breasts cover the lower ribcage or upper abdominal area where you need to work, use the lower edge of the breast drape to lift her breasts away from the area. Do this by holding the two side edges of the drape, and pressing the drape against her lower ribs while scooping the drape under her breasts, in order to lift them toward her clavicles. Keep your tension on the fabric as you tuck each end under her, near her armpits. She should then be able to release the drape, comfortably letting her arms and hands rest wherever she prefers. Of course, another alternative is to ask her to lift and hold her covered breasts for those few minutes of your session.

To redrape her, just bring the sheet back over the breast drape. You can remove the breast drape then, or when she changes position, or just leave it in place until you are finished with your session.

Sidelying

Depending on where you want to work, use one of the following sequences to uncover that area while protecting your client's modesty. In each case, arrange the sheet lengthwise along her body, aligning its edge with the edge of the back side of the table, which will mean there is more sheet over the anterior side of her body.

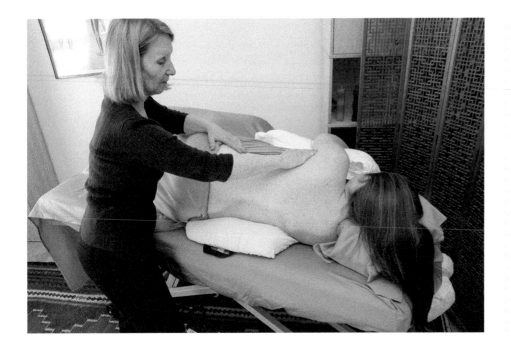

Figure 3.6
Sidelying draping for the back. Notice the sheet tucked between hip and table, and across the ilium and along the ribs, creating a backward letter "L."

Undraping the Back (the "L" Drape)

1. Stand behind your client at pelvis level, facing her head.

2. With your outside hand, tuck the edge of the sheet between the table and the table-side buttocks, at the level of her greater trochanter. With the hand closest to her, gather the sheet to the ceiling side of her pelvis, thus undraping her back.

3. Roll the sheet into the waist of her underpants, or if she is not wearing underpants, just superior of the gluteal cleft.

4. Roll or fold the sheet that remains against her back, so that her back is fully undraped. Press that rolled or folded portion firmly against her ribcage, so she feels it along the midline of her torso. The drape will now be shaped like a backward letter "L" – allowing access to her entire back and sacral structures (Figure 3.6).

5. Finish securing the drape by tucking the remaining back edge of the sheet between the table and her buttocks and thigh, with your palm facing the table as you tuck.

Undraping the Ceiling-Side Hip and Leg (the "U" Drape)

1. Again, stand behind her at pelvic level, but now face her feet. With the hand closest to the bottom of the table, reach across the table and take the far corner of the sheet (Figure 3.7A).

2. Bring that corner toward your body to expose her ceiling-side leg and knee (but no higher). Starting at the back of that leg, thread that corner between the leg and the pillow beneath, just proximal of her bent knee, moving from posterior to anterior (Figure 3.7B).

3. Switch which hand holds that corner and pull only 2 to 4 inches (5 to 10 cm) of the sheet to the anterior side of her knee. Use your outside hand to shape the sheet into a deep "U," thus uncovering her lateral thigh, and keep that hand there. Pull gently, alternating one hand with the other, moving that "U" proximally until you have exposed the muscles just proximal to her greater trochanter (Figure 3.7C).

4. If her underwear will allow for it, ask if she would be comfortable with you continuing the undraping to bikini height. If she says no, stop where you are

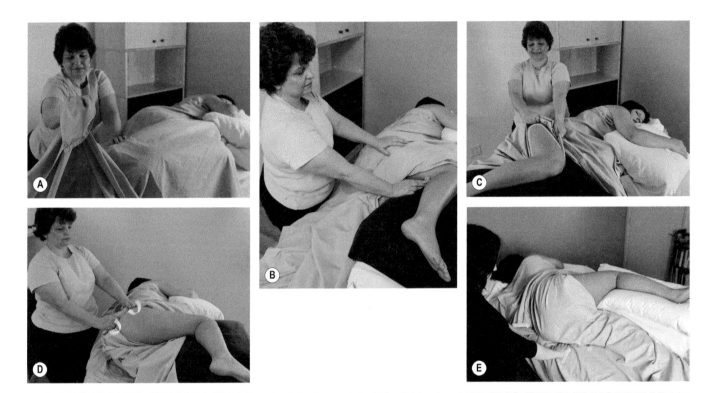

Figure 3.7A–E
Sidelying draping for the ceiling-side hip and leg. The sequence proceeds from **(A)** reaching across the table for the opposite corner of the cover sheet; **(B)** slipping that corner between the ceiling-side knee and its supports; **(C)** alternating pulling a U-shape up the lateral thigh while sliding the sheet along the medial thigh; **(D)** tucking the end of the sheet around the lateral pelvis; and **(E)** tucking drape under gluteals and thigh to ensure that she feels covered.

and tuck the corner of the sheet under the most anterior portion of the "U." If she okays a higher drape, continue alternating your pull with each hand until the entire ceiling-side gluteal area is also accessible, and then tuck the end near her lateral iliac crest (Figure 3.7D).

5. Throughout, monitor the portion of sheet covering her abdomen and genital region. Make sure to tighten or rearrange the sheet as you go to ensure she does not feel exposed; as you do so, avoid tucking into the genital region or into the gluteal cleft.

6. Finish by securing the posterior drape between the table and her table-side buttocks and upper thigh, with your palms facing the table (Figure 3.7E). The propping of the leg in the sidelying position can make

some clients feel exposed, even when they are not. For this reason, always secure in this way.

When you no longer need the ceiling-side hip and leg exposed, unfurl the sheet to her knee. Reverse the previous directions, gently sliding the sheet out from under her thigh as you move the sheet over her leg again, making sure to avoid exposing her groin or abdomen as you do so.

If moving her legs for passive moves and stretches, you will probably find it easiest to redrape her ceiling-side leg only halfway, keeping the drape loose but secured just above her knee, allowing you access to the part of the leg you need to hold without exposing her genital region. This is especially important with any larger movements (circumduction of the hip and other hip movements).

What would you do?

Your 38-week-pregnant client comes into your office breathing heavily, red-faced and sweaty from the 90-degree heat outside. You notice that her feet and ankles are very swollen, but all else seems normal with her pregnancy. When you return to the room, she's on the table, wearing only her underpants; all supports except her head pillow and the cover sheet are pushed aside. She comments gratefully about cooling off. How will you handle positioning and draping this client for her session? 🌐

Undraping the Table-Side Leg

1. Again, stand behind her, at the level of her knee. Check that the sheet is tucked securely under the table-side gluteal area. Shift the sheet off her medial foot and lower leg, tucking it between the table and the leg supports for the other leg.

2. Keep tucking until mid-thigh. Be sure that it is secure against her leg. To redrape, simply pull the sheet from under the supports and back over her table-side leg.

Undraping the Ribcage and Abdomen

1. Remove the pillow beneath your client's ceiling-side arm. Standing behind her, cover her breasts with a folded pillowcase (placed over the sheet and under her ceiling-side arm). Ask her to hold the pillowcase

in place, then shift the sheet down to waist level and tuck it under the table-side pelvis (Figure 3.8A).

2. Ask her to roll back toward you and to tuck the pillowcase under the table-side breast and ribcage, if possible (Figure 3.8B).

3. Hold the untucked end and gently scoop the bottom edge under her breasts, both to give her a sense of security and to lift the breast tissue slightly so you can access the distal ribcage. Tuck the end between her back and the table (Figure 3.8C).

Seated

Many therapists find seated massage easiest with the client clothed, or with a sports bra and loose or spandex pants. This is a very viable option, although it limits you to those techniques that do not require lubricant. Another option is to use your cover sheet evenly arranged widthwise around your client at armpit level. Bring each end completely around her shoulders from front to back to front, and tie it securely at her upper chest. That keeps her breasts and gluteal area covered, leaving her upper back and chest accessible. A garment that opens in the back also works.

Making Transitions

In a typical 50- to 60-minute prenatal massage session, you will likely need one change in position on the table, though additional transitions may disrupt the session's serenity. Of course, the comfort and safety of some clients might require additional changes, or may limit you to only one position. Sometimes you might want to concentrate on one area, and a position change is not necessary.

When it is time for your client to transition to a different position, a bit of organization and direction goes a long way. Clearly tell her where and when you want her to move. (For those clients with symphysis pubis discomforts, encourage them to keep their knees together whenever possible for all transitions; see Chapter 4 for more instructions.) With clear directions and efficient management of your equipment, your clients will usually manage these transitions just fine.

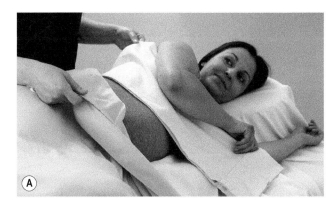

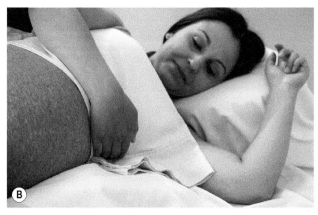

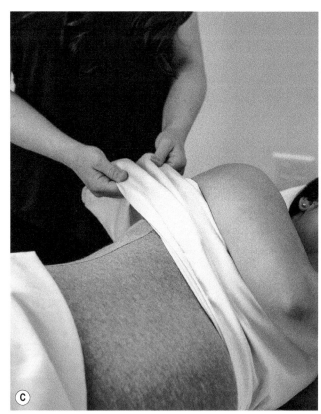

Figure 3.8A–C
Sidelying draping for the breasts.

Supine/Prone Switches

Switching from supine to prone, or the reverse, is almost exactly the same as with non-pregnant clients. You will only need to remove, or insert, the small wedge under her right hip (or other bolsters suggested in the earlier positioning sections). If she has symphysis pubis pain, suggest that she use her arms to push up while keeping her knees together, and then turn.

Supine or Semireclining/Sidelying Switches

Moving from supine to sidelying requires a pause for placement of the supports. Ask her to use her arms or assist her to sit upright, facing the foot end of the table, and help her keep her torso drape in place. Position the head and torso supports with the edge lined up along the side of the table where her back will be. Instruct her to maneuver so that she lies on the supports as described in

the sidelying positioning section above. Once you have adjusted her position so that there is adequate space for her entire scapula to lie between head and torso supports and to be centered on those, add any necessary additional belly support, level her leg and carry out any other adjustments needed to make her content.

If the client feels dizzy or has heartburn, you will need to transition to a semireclining position. Ask her to push up to a seated position while you gather the cover sheet to keep her covered. Once she is seated, ask her to hold the drape with her arms against her torso or with her hands if she can reach. Take your time to build a sturdy, sufficient support. As you help to keep her modestly covered, ask her to scoot her buttocks back into position against your supports, using her arms to avoid straining the abdominal muscles as she settles back.

Side-to-Side Switches

One of your most common transitions will be from one side to the other (Figure 3.9). The details of how to do this well vary slightly, depending on your support equipment. Here is how to ensure it goes smoothly if using just pillows. First, loosen any tucked areas and arrange the sheet evenly over your client. Ask her to stay on her side while you move some of the pillows out of her way. Remove the pillows in the opposite order that you placed them: arm, leg and then belly, leaving the head and torso pillows in place. Place these removed pillows by the other side of the table, where you will be using them next. Then, standing on the side of the table at her back, secure the sheet between the edge of the table and your thighs, hold the sheet just above her body, and ask her to turn over.

Most clients tend to roll onto their back (rather than onto hands and knees). Ask her to pause on her back while you move to the other side of the table. You will now be in position to ensure that she moves safely to that edge of the table. If necessary, reposition the head and torso pillows in preparation, then instruct her to scoot towards you and turn onto her other side. Readjust, if necessary, so that her entire scapula rests on the table between the head and torso pillows. Then replace the other supports: first belly and then leg, arm and other fine-tuning items.

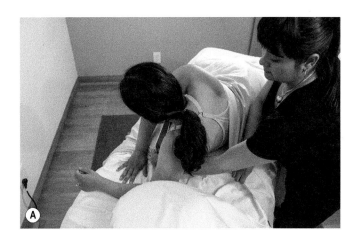

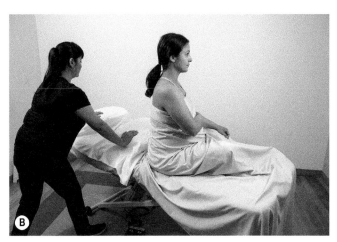

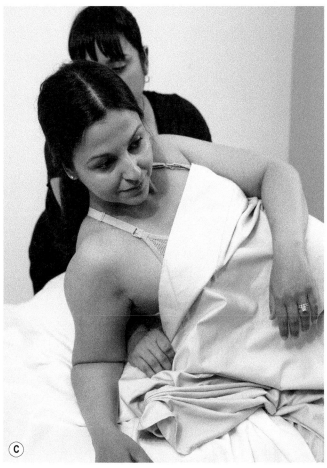

Figure 3.9A–C
Turning from side to side. Help your client to turn over by giving clear, simple directions, moving supports efficiently and managing the cover sheet.

If she turns in the opposite direction, toward her abdomen, direct her to push up onto her hands and knees, and then ask her to pause. Then reposition the torso and head pillows, if necessary, shift to the other side of the table, and proceed as above.

The procedure is a little different when using either the Side Lying Positioning System or the bodyCushion (though you can also follow this same procedure if using just pillows). Remove the arm and leg supports. Have your client push up to a seated position with her arms while you keep her covered (see Figure 3.9A). As she sits facing the foot end of the table, simply slide the torso and head cushions to align with the opposite edge of the table (see Figure 3.9B). Then move to that side of the table, have her turn onto her other side, and help her settle in, adjusting as needed so that she is centered in the cushion and her entire scapula is resting on the table (see Figure 3.9C). Then replace the remaining supports.

Caring for all

We are adamant – and hope you will be, too – that pregnancy is *not* a disability, just as it is not an illness. That said, a prenatal, birth or postpartum client – just like any of your clients – might have a disability or be differently abled. For some clients, that might mean they have a pre-existing condition (such as cerebral palsy, rheumatoid arthritis or multiple sclerosis); for others, their mobility restrictions might emerge from childbearing (see Chapter 7). In response, and especially during intake, ask sufficient questions to fully understand their needs. If your inquiries are thoughtful and made without judgment or assumptions, your clients will appreciate how more complete information will make your sessions more effective. Make your workspace as navigable as possible – whether for a wheelchair or crutches, or just an unsteady client. Slow down whenever and however possible. When a client feels accepted, rather than rushed along, she will feel more at ease, regardless of any body restrictions.

Helping the Client off the Table

At the end of the session (or if she needs to use the bathroom mid-session), determine whether she would like your help getting off the table. If not, give her the option for you to remove all of the supports except whatever is beneath her, or for her to rest awhile with all supports in place. Remind her to note where the edge of the table is and to push from her side to a seated position. Suggest that she pause and let her legs dangle for 30 to 60 seconds. Move the footstool to an accessible spot, remind her of it, and then leave her to rise on her own.

If she prefers assistance, help her to push up from her side, as when turning over. If she needs more help up from the semireclining position, stand at her side, interlocking whichever of your arms is closest to the table with whichever of her arms is closest to you, forearm to upper arm. Place the palm of your remaining hand over her scapula, and ask her to do likewise on you. Shift your weight toward the head end of the table. Tell her to sit up slowly; as she starts to move, shift your weight back, and you will easily help her to sit up without any engagement of her abdominal muscles. She can sit for a few moments before easing down to the footstool, with you bracing her at the forearm if necessary.

Therapist's Body Mechanics

To perform effective bodywork, you must use your body as a tool. We will end this chapter with an exploration of body mechanics (see Figures 3.10 to 3.12) – how you align and use your body to generate the pressure, power, rhythm and sensitivity your client needs. Coupled with a keen kinesthetic awareness, good body mechanics means that your work will be less effortful, your touch more easily received, and your outcomes more satisfying for your client and for you. An internal awareness of how you use your body can help protect you from injury and improve both your sensitivity and your ability to stay present in the session.

The concepts in this section are rooted in the ancient martial art of **tai chi chuan** (Cheng 1999) and in the twentieth-century structural integration modality of Rolfing, as taught by Edward Maupin (2005). Tai chi offers insight into alignment principles, weight direction and transfer, and the "rooting" and "generating" of body energy. Maupin's approach, centered around a concept of both vertical polarity and horizontal expansion, lends space and grace to organization at the table. Synthesized from these two systems, and refined in over 47 years of bodywork practice, the principles below can direct you to more gratifying and less effortful work.

Because you will work most extensively with your expectant clients on their sides, this section focuses on applying these principles for sidelying sessions. (That said, if you hurt or feel depleted when you work, the guidance below might give you some insight into how to change your prone and supine work, too.) The sidelying position usually requires directing the force of your touch horizontally and diagonally into your client, rather than primarily down toward the table. Many therapists struggle to use their body with sidelying clients because they do not modify their approach for this fundamental difference.

Basic Principles of Alignment

Imagine a vertical line dropping from the crown of your head directly down to your feet. See the subtle curvatures of each spinal segment softening that line. Visualize your ear, shoulder joint, hip joint, knee and ankle bisected by that vertical line. Now imagine a horizontal ring at your shoulder joint, diaphragm and pelvis. Imagine any lateral movement at these rings reaching out from your core, into the related joints and structures. You now have a simplified vision of a dynamic way of being in your body. This **expansional balance** concept complements the vertical polarity and expands the thrust of your bodywork to be directed from your core and then out into your arms and hands (Maupin 2005).

There is a bit more symbolism in how tai chi principles illuminate similar alignment concepts. Imagine a string from the crown of your head extending up to the heavens above. Think of another string, tied to a weight, hanging from your coccyx and stretching down into the earth. Now, allow your body energy to move freely through your joints, feeling them open like a silk thread through a string of pearls (Cheng 1999). These and other metaphors are central to tai chi, and help us inhabit a body that is both stable and dynamic. Using

your body with these images in mind can help every type of contact you make, from palpation to compression to cross-fiber friction, and can foster some of the other skills of therapeutic touch, including breathing, engaging your mind and directing your energy. Keeping these principles in mind, and exploring them as you work, will make your sessions easier for you and more effective for the client, and will probably help to reduce career-limiting injuries.

Stance, Weight, Alignment

Most styles of tai chi are built on three basic stances: bow, horse riding and "tee." Many therapists already use some version of the **bow stance**, which is often called a lunge, archer or one-foot-forward stance. The front foot is positioned two to three foot-lengths forward of the rear foot, with a shoulder's width between the feet; the knees and hips are flexed slightly. This stance is often used for effleurage-type strokes: weight shifts from foot to foot and into the working tool while the spine stays lifted and aligned (Beck 2017).

The **horse-riding stance**, what we usually call a parallel stance, will also be familiar to some therapists. Feet are a shoulder's width apart but aligned with each other directly under the flexed ankle, knee and hip joints. This works well as a stationary stance or when alternating hand motions, such as in petrissage techniques. Weight can easily slide from foot to foot to power the momentum and pressure of the hands. Both lunge and parallel stances can be effective with the client prone, supine or semireclining.

In this section, we focus on modifying the less frequently used **tee stance** or "white crane" stance, which makes a very effective base for most forms of massage and bodywork, and is especially useful for the sidelying position (Figure 3.10). In this stance, point your front foot in the direction of your work's movement. Place the back foot shoulder-width apart, but with the toes even with the heel of the front foot. Allow your rear leg to externally rotate slightly, to no more than 15 to 20 degrees, so that the rear hip joint is freer for movement. (This is one of the main modifications to the tai chi bow stance, where the rear foot is externally rotated 45 to 90 degrees.)

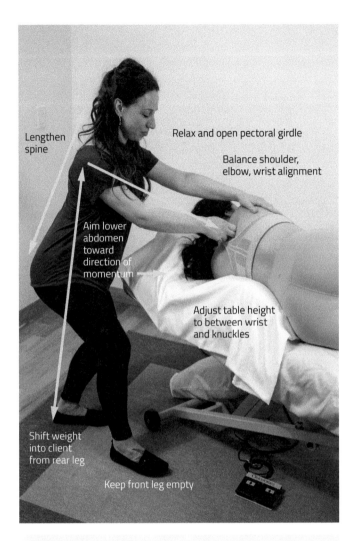

Lengthen spine

Relax and open pectoral girdle

Balance shoulder, elbow, wrist alignment

Aim lower abdomen toward direction of momentum

Adjust table height to between wrist and knuckles

Shift weight into client from rear leg

Keep front leg empty

Figure 3.10
Optimal body mechanics in the modified tee stance.

The other difference is in weight shift and distribution. Rather than distribute your weight between your feet, as in the lunge or parallel stances, gather all of your weight into your rear leg, sinking down into your slightly flexed knee and hip. This empties the pressure on your front foot and leg, so that only the weight of the leg itself rests on the floor, with no tension in it: thus the image of a standing white crane, effortlessly balanced on one leg.

Now, imagine using this starting position in a session. Visualize yourself standing at the head end of the table,

behind your sidelying client, and placing your fist on her mid-trapezius. Instead of creating the pressure by pushing your arm into the client, think of pushing into the ground with the rear leg (but do not lock that knee in doing so). Then lean forward, allowing your body weight to transfer through your pelvis, spine and shoulder girdle into your fist. Direct your weight into your working tool, rather than into your front leg, which should remain empty, relaxed and free to step if needed. Your center of gravity will then be somewhere between you and your client as you lean into her. You should be able to lift your front leg from the floor without any weight adjustments. Increase your pressure by pressing into the ground and leaning more of your body weight into your fist; lighten it by subtly shifting back into the rear leg.

Remember those expansional polarities and open, silk-threaded joints discussed above? As you lean from your rear leg, let your spine extend downward and upward, keeping your head centered over your spine. Notice and correct any collapse or sidebending of your head or torso. Look downward when necessary to locate structures and monitor client reaction, but otherwise maintain your head long on your spine, establishing a gentle cervical curvature, with your chin gently tucked in.

Release all unnecessary contraction of the pectoral girdle muscles, so that your shoulders remain down and relaxed, balanced horizontally on the torso. Avoid hunching or rounding of the shoulders by allowing your sternum to press forward rather than collapse between your ribs. Pay particular attention to releasing excess tension in your trapezius, levator scapulae, supraspinatus and rhomboids. With each contact, lean with your body weight to create the pressure your client needs, rather than overusing your deltoids, pectoralis major, biceps, triceps, latissimus dorsi and trapezius (see Figures 3.10 and 3.11A).

Reminder

Lift the crown of your head, extend your lower spine downward, allow your sternum to press forward and balance each joint.

As you shift your weight into your client's body, remain as relaxed as possible by stabilizing your shoulder and scapulothoracic joints, rather than straining them. Think of the paired muscle groups all working together in balance – the serratus anterior/rhomboids and the latissimus dorsi/upper trapezius, along with the humeral stabilizers (teres minor, infraspinatus and subscapularis). Allow your pectoral girdle to relax downward and open horizontally throughout your work, with serratus anterior actively engaged against the press of your weight into your client. This care of your shoulder and scapulothoracic joints helps to avoid injuries such as rotator cuff syndrome, shoulder bursitis, muscular strain and kyphosis.

In addition to your shoulder girdle, you must protect the integrity of your fingers, wrists and elbows. Whatever technique you apply, perform it with as much open, balanced alignment of these joints as possible. Work with a slight flexion in your elbow but a straight wrist whenever possible. If you repeatedly hyperextend your wrist, you put yourself at higher risk of carpal tunnel syndrome, tendonitis and/or ligament strain in the wrist. Excessive pressure on your fingertips, particularly on the thumbs, can hyperextend or hyperflex the metacarpal–phalangeal joint. The resulting ligament strain and stretching can cause pain, swelling and instability in the affected joints.

Avoid these problems by bracing or supporting your fingers and hands to create additional protection for the joints sustaining the greatest pressures. Use smaller tools such as these for thin and small muscles and specific sites of tissue disorganization. Broader tools, such as your forearm and loosely fisted hand, deliver a more generalized, broader effect to larger areas of tissue. Not only do they tend to be less penetrating and painful, but also their structure better supports heavier pressure without risking damage to your body (Osborne 2002). No matter what tool you are using, like a silk thread through pearls, let your weight and energy slide from that tool into the client (Barrett 2006). At the end of each technique, release your pressure by smoothly and slowly returning your body weight into your rear leg.

What would you do?

Fifteen minutes or so into a session, you feel your back and neck tiring and beginning to ache. You realize that your client's upper body, where you need to work, is not lined up with the back of the table; instead, it is at an angle so that you need to reach far in order to work on her mid-back. Your client seems to be almost asleep. What measures can you take to attend to your body mechanics with the minimum disturbance to your client? 🌐

For this to be a light, easy posture rather than an effortful stance, adjust your table so that the top is level with your wrist when you are standing upright beside it, your weight on both feet. Otherwise, the hip and knee flexion of the tee stance will be deeper and more demanding than most can manage. With the right table height, and following a few other guiding principles, therapists who adopt the tee stance often become enthusiastic about its benefits and have fewer occupational injuries and more satisfied clients. Others will continue to find the bow stance works for them so they keep their tables lower, and they are hopefully very attentive to not bending their torso or twisting their neck.

Positioning and Stabilizing Yourself

In tai chi, it is said that energy and its movement begin in the legs, find direction through the lower abdomen and pelvis, and complete its expression through the arms and hands (Barrett 2006). Here is how to direct your weight and energy in this way. Think about how you use a flashlight when you walk in darkness: pointed in the direction that you want to see. Now, imagine that your lower abdomen is like a flashlight, shining with your vital energy. Direct that light toward your work: point your feet – and, in turn, your abdomen and torso – in the direction that you want to shift your weight (Figure 3.11A). Each time you contact the client, think of leaning – or "pouring" – your body weight into your client, rather than pushing with your

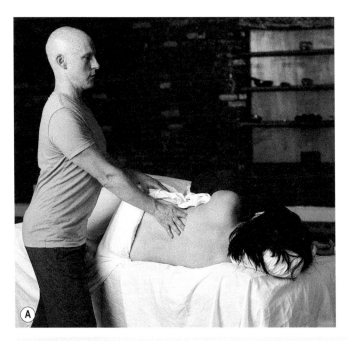
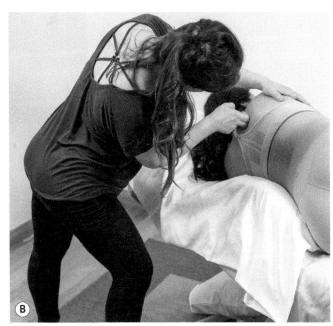

Figure 3.11A–B
Body mechanics comparison: modified tee stance. Notice the ease of **(A)** the therapist who is upright and aligned, compared to the strain of **(B)** the therapist who sidebends and slumps.

muscles. When you are not pushing each stroke with your arms and shoulders, your work can originate in your lower body, flow into your relaxed torso, and from your core into your hands (Lobenstine 2016a).

One common detrimental tendency of therapists unaccustomed to sidelying work is to sidebend the head and upper body rather than staying upright (Figure 3.11B). Perhaps this occurs in an effort to align the eyes with the spine so that things look "normal," as when the client is prone. Sustained sidebending quickly becomes tiring and damaging, and you cannot as readily focus your weight and energy into your hands. Remember to stay upright as you work. Move your eyes rather than your head and neck. Bend at your hips or knees – and not at your lower back or the sides of your ribs – so that you create each stroke by sinking with your whole body rather than muscling from your upper body (see Figure 3.11A).

From this modified tee stance, you can accomplish movements away from the client's center, too, such as many traction stretches and return effleurage. Just start with your weight in your front foot instead. Gradually shift weight from your front foot to your back foot, again emptying your front foot. To obtain a fuller traction, bend deeper into your hip and knee joints to leverage more of your weight (Lobenstine 2016a).

Other Pointers

The horizontal direction of your work on the sidelying client means that you will sometimes need to modify techniques so that she remains safely and comfortably aligned. For example, when effleuraging up the lateral thigh, anchor her knee with the other hand, exerting a slight traction toward you. This will counterbalance the force of your stroke, which is pushing her leg and pelvis toward the back of the table. Another useful stabilizing placement, when standing at the client's back, is to gently mold your inside hand around the ceiling-side ilium to prevent the pelvis rotating forward as you work along the sacrum with your outside hand.

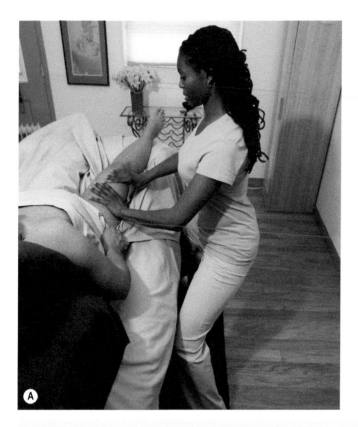
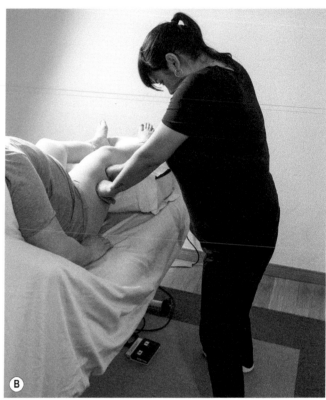

Figure 3.12A–B
Body mechanics comparison: the horse-riding stance. Pouring from your whole body **(A)**, instead of pushing from your shoulders **(B)**.

You will sometimes do procedures that require you to squarely face the side of the table, such as petrissage. This is when the parallel or horse-riding stance is more efficient (Figure 3.12A). With the table higher for side-lying, you will not need to sink as low into your knees and hips as when at a lower table. Create your power by shifting your weight between your feet, while also creating a torso-twisting motion that flows through your core and into your arms. As with sidelying, use your whole body to create each stroke, rather than trying to push with just the muscles of your arms and shoulders (Figure 3.12B).

Parallel position is often best when you need to lift an arm or leg for passive movements. Remember to use your legs rather than your back to lift. Bend into your knees, encircle the thigh or arm, and then straighten your knees to lift. But even the strength of your leg muscles might not be sufficient with a large client. When your client's size is too large for you to safely lift, eliminate these types of techniques and address her needs with techniques that will not be risky for you (Beck 2017).

Particularly when working on the table side of the back, a seated position can be efficient. Use an adjustable stool so that you can keep your hands level with your work without elevating your pectoral girdle. Plant your feet firmly on the floor to stabilize your body. Then, shift your weight by pressing your ischial tuberosities into the stool and leaning forward, allowing your hips to function as the feet do when standing. As always, maintain expansional balance and spinal alignment from hips to head. An awareness of your own body mechanics will continue to benefit you and your prenatal clients, especially if you decide to work with them during labor and postpartum, where you will encounter a variety of other positioning dilemmas (see Chapters 5 and 6).

Your self-care in the rest of your life is as important as your body mechanics. Maintain your flexibility and strength with regular stretching and exercise. Replenish your energy with rest, healthy nutrition, recreation, and other activities that bring you peace and rejuvenation.

From the treatment room

I strongly believe the prenatal work I do has helped me to thrive in private practice for 10 years (and going!). Sidelying positioning is a break for my body from the supine- and prone-positioned clients. My own comfort and skill with sidelying positioned clients has improved my work with the full spectrum of clients in any position. Prenatal bodywork brings me a steady stream of clients, many of whom continue to see me for years after they deliver. They bring their partners, parents and children to be clients as well!

I've chosen to work within my passion to support growing families – working from my heart motivates me to stay strong, to use techniques that feel good in my own body to maintain longevity, and to continue learning so that I can remain in this work for many years to come.

– Faith Davis, therapist

Body mechanics are about the efficient organization and use of your body's energy and structure to perform your work (Box 3.3). The goal is not a static posture, but rather a dynamic flow of how you use pressure, speed, strength, direction, subtlety and energy. Body mechanics are not just what you are doing to the client but what you are feeling from the client and your sensitivity in responding to those signals. Equipment, stance, weight shift and alignment are all useless if you forget to do one other thing: breathe! Engage your diaphragm fully for maximum oxygen and waste exchange. Focus on slowing your breathing and letting your diaphragm create the inhale, without any excess effort from the secondary

---

Box 3.3
Body mechanics principles

- Relax and expand into each joint.
- Guide the direction of weight by pointing the lower abdomen in the direction of work.
- When in modified tee stance, gently flex the ankle, knee and hip. Shift weight from the rear leg into the client. The front leg remains "empty." (For traction techniques, reverse.)
- When in horse-riding or bow stance, fluidly shift weight from leg to leg.
- Align the spine and lengthen downward and upward, with no excessive spinal curvatures.
- Lift the head at the occiput to tuck the chin in.
- Allow the sternum to press forward without overinflating the chest.
- Maintain a horizontal pectoral girdle with balanced engagement of related muscle groups, paying particular attention to the serratus anterior's stabilizing potential.
- Maintain open and balanced shoulder, elbow, wrist and finger joints.
- Breathe fully from deep in the abdomen, expanding/ compressing in all directions on each breath cycle.

---

muscles of respiration in your shoulders, neck and back. Your breathing will be less effortful and your upper body more relaxed, which, in turn, translates into touch that is softer and more powerful. Fuller breathing means more rhythmic and dynamic movement, more parasympathetic effect that you can transmit to your client, and more energy for you (Lobenstine 2016b).

Chapter Summary

A cozy, well-equipped room; a client safely positioned and comfortably draped; and a dynamic, focused therapist: as we moved from theory to practicalities, this chapter has equipped you to achieve all of these. You are now ready to make your way through the trimesters of pregnancy and learn specific techniques to meet the needs of each client, both during pregnancy and beyond.

Think it through

To deepen your knowledge, go to our online resources, answer the test questions for this chapter and explore further. 🌐

References and Further Reading

ACOG (American College of Obstetricians and Gynecologists) (2015) Physical Activity and Exercise During Pregnancy and the Postpartum Period. Committee Opinion 650. December.

Barrett R (2006) Taijiquan: Through the Western Gate. Berkeley: Blue Snake.

Beck M (2017) Theory and Practice of Therapeutic Massage, 6th edn. Boston: Milady.

Cheng M (1999) Master Cheng's New Method of T'aichi Ch'uan Self-Cultivation. Berkeley: Blue Snake.

Lobenstine D (2016a) Pour don't push: how to massage with greater depth and ease. Massage & Bodywork. November/December.

Lobenstine D (2016b) Breath: your most powerful tool. Massage & Bodywork. May/June.

Lobenstine D (2017) Rock on! Soothe clients with satisfying contact. Massage Magazine. June.

Maupin E (2005) A Dynamic Relation to Gravity, vol 1. San Diego: Dawn Eve Press.

Osborne C (2002) Deep Tissue Sculpting, 2nd edn. San Diego: Body Therapy Associates.

Osborne C (2008) Health maintenance: preventive care for hands and bodies, July 31. Available at: https://bodytherapyeducation.com/health-maintenance-preventive-care-hands-bodies/ [accessed April 29, 2020].

Studying this chapter will prepare you to:

1. apply guiding principles as you adapt your therapy sessions for pregnant clients

2. consider how typical pregnancies progress through the three trimesters so that you can better meet your clients' needs

3. choose safe positioning options and techniques appropriate for each client in each trimester

4. perform specialized massage and therapeutic bodywork techniques that address typical prenatal discomforts.

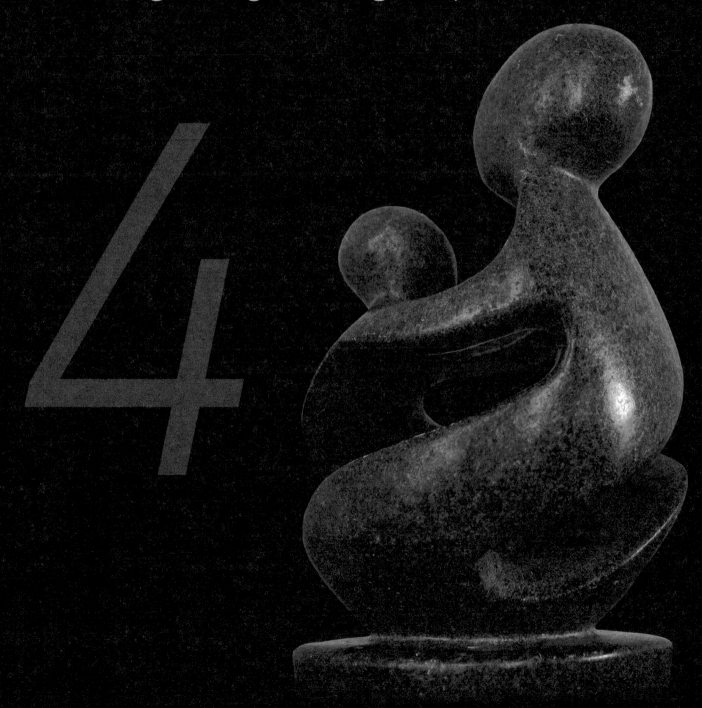

Prenatal Techniques
Nurturing Throughout Pregnancy

4

Chapter 4

Chapter Overview

In Chapters 1 and 2, you learned how and why therapeutic massage and bodywork can benefit pregnant people. You read our evidence basis for those claims and for our guidelines and precautions to maximize client safety while she is in your care. Then, in Chapter 3, you learned how to manage many practicalities of prenatal massage therapy. Now you are ready to actually put your hands on your expectant clients and address their individual needs.

This chapter starts with our general guidelines for client-centered prenatal massage therapy. Next, we overview pregnancy's three trimesters to further prepare you for your clients' ever-changing experiences.

Within this overview, we suggest specific techniques for your clients' most common complaints and needs during those months. Many of them have been used with pregnant clients in at least two small research studies, both of which showed positive effects (Field et al. 1999; Çakır Koçak et al. 2018). All of these techniques – developed and clinically applied across four decades – are collected into the Technique Manual that makes up the majority of this chapter.

Our focus throughout is to succinctly convey the intended outcomes for each technique, how to do it, and ways to enhance its effectiveness while remaining safe. As you assimilate this knowledge, you can then intersperse these procedures into whatever routines you are already comfortable performing. Later chapters also will guide you in creating your own session flows (Chapter 8) and in adapting during labor (Chapter 5) and postpartum (Chapter 6), and for special needs clients (Chapter 7). We are confident that many of these techniques will become favorites as you deliver thoughtful, targeted therapy.

Guiding Principles

About 80 percent of babies gestate healthily and long enough, and their moms' bodies support that process without compromise or medical complications, a fact that should give confidence to all prenatal massage therapists (DeCherney et al. 2019). As a facilitator of well-being and physical and emotional comfort, you are uniquely positioned to support this "normal" reality of pregnancy.

Your words, body language and sessions can exude this confidence and strength that we want all our pregnant clients to have.

As presented in Chapter 1, massage therapy can provide powerful support for maternal and fetal well-being. Wherever your client is in her prenatal journey, her steps will be easier when you work toward the aims summarized in Box 4.1. Your own current repertoire of modalities surely offers you many ways to accomplish these goals (use the guidance presented in Box 2.4 as you determine how to safely adapt those modalities). This chapter, in turn, will further your understanding and skills for achieving these possibilities during pregnancy.

> ### Box 4.1
> #### Goals of bodywork throughout pregnancy
>
> - **A supportive, caring experience** that helps create autonomic sedation, internal focus and awareness to illuminate her body's amazing adaptations
> - **Education** in fuller breathing, pelvic positioning and other structural balance
> - **Reduction of pain** from tense and bound myofascial tissues, strain to joint and uterine ligaments, compression of nerves and trigger point referrals
> - **More torso space** for baby and mother by interrupting imbalanced holding patterns and increasing tissue pliability
> - **Support** for the normal and unfolding prenatal physiological processes, including promoting restorative sleep and reducing nausea and other digestive disturbances
> - **Increased awareness** (and, if within scope of practice, appropriate strengthening) of abdominal, iliopsoas and pelvic floor muscles
> - **Prevention of and/or relief** from varicose veins, cramps and fluid buildup
> - **Assimilation of feelings** and emotional issues that she may be experiencing (providing appropriate referrals to counseling or mental health professionals, as needed)

Whatever your client's goals, each session you create should be built upon the following primary therapeutic principles:

- **First, do no harm**: apply the safety parameters (see especially Chapters 2 and 7) that are relevant to your client. Explore any concerns through detailed intake and assessments, and update those at every session. (See Chapter 8 for more on intake and record keeping.) Work within your skill and knowledge base, and readily refer to others when needed.

- **Create safe, comfortable and stable positions**: use sufficient, sturdy equipment, arranged according to Chapter 3's guidelines. Be responsive to your pregnant client's needs and requests, as long as they do not compromise safety (see Chapter 2).

- **Prioritize autonomic sedation**: adjust speed and depth of pressure to avoid sympathetic nervous system arousal. Too light and brisk can be annoying; quick, forceful contact can prompt defenses. Reach your client's "just right" through gradual weight shifts into relaxed arms and hands, and with exquisite attention to your client's receptivity.

- **Communicate to find your client's preferences:** ask "What's happening for you with this work?" rather than a vague "How's this pressure?" Use simple feedback systems to find the needed depth, speed and type of touch. (See Chapters 2 and 8 for more on client communication.)

- **Respond to your client's goals**: when clients desire rest, skip techniques requiring their participation. Clients seeking "something to do" about their discomforts are more likely to enjoy active movements and instruction in self-care.

- **Make needed variations**: use this chapter's techniques and/or carefully consider and adapt others to safely meet pregnancy's demands.

- **Maintain scope of practice**: avoid giving advice about how, where and with whom to give birth, what to eat or supplements to take, and other relevant but non-massage concerns (see Chapter 8 for more on boundaries and ethics).

- **Collaborate with medical professionals**: "What does your midwife have to say about that?" and "Shall we consult with your doctor before our next session?" should become regular questions for you. Work with your clients' medical care teams.

- **Accommodate her changing body**: remember that the pregnant client might move more slowly; try not to rush her. Adopt techniques that meet her at her slower, more fluid state and use sufficient yet pleasurable therapeutic depth.

You will be most able to apply these therapeutic principles – and your work will be most effective – if you understand what is happening in your clients' bodies. While each person's experience of each pregnancy is unique, the 37 to 42 weeks of pregnancy generally follow a predictable progression. This next section highlights that typical progression in three-month groupings, or trimesters, and explains how maternal and fetal developments will inform our thoughtful work.

First Trimester (Weeks 1 to 13) (Box 4.2)

Most women have hints of their pregnancies beyond a missed menstrual period – tender, swollen breasts, a queasy stomach, frequent urination, deep fatigue. An at-home pregnancy test usually first confirms what is

---

Box 4.2
First-trimester overview

Common Maternal Developments

- Enlarged, tender breasts
- Emotional and hormonal adjustments
- Fatigue
- Frequent urination
- Morning sickness or all-day nausea and/or vomiting

Recommended Positioning

- Supine
- Sidelying

happening: the initiation of extensive hormonal communications that prepare for the 9 to 10 months of gestation ahead. Newly pregnant people, and their babies, can benefit greatly from knowledgeable massage therapy (O'Hair et al. 2018). These benefits are often withheld because of employers' and therapists' concerns regarding the safety of first-trimester sessions. The sections that follow will help you to think your way through this precaution for each individual situation and client.

Maternal and Fetal Development

Although enlarged breasts are often the only visible sign of early pregnancy, internally embryonic cells are dividing wildly, becoming specialized structures and body systems in this most developmentally critical trimester. Within two weeks, the placenta forms. Vascularly intertwined with the uterine blood vessels, the placenta is the fetal conduit for nourishment and oxygen, as well as its waste removal system. By trimester's end, it fosters the embryo's growth into a fetus with recognizable human shape about 3 inches (7.6 cm) long and weighing 1 ounce (28 g). It has eyes, ears and a beating heart. The placenta, usually firmly implanted on the superior uterine wall, is also a primary manufacturer of estrogen, progesterone and other pregnancy-specific hormones. During these first 13 weeks, the uterus expands to one-third larger than normal, from plum to grapefruit size, often reaching halfway to the umbilicus (US Dept. HHS n.d.) (Figure 4.1).

Although their abdomens may not yet look identifiably pregnant, most expectant mothers notice a wider waistline and sensitive breasts. Many feel they would just like to sleep through these first months and need one or two naps daily and 9 or 10 hours of nightly sleep; unfortunately, frequent urination – brought on by hormonal influences and the enlarged uterus pressing on the bladder – will probably interrupt this much-needed sleep (Merck Manuals 2019).

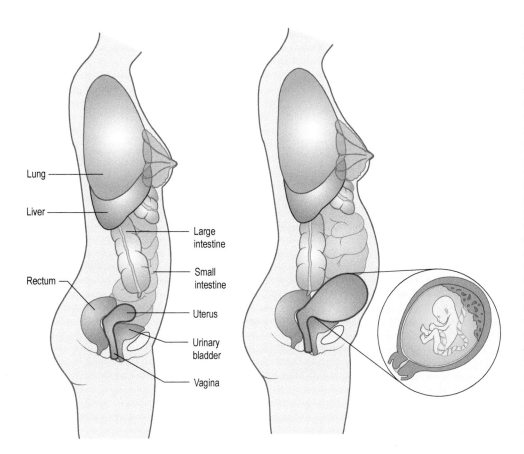

Lung

Liver

Rectum

Large intestine

Small intestine

Uterus

Urinary bladder

Vagina

Figure 4.1
First trimester of pregnancy. Left: the non-pregnant uterus *(outlined in red)*. Center: growth by 13 weeks. Right: fetal gestation by 13 weeks.

Some experience no nausea; however, 60 to 80 percent of pregnant people have a very queasy stomach in the morning or throughout the day, and many are hypersensitive to smells. When individuals suffer severe nausea and/or vomiting, they may need medical care (see Chapter 7) (Merck Manuals 2019).

Structural stresses to the newly pregnant body are minimal in these first 13 weeks. The thoracic spine and ribcage may begin to sink slightly with increased breast weight and as a protective posture for sore breasts and upset stomach. The pectoral girdle may tend toward anterior rotation, further compressing the ribcage. The head shifts forward with the chin more lifted. This can put pressure on the all-important vagus nerve, with negative impact on its parasympathetic functions (Alexander 2017a). As the body makes these postural adjustments, those whose pre-pregnant posture is swaybacked may begin shifting even farther forward into lordosis. Ramped-up relaxin production can create additional discomforts for those who already have ligamental laxity and hypermobility.

You will have some clients who have supreme trust in their body's natural wisdom and power to grow and birth their baby. They seldom fret or become anxious, and glide through their pregnancies in a gestational euphoria. Yet even the most desired pregnancy may prompt fear, worry, regret, or sometimes anger or fatalism. Especially in the first trimester, fear of miscarriage or debate about continuing the pregnancy or not may cause anxiety. Guilt about prior drug use, lifestyle choices or health issues may diminish happiness. Even this early, typical worries about the actual birth might begin to percolate.

As estrogen, progesterone and other pregnancy-generated hormones increase, so can emotional **lability**. This creates frequent, steep fluctuations between these highs and lows, and heightened emotions in general. Be alert and aware that clients may want your empathetic ear to explore these feelings and issues. Some 10 to 20 percent may need more support from their providers, including referrals to pre- and perinatal mental health professionals, to explore and resolve their concerns (Ricci 2017).

For those clients in relationships, their partners are hopefully happy and anticipating their baby's birth; however, remember that they also might need support

and nurturing, particularly if they feel isolated, trapped, jealous, angry, disconnected or fearful. Some partners are worried about failure, financial stresses, rejection and older children. Their own memories and traumas can begin to stir while expecting (Simkin et al. 2018).

Reminder

Listen empathetically and objectively to the full spectrum of emotional responses that a newly expectant client may have.

Caring for all

Throughout this book, we use this "Caring for all" feature to explore various strategies for including all pregnant people and families. But what if you do not want, or are unable, to care for all? Diversity and inclusivity are ideals with multiple manifestations. There are meaningful reasons to *not* "care for all," and they do not mean that you do not care! Not every therapist is equipped for, has access to or is non-judgmental about certain groups. You might serve these populations exclusively, or any other that you can offer very individualized care to – and maybe that is your own demographic, however broad or narrow it is. While we must be respectful of all, we must not confuse discernment with discrimination. Instead, acknowledge your limitations. Determine who you will provide with the utmost quality of care, and how you will offer thoughtful referrals to those who you cannot or choose not to care for.

Guidelines and Considerations

Working with a client in their first trimester can help launch a healthy pregnancy. Your sessions have considerable potential to reduce the negative effects of stress during these early weeks (see Chapter 1 for stress's many impacts). First, a review of why that is so: blood shifts to her extremities when a pregnant woman is stressed, resulting in less oxygen, nutrients and waste-product removal in her uterus. During this critical time, when organs and systems are rapidly forming and are most vulnerable to malformations, reduced uterine blood supply is particularly detrimental to fetal growth.

Parasympathetic activation – just what you are highly skilled in – corrects that endocrine and circulation imbalance. When feeling relaxed, her fetus is amply supplied for optimal growth. As you carefully respond to her changing needs, you can be a reassuring resource on issues of stress reduction, comfort, kinesthetic awareness and functional activities. (Of course, some clients may choose not to see you until the second trimester, because they are too nervous, too nauseous or just too tired.)

Interestingly, the first trimester is both a high-stress time for many, and the most common period for pregnancy losses (see Chapters 2 and 7) (ACOG 2015; Mayo Clinic 2019). Many causes of miscarriage, of course, are unrelated to any possible effects of massage therapy, and most pregnancies proceed normally. Yet some people have an excessive caution and anxiety about "forbidden" times to have a massage, especially the first trimester, and body areas to be touched. This view – not based on evidence – suggests that pregnant people are fragile, and it can contribute to fears your client may already have – that the pregnancy is so vulnerable that she is a miscarriage waiting to happen. What if massage therapy's calming effects could actually *reduce* the frequency of first-trimester miscarriage? No research has explored that specific potential, but it is a possibility worth considering.

As you assuage your client's worries, you must also resolve your own. Commit to careful critical thinking about first-trimester appropriateness for each individual client. Consider the following to determine if waiting until later in the pregnancy would be more prudent:

- **Is the pregnancy low risk and proceeding normally, or does it involve medical complications or high-risk factors?** If there are conditions that make miscarriage more likely, in addition to the risks inherent in the first trimester, waiting until those resolve or the client is past 13 weeks may reduce any worries about possible liability implications for you and/or for your employers (see Chapters 2 and 7).

- **Is your own knowledge base sufficient and your intake process robust?** If not, delay massage therapy. If you do proceed, thoroughly and conservatively apply whatever intake information you have received to reinforce the safety of your first-trimester work (see Chapter 8 for more on intake).

- **Do you have sufficient understanding and supports, as well as the decision-making authority, to create recommended first-trimester positioning?** If you are unable to ensure that your positioning will not increase intrauterine pressure, then you may want to say "no" (see later sections here and in Chapters 2 and 3).

- **What is your (and, if you are employed, your employer's) level of risk tolerance?** If your client does have a miscarriage or pregnancy complication at any time after your session, are you prepared for the possible legal implications? (See Chapter 2's discussion of first-trimester massage risks and Chapter 8's section on liability.)

- **Would it be helpful to you or your prospective client to seek advice from her maternity healthcare provider?** If she has already selected her physician or midwife, she can convey their input to you. When you are working under direct medical supervision, you can seek consultation and/or require orders from her physician or midwife prior to your first-trimester work. In most cases we consider this an unnecessary precaution, but you or she may prefer to consult.

Once you are ready to massage a first-trimester client, remember to observe all contraindications and precautions detailed in Chapter 2, especially the following:

- Delay abdominal techniques – however lightly performed – as a liability precaution.

- Stay broad and light with touch over potential contraction stimulation points on the lower legs, feet, hands, sacrum and upper back (see Figures 2.8 and 2.9).

- Schedule sessions at the time of day when she is least nauseated. Monitor her response to rhythmic rocking movements. Be particularly careful to not increase nausea with strong scents in your lubricants, in your environment or on you. Suggest that she stimulate the nausea relief points near her wrists (see Figure 7.3) during the session.

- Although compromise of femoral veins is usually minimal in the first trimester, blood-clotting factors do change early in pregnancy (DeLoughery 2015). Especially for those whose activity level has decreased, begin to limit techniques on the medial leg and inguinal area to soft, whole-hand pressure.

- Use a gentle, yet firm touch with all techniques, moderating them so that she experiences no more intensity than pleasure on the borderline of pain. Massage that is too deep or painful can trigger sympathetic nervous system arousal and its detrimental effects (see Chapter 1).

Points of view: Sacral and lumbar work

Yet another area of discrepancy among pregnancy massage instructors (Stager 2010; Stillerman 2008; Yates 2010; Rattray and Ludwig 2000) involves work to the sacrum and lumbar areas, particularly in the first trimester and up to 18 to 20 weeks. Some instructors teach that deep massage in these areas can cause miscarriage. One argument is that deep stimulation of the sacral nerves might affect the uterus negatively. This seems unfounded as these nerves are deep to the sacrum. Another argument is that gliding over acupuncture points below the first lumbar vertebra could create a "downbearing" effect.

Review Chapter 2 for discussion about similar fears that are perpetrated about foot and lower leg points. All this seems like a misconstruing of what is required to affect an acupuncture point.

A less alarmist and reasonable precaution is to avoid deeply focused, pointed pressure into Urinary Bladder 31–34, points near the sacral sulci (see Figure 2.9). This protects those clients whose pregnancies and general health might make them more vulnerable to strong stimulation of these points, particularly in the first trimester. Broader pressure to the sacrum is not only safe but often indicated for expectant clients, depending on their posture, activity, gait and injuries.

One maternity massage instructor additionally cautions against quadratus lumborum and piriformis work, particularly in the first eight weeks, due to the proximity of these muscles to the now-enlarged uterus. This seems unfounded as the piriformis is on the posterior side of the pelvis, not the anterior. Regarding the quadratus lumborum, the uterus begins to outgrow the full protection of the pelvis only *after* the first trimester – the rule of thumb being that it is not until approximately 20 weeks that the fundus is usually at umbilical height. It does not fill the abdomen laterally to the quadratus lumborum until sometime after 20 to 26 weeks. Certainly, after that point, you must be precise in locating the quadratus lumborum posterior of the midline of the torso and compressing into it without also compressing the lateral side of the uterus.

Positioning

Most positions, if bolstered properly, are possible for the first trimester: supine, sidelying, semireclining, seated and maybe even prone. But if you are considering the prone position, review these factors. First, there is limited evidence to confirm or refute the position's potential dangers, whether with special equipment or without; however, the greater likelihood of miscarriage in the first trimester is established. Although miscarriage is more often due to genetic or hormonal causes, consider the many possible impacts of a client's loss if it came after being massaged in the prone position. Second, look for a "baby bump." If you can see one, then it is unlikely that her pubic bone and anterior superior iliac spines will entirely protect the uterus from the likely increase in intrauterine pressure during prone massage (see Chapter 2). Third, some prone positioning options may provide sufficient space for the relatively small first-trimester uterus to hover above the table without excessive strain to its ligamental supports; however, often clients' breasts will be too tender for lying face down, even with additional support. For all these reasons, the sidelying and supine or semireclining positions will likely be better choices. Use Chapter 3's guidance for creating comfortable, secure sidelying and semireclining support.

From the treatment room

My work with Ashley began in the 18 months prior to her first successful pregnancy. She had just miscarried again after 10 years of trying to get pregnant, including extensive fertility treatments. She asked for my help to become more in tune with herself and be more receptive to her natural fertility.

Over the course of our bimonthly sessions and with committed lifestyle changes, she conceived again. Together we developed a visualization of her breath holding this baby protectively inside her. We focused on relaxation, particularly in her legs, pelvis, and computer-cramped neck and upper back. What an achievement and joy for her to give birth to her naturally conceived daughter later that year!

– **Carole Osborne**, therapist

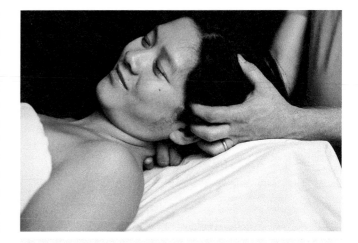

Figure 4.2
Prioritizing autonomic sedation during the first trimester.

Box 4.3
Summary of first-trimester bodywork

Pregnant clients in weeks 1 to 13 will derive benefit and enjoyment from your focus on the goals listed in Box 4.1. In addition, focus on these following first-trimester-specific priorities:

- Promoting sleep through autonomic sedation and pain reduction
- Reducing nausea through autonomic sedation and teaching reflexive point on forearm
- Preparing for the functional challenges ahead with structural balancing and breathing education

Selecting Effective Techniques (Box 4.3)

Use the general goals listed in Box 4.1 as you work with your first-trimester clients. In addition, here are some specific first-trimester priorities, followed by specific techniques that will help with those issues.

In these early weeks, guide the client in creating comfort during daily life and in participating in and receiving your work. Focus on relief for stress, fatigue, nausea and other physiological adjustments, and on improved sleep (Figure 4.2).

- Autonomic Sedation Sequence 3-1-1 (see Figures 4.8–4.10)
- Breathing Enhancement (see Figure 4.11)
- Cervical Transverse Rocking (see Figure 4.12)
- Grounding Hold (see Figure 5.11)
- Occiput Traction and Rocking (see Figure 4.14)
- Pectoral Girdle Mobilizations (see Figures 4.24–4.25)
- Foot Reflexive Zone Therapy (see Figure 4.13)
- Wrist Acupressure (see Figure 7.3).

In anticipation of uterine and fetal enlargement, choose techniques that help the mother's body to accommodate the progressively enlarging uterus. You can encourage more space in the pelvis and torso with techniques that increase flexibility and function in the pelvic stabilizers and the muscles of the spine and ribcage:

- Anterior Hip Deep Tissue Sculpting (see Figure 4.43)
- Lateral Pelvis Deep Tissue Sculpting (see Figure 4.20)
- Lumbar Lengthening (see Figure 4.21)
- Paravertebral Deep Tissue Sculpting (see Figure 4.23)
- Pelvic Alignment Education (see Figure 4.32)
- Pelvic Girdle Decompressions (see Figure 4.33)
- Ribcage Deep Tissue Sculpting (see Figure 4.34)
- Ribcage Trigger Points (see Figure 4.35)
- Spinal Rocking (see Figure 4.40)
- Structural Balancing Education (see Figures 4.15–4.17).

Also integrate techniques you already know – after answering the questions in Box 2.4 – to further assist first-trimester needs.

There also are educational activities and other ancillary ways to help clients with common prenatal discomforts. We have collected strengthening and stretching exercises, for example, and other such suggestions in our online resources. For possibilities outside of your scope of practice, present them not as prescriptions, but as ideas for clients to explore and discuss. ⊕

What would you do?

An established, very athletic client of yours comes in for their quarterly massage and happily announces that they are nine weeks pregnant! They usually enjoy a very deep Swedish and deep tissue massage, particularly addressing their tendency toward constipation and an extreme lumbar lordosis. They have also recently increased their preparation for a 10K race next month that they still intend to run, as long as the fairly intense nausea eases up by then. This is the third pregnancy for this 28-year-old person. They have no high-risk factors and have had no problems with previous pregnancies. Their midwife expects this to also be a low-risk, uncomplicated pregnancy.

What changes in your usual positioning and techniques to address their constipation and lumbar lordosis are advisable? Staying within your scope of practice, what might you teach them and what techniques might be effective in helping them be more comfortable with their pregnancy-related discomforts? ⊕

Second Trimester (Weeks 14 to 26) (Box 4.4)

Most pregnant people usually enjoy this middle third of their pregnancies. Some feel these are the most vibrant and vital months of their lives. By this point, they usually have adjusted hormonally, adopted well-considered nutrition, exercise and daily routines, and chosen a midwife or physician. They also may begin to feel additional structural stresses on the weight-bearing joints and the myofascial structures that massage therapy can often reduce – or, at least, help to prevent worsening.

Maternal and Fetal Development

Fetal development accelerates and sensory systems become active, especially touch and hearing, during these weeks. Babies grow to between 11 and 14 inches (28 and 35 cm), weighing about 1½ pounds (0.7 kg). Increased to melon size, the uterus reaches the umbilicus, and fills most of the pelvic region laterally.

By now, hormonally softened joints prompt postural adjustments for increased weight and a definite anterior shift in the center of gravity. Abdominal and spinal extensor muscles may become fatigued, and chronic lumbar shortening develops throughout the posterior myofascial sheath. Prenatal postural changes can influence balance and functioning anywhere along the back of the body, from heels to skull. As normal balance diminishes among the abdominal, iliopsoas and paravertebral muscles, maintaining good posture is more difficult, and often results in some pelvic and back pain.

Relaxin and other hormones have been accomplishing their softening job, allowing gradual maternal adaptation to this trimester's increase in fetal size (Ricci 2017). The uterus not only grows in the second trimester, it also lifts superiorly into the abdominal cavity (Figure 4.3). This change usually allows more room for the urinary bladder to fill, bringing some relief from

---

Box 4.4
Second-trimester overview

Common Maternal Developments

- Pregnancy seems more real
- Increased weight and anterior center of gravity
- Back, pelvic, hip and leg pain
- Round and broad ligament pain
- Stretch marks and other skin and hair changes
- Varicose and/or spider veins, lower leg edema
- Constipation and/or heartburn, some urinary incontinence

Recommended Positioning

- Supine, with pillow under right hip, up to 22 weeks
- After 22 weeks, switch to semireclining rather than extended supine work
- Sidelying
- Seated

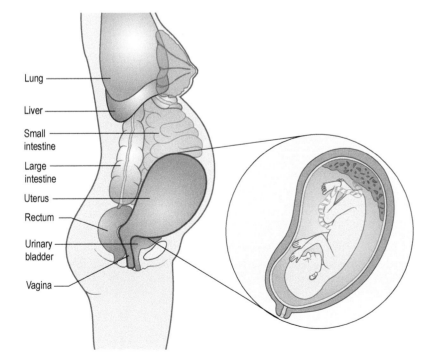

Lung
Liver
Small intestine
Large intestine
Uterus
Rectum
Urinary bladder
Vagina

Figure 4.3
Second trimester of pregnancy. Left: the uterus by week 26 *(outlined in red)*. Right: Fetal growth.

the first trimester's frequent urination. Unfortunately, this growth also may produce intermittent, sharp pain in the lower abdomen, groin and perhaps down the anterior/medial thigh as the uterine round ligaments stretch. Some describe this as feeling as if a rubber band is snapping in their groin. It most often occurs with sudden movements like standing from sitting, or uncrossing the legs, or when driving. Diffuse, achy pain in the lumbar, gluteal and posterior thigh areas – referred from the uterine broad ligaments – is also common (see Figure 1.7).

With this growth, mothers often compensate with an anterior shift in their center of balance and a broadening of their standing base. The external femoral rotation involved creates a bit more space in the pelvis and stabilizes her, but muscles and ligaments around the hip joints may begin to strain and develop trigger points as a result (Werner 2015). Many women feel compressed in these joints, and in the knees and feet, depending on weight gain, gait and sedentary lifestyles – especially excessive sitting – as well as the body that she brought into the pregnancy.

Reminder

The second trimester is often a robust three months for pregnant clients. Enhance their enjoyment of this trimester with guidance and techniques that support postural integrity.

Progesterone's continuing relaxation of smooth muscle keeps the uterus calm and quiet; however, it also produces some potential challenges. Its effects extend to the pelvic floor muscles, which are half smooth and half striated muscle. Combined with the increased uterine weight that also stresses these muscles, some women have urinary stress incontinence. Others may hyperventilate and/or experience heartburn.

Many also notice other progesterone- and estrogen-related effects to their skin, mucous membranes and blood vessels. Facial and abdominal pigmentation may darken. Stretchmarks may appear on the abdomen and elsewhere. Sinus congestion and vaginal secretions may increase (one reason why some clients keep undergarments on during sessions). Many develop spider veins and/or varicose veins in their legs, vulva or rectum (hemorrhoids), or constipation or strained bowel movements (Nievenberg 2015).

Often, the emotional highlight of the second trimester is feeling baby's first movements and hearing the heartbeat. These experiences usually make pregnancy more real and more personal. But this reality may also generate changes in roles and relationships with the spouse, family and friends, and cause financial concerns and health worries. Many women delight in their full, rounded appearance during pregnancy. They discover a new bodily sensitivity and perhaps relish their heightened sexual responsiveness, more typical in this trimester. Others may feel unattractive. Some may also endure rejection by partners as their body rounds, or because of fears of "hurting the baby" during sexual activities (Simkin et al. 2018).

Guidelines and Considerations

Interview every client thoroughly before your first session. Update yourself with their developments and most recent checkups at each subsequent appointment (see Chapter 8). If their maternity healthcare provider has no concerns about their progress, then be assured of the pregnancy's normalcy. If any signs of complications have occurred in the meantime, communication and consultation are prudent (see Chapter 7).

Observe all of the precautions and guidelines detailed in Chapter 2. Some specifics relevant to the second trimester to remember are:

- First-time mothers are more likely than others to develop gestational hypertensive disorders, perhaps as early as the twentieth week (Simkin et al. 2018). Be alert for those symptoms and adapt accordingly (see Chapter 7).

- Increased urination in the second trimester, when less frequent urination is the norm, can indicate gestational diabetes. Be sure to adapt your work accordingly (see Chapter 7 for more on gestational diabetes).

- Note symptoms of other complications and refer these clients to their medical healthcare providers (see Chapters 2 and 7 for more on pregnancy complications).

After the first trimester, light abdominal effleurage and rocking is usually soothing and safe (Although most miscarriages occur in the first 13 weeks, later miscarriages and non-viable early births can happen in the second trimester.) Of course, you will not massage the abdomen if specifically contraindicated by your client's healthcare provider. If the risk of miscarriage or preterm birth is high, you may be more comfortable skipping even light abdominal massage, although this is only a liability precaution.

Even though strain to the abdominal and iliopsoas muscles and sluggishness in the colon are common, observe strict contraindications to massage therapy techniques requiring deep abdominal pressure. Use foot and hand reflexive techniques to promote safe relief in these areas and encourage iliopsoas and abdominal strengthening and stretching. Techniques that address the quadratus lumborum and the iliolumbar ligaments become more relevant in the second trimester; however, remember to apply those techniques posterior of the midline of the lateral torso. Avoid deep anterior-directed pressure when working on any structures between the ilium and lower ribs.

In the second trimester, uterine size and weight may begin to restrict fluid flow from the lower extremities. This increases edema and femoral venous pressure, making varicose veins more likely. Remember that when varicose veins are visible in the more superficial perforator veins, deeper veins may be similarly weakened and harboring potentially dangerous blood clots (see Figure 2.6).

As a result, avoid all techniques that can potentially dislodge these thrombi and cause embolisms, particularly throughout the medial leg (detailed in Chapter 2). Usually, the closer to the pelvic bowl a clot forms, the more serious the consequences, so exercise special caution in the femoral triangle and throughout the inguinal region. It is safest to assume that all of your pregnant clients have asymptomatic thrombi. Refresh your memory on

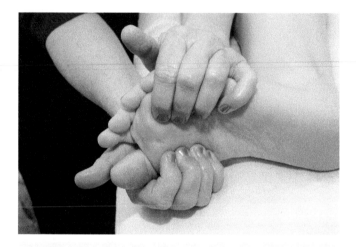

Figure 4.4
Calf cramp prevention.

symptoms and the factors that increase clot risks, the most common being decreased exercise and activity, and moderate to severe varicose veins (see Chapters 2 and 7 for more on health conditions that are also relevant) (Devis and Knuttinen 2017).

Movements that you might regularly use can be problematic due to ligamental laxity. Avoid overstretching by keeping all movements well within normal joint ranges, even if a client's flexibility exceeds the norm. Symphysis pubis dysfunction requires additional precautions. It is more common in the third trimester, although those with multiple gestations or who have had several babies can be affected sooner (see Chapter 2 and this chapter's third-trimester guidelines). Also, maintain ankle neutrality or dorsiflexion (Figure 4.4) to prevent possibly inducing a calf cramp, increasingly likely in this and the third trimesters.

What would you do? (?)

After receiving the results of diagnostic genetic testing, your client decides to terminate the gestation of her fetus. What strategies will help you to stay present, non-judgmental and supportive of your client, despite your own personal beliefs, feelings and values?

Positioning

Adjustments for increased uterine size are now a primary concern. The uterus has usually outgrown the pelvic bowl's protective borders. When in prone position and with pressure applied, increased intrauterine pressure probably occurs. More uterine weight further strains uterine ligaments – another reason to avoid prone positioning from here on. This is why we recommend the sidelying and semireclining positions at this point. With the client positioned securely on her side with a small wedge pillow supporting her abdomen, uterine ligaments are well supported. You can safely apply the deep pressure that is often necessary for relieving the posterior structures without concern about increasing intrauterine pressure (see Chapters 2 and 3).

As for the supine position, you must now prevent supine hypotensive syndrome with bolstering and/or semireclining positioning (see Chapter 3). Of course, when there are twins or triplets, you will have to make modifications for all positions earlier in the pregnancy.

From the treatment room

One of my clients had an unexpected pregnancy a few years after she turned 40. She was a physical therapist and, though she had helped many people deal with chronic pain, she had never experienced it herself. As she moved into her second trimester, she began waking up at night with fiery, electric arm and hand pain. Her obstetrician diagnosed pregnancy-related carpal tunnel syndrome, and then he prescribed bed rest because of placenta previa.

At our next session, this very active woman was quite upset and concerned that the carpal tunnel syndrome would last beyond pregnancy. After our work, she was relieved that her pain diminished dramatically. In subsequent sessions at her home, I also instructed her husband in basic arm massage for between our sessions. Her carpal tunnel syndrome discontinued when she finished breastfeeding.

– Liz Ellis, therapist

Box 4.5
Summary of second-trimester bodywork

Pregnant clients in weeks 14 to 26 will derive benefit and enjoyment from your focus on the goals listed in Box 4.1. In addition, focus on the following second-trimester-specific priorities:

- Teaching and reinforcing upright alignment
- Improving breathing dynamics
- Reducing strain and pain around spine, hips, and pelvic and pectoral structures
- Maximizing space throughout the mother's torso
- Relieving pain patterns originating from uterine ligament strain and from nerve compressions
- Assisting in preventing and/or relieving developing varicose veins, cramps, and fluid buildup in the feet and legs

Selecting Effective Techniques (Box 4.5)

Use the general goals listed in Box 4.1 as you work with your second-trimester clients. In addition, here are some specific second-trimester priorities, followed by specific techniques that will help with those issues. If you are trained in functional assessment, use those tests to make your technique choices more targeted (Zulak 2018).

- Begin and complete sessions with guidance in structural balance. Encourage her daily usage of these lessons:
  - Lumbar Lengthening (see Figure 4.21)
  - Pelvic Alignment Education (see Figure 4.32)
  - Structural Balancing Education (see Figures 4.15–4.17).
- Deepen her breathing, reduce tension and create more ribcage space:
  - Scalenes (see Figure 4.28)
  - Pectoralis Major (see Figure 4.29)
  - Pectoralis Minor (see Figure 4.30)

- ○ Ribcage Deep Tissue Sculpting (see Figure 4.34)

- ○ Spinal Rocking (see Figure 4.40).

- Maximize torso space to accommodate the enlarging baby by emphasizing work for fascia, superficial and deeper intrinsic muscles and each joint of the spine, pelvic and pectoral girdles. This will also help to relieve torso tension and pain.

  - ○ Paravertebral Sculpting (see Figure 4.23)

  - ○ Spinal Rocking (see Figure 4.40)

  - ○ Lumbosacral Joint Decompression (see Figure 4.22)

  - ○ Pelvic Alignment Education (see Figure 4.32)

  - ○ Lumbar Lengthening (see Figure 4.21)

  - ○ Pelvic Girdle Decompressions (see Figure 4.33)

  - ○ Sacroiliac Joint Decompressions (see Figures 4.36 and 4.37)

  - ○ Sacroiliac Joint Rhythmic Deep Tissue (see Figures 4.38 and 4.39)

  - ○ Hip Joint Decompression (Figure 4.46)

  - ○ Lateral Pelvis Deep Tissue Sculpting (Figure 4.20)

  - ○ Pectoral Girdle Mobilizations (see Figures 4.24 and 4.25)

  - ○ Pectoral Girdle Deep Tissue Sculpting (see Figures 4.26–4.30)

  - ○ Pelvic Girdle Decompressions (see Figure 4.33)

  - ○ Ribcage Deep Tissue Sculpting (see Figure 4.34).

- Relieve fascial pain from uterine ligament strain (see Figure 1.7):

  - ○ Lateral Pelvis Deep Tissue Sculpting (see Figure 4.20)

  - ○ Hip Infinity Mobilization (see Figures 4.44 and 4.45)

  - ○ Lumbosacral Joint Decompression (see Figure 4.22).

- Reduce nerve compressions (more common in third trimester; detailed below).

- Reduce fluid congestion in the extremities with appropriate positioning (see Chapter 3 for instructions) and the following techniques:

  - ○ Abdominal Massage (see Figure 4.18)

  - ○ Hip Infinity Mobilization (see Figures 4.44 and 4.45)

  - ○ Hip Joint Decompression (see Figure 4.46)

  - ○ Thigh Adductors Passive Relaxation (see Figure 5.14)

  - ○ Leg Swedish Massage (see Figure 2.7)

  - ○ Foot Reflexive Zone Therapy (see Figure 4.13)

  - ○ Consider also taking an in-person workshop, where you will learn additional more advanced abdominal and pelvic techniques.

- Encourage frequent leg elevation when sitting or lying to alleviate circulatory fluid pooling and ease edema and varicose vein pain.

- Prevent and/or relieve calf cramps and plantar fasciitis brought on by fatigue, postural changes and physiological imbalances. Both the gastrocnemius–soleus complex and/or the peroneals may spasm, causing almost 50 percent of expectant people nightly pain. These cramps may begin now, but more often occur in the third trimester (Simkin et al. 2018). ⊕

- Ease aching, tired feet with Swedish and joint mobilization techniques. Foot Reflexive Zone Therapy also may help to alleviate many common complaints: constipation, heartburn, headaches, hemorrhoids and musculoskeletal pains.

- Encourage and teach your clients, if appropriate, to do essential maternity exercises, like pelvic tilting, abdominal strengthening and pelvic floor awareness (Simkin et al. 2018; Calais-Germain 2003). Help your clients to find other self-exploration modalities and daily exercise that can also increase their comfort and make room for baby. Some popular ones are modified prenatal yoga classes, belly dancing, walking, swimming and other aerobic conditioning.

Also, integrate techniques you already know – after answering the questions in Box 2.4 – to further assist second-trimester needs.

There also are educational activities and other ancillary ways to help clients with common prenatal discomforts. We have collected strengthening and stretching exercises, for example, and other such suggestions in our online resources. For possibilities outside of your scope of practice, present them not as prescriptions, but as ideas for clients to explore and discuss. ⊕

Third Trimester (Weeks 27 to 40+) (Box 4.6)

The most common musculoskeletal and physiological discomforts of pregnancy usually occur, or get worse, during these final weeks of pregnancy. Review descriptions of these third-trimester changes and our potential to help with them in Chapter 1. Also consult Chapter 2 for important safety and efficacy considerations.

Maternal and Fetal Development

Pregnancy's final months are often both exciting and bittersweet. The pregnant person may be reluctant to move ahead to parenting even while the longing intensifies to hold and see the baby whose movement delights them so. This anticipation and the fetus both grow dramatically in the third trimester. Fetal weight triples to a typical 7½ pounds (3.4 kg) by birth, and length almost doubles, to 20 inches (51 cm) on average. All organ systems are developed by the eighth month, with the exception of the lungs. These almost-newborns respond to bright light and familiar sounds, and often choose a favorite uterine position for their sleep/wake cycles (Figure 4.5). This dramatic fetal growth increases anterior weight load and

---

Box 4.6
Third-trimester overview

Common Maternal Developments

- Eagerness and anxiety
- Further weight gain
- Increased back, ribcage, pelvic and hip pain
- Diastasis recti
- Wrist or hand pain
- Hyperventilation
- Heartburn, constipation or hemorrhoids
- Edema in feet and legs
- Leg cramps and restless leg syndrome
- Varicose veins
- Urinary frequency
- Braxton Hicks contractions
- Lightening

Recommended Positioning

- Sidelying
- Semireclining
- Seated

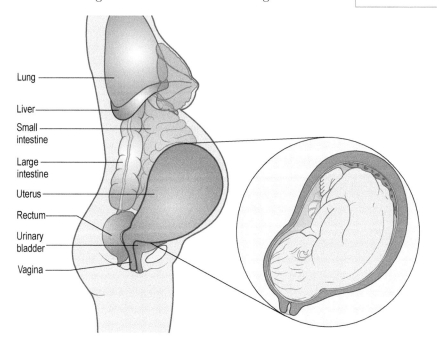

Lung
Liver
Small intestine
Large intestine
Uterus
Rectum
Urinary bladder
Vagina

Figure 4.5
Third trimester of pregnancy. Left: the uterus by the end of the ninth month *(outlined in red)*. Right: the nine-month fetus.

prompts further maternal weight gain – 35 pounds (16 kg) is typical, but up to 80 pounds (36 kg) is not uncommon.

Ideally, she maintains her alignment close to that shown in Figure 4.6B. If spinal curvatures collapse, she may have more pain and movement limitations. The typical musculoskeletal strain and discomforts (see Chapter 1) are:

- excessive lumbar lordosis

- sacroiliac, lumbosacral and other lumbar joint and myofascial pain

- uterine ligament strain, particularly broad and sacrouterine, causing referred pain in the buttocks, lower back and posterior thigh (and, less frequently, the groin from the round ligament)

- diastasis recti that further weakens the already stretched abdominal muscles, adding more strain to the iliopsoas, back pain, and sometimes abdominal tenderness too

- increased gluteus medius recruitment for walking, with resulting chronic tension and trigger points

- hip joint compression and increased lateral femoral rotation with painful chronic tension in the deep lateral rotators

- pelvic joint instability, particularly for some symphysis pubis dysfunction, causing sharp anterior mid-pelvic pain, especially when walking, climbing stairs, rolling over, standing from a seated position, and getting in and out of a car

- ribcage pain and soreness from fetal activity and trigger points in intercostals and abdominal muscle attachments.

Throughout pregnancy, but especially as effects of anterior weight load dramatically increase, compensatory changes (Figure 4.6A) may significantly affect the functions of the vagus nerve. These include regulation of the lung, heart, pancreas and digestive organs, as well as a promotion of calmness – all critical to fetal and maternal well-being. The vagus nerve travels from between the occiput, atlas vertebra and mastoid process, anterior of the cervical transverse processes, through the thoracic outlet and diaphragmatic hiatus – all possible places for pregnancy's shifting alignment to negatively impact vagal activity (Alexander 2017a; Howland 2014).

Changes in structural balance throughout the body may also increase pressure on various other motor and sensory nerves. The most common such prenatal nerve entrapments are:

- Sciatic nerve compression caused by chronic tension in the piriformis and other lateral rotators and/ or by pressure from the fascial hoods of the anterior iliolumbar ligaments, which leads to neurological buttock and leg sensations, including pain, burning and/or numbness, known as piriformis syndrome and often generalized as "sciatica" (Klein 2013; Dalton 2020).

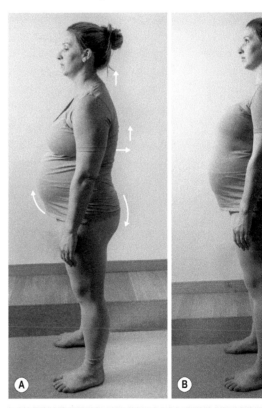

Figure 4.6A–B
Prenatal postural changes. **(A)** Collapse of the spinal curvatures may cause pain and movement limitations unless the client adjusts in the direction of the arrows shown. Those adjustments can result in more vertical alignment **(B)** and help to relieve these discomforts.

- Lateral femoral cutaneous nerve compression from fetal pressure and/or the fascial structures related to the inguinal ligament, which creates numbness and pain along the anterolateral thigh, known as **meralgia paresthetica** (Patijn 2011; Klein 2013).

- Femoral nerve compression caused by fetal pressure, fascial restrictions or edema at the inguinal ligament and creating weakness and limited leg movements (Klein 2013).

- Pressure on the brachial plexus (and/or arm blood vessels), known as thoracic outlet syndrome, from scalene, pectoralis major and minor chronic tension, which causes pain, numbness and weakness in the affected arm and hand (Klein 2013).

- Median nerve compression from fluid and/or fibrosis in the carpal tunnel that results in the thumb and pointer or middle fingers feeling numb, and similar such effects in the tarsal tunnel (Klein 2013).

- Other pelvic nerves that may be affected include the genitofemoral, obturator, pudendal and saphenous nerves. All the above nerves can be negatively impacted from a stretch injury or trauma, in addition to compression (Klein 2013).

As if these musculoskeletal and neurological discomforts were not enough, it is normal for edema to develop in the lower extremities, contributing to varicose vein tenderness and achy feet (Simkin et al. 2018). As the fundus reaches the ribcage, it pushes abdominal organs out laterally and superiorly, contributing to constipation, hemorrhoids, shortness of breath, heartburn and hiatal hernia (see Figure 4.5). Rapid growth can cause uncomfortable stretchmarks and diastasis recti. Normal activities may become difficult; sleep may be interrupted.

Pregnancy's last weeks or days may bring some welcome relief from shortness of breath and the ability to eat more than a few bites at a time. This comes as the baby prepares for labor by dropping lower into the pelvic bowl, its head engaging further into the pelvis. It is called "lightening" but often feels like the opposite; some describe it as like having a bowling ball in their pelvis. Increased urinary frequency may also result as the baby's head compresses the mother's urinary bladder to less than one-third of its normal size.

Reminder

Emphasizing breath awareness and capability can increase your client's enjoyment of pregnancy and her ability to cope with its challenges. In the third trimester, it can help prepare her for the work and breath needed for labor.

As the **estimated due date** approaches, hormonal balances shift, and the uterus "wakes up" to the bigger baby's weight and movements. The uterus will begin contractions as the uterine muscle fibers "practice" and tense irregularly for 15- to 30-second intervals. Although these contractions are usually light and often unnoticeable, some people find them mildly painful. The contractions are irregular and usually brief so that they accomplish only minimal cervical changes, but they often begin to psychologically prepare the woman for labor. While this is referred to as "false labor," most mothers find these contractions quite real! If these practice contractions become more rhythmic and regular and begin to make cervical changes, then labor may have started, regardless of the due date (see Chapter 5 for more on labor signs and progress).

With labor and birthing imminent and hormonal shifts preparing her for giving birth, expectant moms often become impatient and/or restless. They will most likely begin to "nest," making final preparations in terms of home, family and self. All of the potential emotional stressors discussed in Chapter 1 often mushroom at this time. While they are excited, fears for the baby's or their own health may dominate their dreams and thoughts. What they are hearing in childbirth education classes, reading about, and discussing with friends and family may ease their fears, or exacerbate them. Often people who had pleasurable – even ecstatic – births are reluctant to share their enviable experiences. Encourage interested clients to seek out empowering birth stories and aim to be a source of reassurance and calm.

The upcoming birth can bring hidden feelings to the surface, creating conscious or unconscious emotional stress or triggering prior traumas (Simkin and Klaus 2011; Simkin et al. 2018). (See Chapter 7 for more on trauma's effect on childbearing.) Most of your clients will be at least somewhat awash in joyous anticipation of their baby. Be respectfully sensitive to the depth and range of all the emotions that can emerge when clients are under your nurturing hands.

Guidelines and Considerations

You will see many of your expectant clients for the first time in this final trimester. This is often because this is when they become uncomfortable enough to seek possible relief. Perform a thorough intake interview and update yourself regularly with results from her increasingly frequent maternity healthcare provider visits (see Chapter 8). If the physician or midwife has no concerns about progress, then be assured of the pregnancy's normalcy. Of course, you and your clients should communicate with their providers if any signs of complications occur.

Observe all precautions and guidelines detailed in Chapter 2 and Chapter 7. During the final weeks of pregnancy, some mothers will be more physiologically stressed, and thus more prone to medical complications such as gestational diabetes and hypertension. Be especially alert to developing signs of gestational hypertensive disorders such as pitting and/or systemic edema. Remember that edema anywhere other than feet and legs is a warning of possible gestational hypertension. Seek a medical consultation if you notice any symptoms of medical complications (see Chapter 7).

Because preterm labor may include the common third-trimester complaint of low backache, ask those clients if they have had other labor signs like rhythmic pelvic or thigh pressure, abdominal cramping or vaginal discharge. Does the pain have them feeling restless? If so, or if back pain persists, regardless of position or activity, these may be indicators of possible preterm labor (or kidney infection) rather than musculoskeletal problems. Typically, referred pain from organs does not change with movement, whereas musculoskeletal pain will usually increase or diminish depending on the client's movements. With any combination of these indicators of preterm labor, evaluation by her maternity healthcare provider is essential. Your reassuring, sedative contact can counteract the negative effects of this stressful situation and may even help prevent preterm birth (see Chapter 7) (Field et al. 1999).

On the other hand, 3 to 12 percent of pregnancies go beyond their calculated estimated due date. What causes gestation beyond 42 to 44 weeks is obscure, and it can be fine, but fetal and maternal problems may develop when it does (Simkin et al. 2018). Help your clients in this seemingly unending wait be more physically comfortable (Kozhimannil et al. 2013). More frequent relaxation massage can reassure them and promote the deep sense of safety and hormonal balance necessary for labor to begin (see Chapter 5). Our clients often benefit from exploring their physical readiness for labor. Ask for their guidance with appropriate, gentle queries, such as "Where in your body feels resistant or reluctant to giving birth?"

Once a client is **post-term** – "overdue" and past her estimated due date – she may look to you to help start labor. There are conflicting data on the effectiveness of stimulating specific points on the hand, calf and foot (see Chapter 5, "Points of view: Induction and augmentation of labor"); however, for better possibilities with these acupuncture points (see Figures 2.8 and 2.9), teach their locations and how she and her partner can work with them.

There are a few additional considerations: although leg pain and edema may have increased by this point, observing precautions while working there is of critical importance. By this time, many clients tend to be less active; be particularly conservative if your client is on bed rest restrictions (see Chapter 7). Fetal pressure on circulation from the legs is also greater and thus thrombi development risks are highest (see Chapter 2 for more on other factors that increase clot risks) (Devis and Knuttinen 2017).

Deeper pressure into the abdomen still is contraindicated and so take particular care at any diastasis recti or when doing quadratus lumborum work. You may feel the baby's distinctive kicks and squirms; that experience – though delightful – should never be your rationale for performing abdominal massage (see Figure 4.18).

Continue to avoid specific reflexive stimulation of uterus-stimulating points on the feet, hands, upper back and sacrum, unless she is past her due date (see Figures 2.8 and 2.9, and Chapter 7). Though uncommon, if nausea occurs, avoid rocking passive movements.

Positioning

As explained in Chapter 3, during weeks 27 to term, position pregnant clients on the therapy table only in the sidelying or semireclining positions. Because many people labor in the semireclining position, familiarizing clients with this position and with how to achieve maximum relaxation here is useful labor preparation. Also, heartburn and shortness of breath may make semireclining some clients' only comfortable position. When the client is optimally aligned with the entire ceiling-side leg level with the hip when sidelying, and feet level with knees when semireclining (see Chapter 3), positioning on the therapy table may help to mechanically assist edema relief.

From the treatment room

When I became pregnant again after a difficult first pregnancy, I was very anxious. Thankfully, my massage therapist was there for me throughout the entire nine months. She knew how to work me through the usual aches and pains, but, more importantly, she offered her healing touch to control my stress and to help strengthen me to feel and be more resilient. Massage therapy increased my connectedness to my baby and to all the changes I experienced.

– Jasmine, client

Selecting Effective Techniques (Box 4.7)

Use the general goals listed in Box 4.1 as you work with your third-trimester clients. In addition, here are specific third-trimester priorities, followed by specific techniques that will help with those issues. If you are trained in functional assessment, use those tests to make your technique choices more targeted (Zulak 2018).

- Use deep tissue, cross-fiber friction, passive movements and other forms of therapeutic bodywork throughout the torso (see Figures 4.19–4.40).

- Relieve fascial pain from strain to the uterine ligaments (see Figure 1.7):
  o Lateral Pelvis Deep Tissue Sculpting for the broad ligaments (see Figure 4.20)
  o Hip Infinity Mobilization for broad and round ligaments (see Figures 4.44 and 4.45)
  o Lumbosacral Joint Decompression for the sacrouterine ligaments (see Figure 4.22).

Box 4.7
Summary of third-trimester bodywork

Pregnant clients in weeks 27 to 40+ will derive benefit and enjoyment from your focus on the goals listed in Box 4.1. In addition, focus on these third-trimester-specific priorities:

- Reducing strain and pain around pelvic structures, spine, hip joints, structures involved in pectoral girdle and head misalignments
- Encouraging pliability in torso to accommodate significant growth
- Relieving pain patterns originating from uterine ligament strain and from nerve compression
- Assisting in preventing and/or relieving developing varicose veins, cramps, and fluid buildup in the feet and legs
- Increasing flexibility in preparation for labor
- Instructing partners in labor massage
- Instructing parents in infant massage and movement routines

- Offer body-use education for pelvic, ribcage and cervical alignment on and off the therapy table (see Figures 4.32 and 4.15–4.17). Encourage repeated, daily attention to these concepts. More balanced alignment can help with shortness of breath, heartburn, hiatal hernia, pelvic pain and other common discomforts.

- Offer instruction in soothing massage for areas of the torso made sore from the baby's heels always rubbing against the same rib. ⊕

- Maximize torso space with special attention to the distal ribcage, quadratus lumborum and all pelvic structures (see list in second-trimester techniques above).

- Assess clients' breathing patterns, address tension and misalignments that compromise fuller breathing, and help encourage relaxed, deep respiration:

  ○ Breathing Enhancement (see Figure 4.11)

  ○ Pectoral Girdle Deep Tissue Sculpting (see Figures 4.26–4.30)

  ○ Pectoral Girdle Mobilizations (see Figures 4.24 and 4.25)

  ○ Paravertebral Deep Tissue Sculpting (see Figure 4.23)

  ○ Ribcage Deep Tissue Sculpting (see Figure 4.34).

- Offer relief from gastrointestinal complaints by stimulating corresponding zones on the feet (see Figure 4.13).

- Offer relief from normal leg and foot edema by encouraging your clients to regularly return to their best possible vertical alignment, to prop up their legs whenever practical, and to enjoy numerous and frequent pelvic tilts.

Use your positioning on the therapy table to mechanically assist edema relief: entire ceiling-side leg level with hip when sidelying, and feet level with knees when semireclining (see Chapter 3). Specific myofascial techniques to the proximal anterior thigh, lymphatic drainage and gentle, modified Swedish techniques on the legs may be helpful for reducing leg edema. (See Chapter 7 "Points of view: Edema.") Acupressure to the medial arch four times daily and to other specific points also may reduce edema in the feet (Mukherjee 2015).

In addition to lower leg edema, calf cramps are common and normal in the third trimester. Relieve cramps as described in the second trimester. Approximately 25 percent of pregnant people also feel restless leg syndrome when still, causing an intense need to shake and/or rub the affected leg. Because both leg cramps and restless legs are primarily manifestations of physiological imbalances in iron and deficiencies in other minerals, nutrients, salt, water and hormones (Simkin et al. 2018), suggest consultation with a nutritionist or healthcare provider to supplement your modified Swedish massage therapy and stretching.

Symphysis pubis dysfunction is more common now than earlier in the pregnancy. There are several ways to prevent increasing this stabbing pain during your sessions:

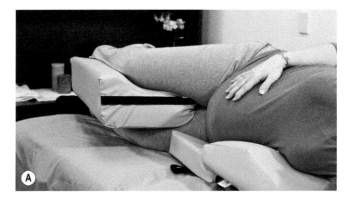

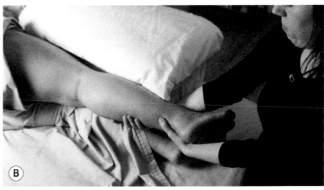

Figure 4.7A–B
Adaptations for symphysis pubis dysfunction. **(A)** Try placing leg bolsters between the legs; **(B)** avoid leg traction, unilateral pressure on the pelvis and large-amplitude movements involving the hip joints.

- Shift the positioning of her table-side leg, placing the bolsters *between* the client's legs, with enough height to level off the ceiling-side leg, as shown in Figure 4.7A.

- Help her to keep the bent knees together as she shifts sides (sometimes a hands and knees rollover is less painful) and minimize position changes on the table.

- Avoid techniques that pull on this joint, such as circumductions or unilateral traction (Figure 4.7B).

- Prevent or reduce this pain by encouraging more upright alignment and try Figures 4.41 and 4.42 for specific symphysis rebalancing.

Many find relief for referred uterine ligament fascial pain, and venous compression from the uterus, by gently cupping their hands under their abdomens just superior to the pubic bone, thus holding the baby's weight. If clients' partners are willing, then teach those couples with no risk factors or complications to do this "baby lift." Other alternatives to accomplish this are supportive undergarments, a prenatal support belt, or fabric wrapped in the styles of many traditional cultures. ⊕

Pelvic nerve entrapments often begin or worsen during the third trimester. When you identify one of the characteristic patterns described above, work to mobilize joints and relax soft tissues to relieve pressure on affected nerves.

If your client experiences hand numbness, pain or weakness, particularly in her thumb and next two fingers, this typically is carpal tunnel syndrome caused by excess fluid. This will need medical diagnosis to confirm, but you can begin to maximize space in the carpal tunnel with gentle, small-amplitude mobilization and traction (see Figure 4.50). Address forearm tension (see Figure 4.49) and restrictions in the retinaculum (see Figure 4.51). Reduce any chronic anterior pectoral rotation that may be restricting fluid flow from the arms and hands (see Figures 4.24, 4.25, 4.28–4.30),

followed by light, rhythmic Swedish or lymphatic drainage strokes, working first proximal then distal areas of the arm. Ice, braces and positioning tips might also be helpful.

For arm and whole-hand symptoms, likely related to thoracic outlet syndrome (Werner 2015), focus on postural realignment activities (see Figures 4.15–4.17) and relief of chronic tension in the neck and pectoral girdle, especially the scalene and pectoralis minor muscles (see Figures 4.26–4.31). Other passive movements to the spine, ribcage and pectoral girdle are also effective (see Figures 4.12, 4.14, 4.24, 4.25 and 4.40). Use the Breathing Enhancement activities (Figure 4.11) to reduce the possible contributions of hyperventilation and upper-chest breathing. Try craniosacral techniques, especially a thoracic inlet release, and strain–counterstrain treatments. Locate and extinguish arm and chest trigger points (see Chapter 6 for more on arm and hand pain).

In addition to providing relief from common pregnancy discomforts, now is the time to focus therapy on labor preparation. The rationale and instruction in such specific techniques are included in Chapter 5. Instructing partners in how touch can enhance the family's ability to support the laboring mom also are included in Chapter 5. You may want to teach simple postpartum massage techniques to her and her family now, too. Plant the seeds for her continued massage therapy by sharing how you can assist her postpartum recovery and enjoyment of mothering.

Also, integrate techniques you already know – after answering the questions in Box 2.4 – to further assist third-trimester needs.

Some clients will appreciate suggestions for self-care that reduce common prenatal discomforts. When these possibilities are outside of your scope of practice, present them as ideas for clients to explore and discuss with their medical care provider. ⊕

You have now arrived at the "fun stuff" – the actual techniques! Perhaps you have even skipped the prior chapters because you are so eager to "just do it"; if so, we urge you to go back. The first three chapters are crucial to making sense of these techniques, to realizing their benefits and maximizing their safety. Be sure you have absorbed the guidance in the previous pages, in order to best integrate the specialized techniques in the pages ahead.

What follows is not a prescribed sequence or protocol. Instead there are five groupings of alphabetized techniques: those with a full-body, integrative effect; those focused on the torso; the legs; then the arms; and finally, those for gastrointestinal complaints. Once you have determined each client's needs, you can choose from these groups. Incorporate a few particularly appropriate techniques into your usual session sequence, as was done in one study (Field et al. 1999); or use primarily these techniques, as the researcher in a more recent study did (Çakır Koçak et al. 2018). The choice is yours.

Note that the online resources contain a few specific sequences, including most of those used in the studies listed above. Using these sequences may offer you a basic session structure until you gain enough experience to confidently design more individualized sessions. Also, the evolution of a full pregnancy's massage therapy treatments is summarized online in the individual session notes of three therapists.

Each of the techniques is described as follows:

- an overlay with the anatomical structures involved
- solid red arrows indicating the vector or direction of your pressure
- dashed red arrows marking the total area to apply the technique
- white arrows showing movement you request of your client
- red dots identifying typical trigger points to locate and extinguish
- an indication of whether to use a professional massage therapy lubricant.

These instructions use the following terms:

- Outside hand = your hand farthest from the table when you are standing beside it. Which hand is "outside" depends on if you are facing the head or the foot end.
- Inside hand = your hand between your torso and the table when you are standing beside it. Which hand is "inside" depends on if you are facing the head or the foot end.
- Ceiling side = the side of your client's body that is highest from the table and usually most available to work with when she is sidelying.
- Table side = the side your client is lying on.

Hints

Tips for ease, variety or effectiveness. These are pointers for your own body use and ways to adapt the technique, including suggested alternatives for creating the same effect.

Precautions

Safety adaptations and guidelines. Certain techniques require specific guidance – in addition to that in Chapter 2 – so that they are not only effective but also safe.

[Name of Technique]

Intentions

The outcome or purpose of the procedure. Understanding this underlying rationale will enable you to be more anatomically precise; to create safe and individualized sessions; and to talk with your clients and alleviate any concerns about your work.

Procedure

Precise written instructions for accomplishing the technique (written with a specified client position in mind), usually accompanied by a photo of a client and a therapist correctly performing the technique. (Note that, for clarity's sake, the client is usually clothed, rather than professionally draped as shown in Chapter 3.) Most figures have some of the following to convey further details:

Full-Body Integration

Each technique in this section can help to reduce stress and promote physical, emotional and mental integration. They also facilitate relaxation; increase kinesthetic awareness; assist the client in being more present with the emotional and physical reality of her pregnancy; and create a conducive environment if she chooses to explore her feelings in more depth.

Autonomic Sedation Sequence 3–1–1

(Adapted from slow-stroke back massage in Jalalodini et al. 2016; Keramati et al. 2019; Longworth 1982.)

Intentions

To induce a sedative, calming state; to lower blood pressure by stimulating the vagus nerve, sacral plexus and spinal parasympathetic nerves; to gather and center the client's awareness around her core.

Procedure

Best performed (and described) in sidelying position; with or without lubricant.

Paravertebral Raking (Figure 4.8)

1. Stand behind the client at about her waist level and facing her head. Rest your inside hand on her side as a stabilizer. Spread the fingers of your outside hand slightly.

2. Beginning at the crown of her head, stroke down each side of the spine with your outside hand, index finger on one side of the spine and middle finger on the other, sinking to the superficial fascial level. Continue paravertebrally down to her sacrum, touching approximately 2 inches (5 cm) on each side of the spine. Stroke gently with your relaxed, flat hand and slightly flexed fingertips to drag through her skin and fascia, creating a reflexive response through the skin dermatomes into the parasympathetic nervous system.

3. Repeat rhythmically at approximately three-second intervals for three minutes.

4. Pay particular attention to the base of the skull and upper cervicals (where the vagus nerve emerges) to increase effects on chest and abdominal organs.

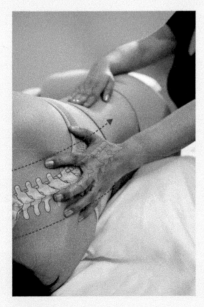

Figure 4.8 Autonomic Sedation Sequence 3–1–1 (Paravertebral Raking).

Sacral Friction (Figure 4.9)

1. Stand just distal of her sacrum and facing her head. Rest your inside hand on her side as a stabilizer.

2. Continue using your outside hand to perform one minute of rhythmic, gentle friction to the sacrum. Use the flat pads of three or four fingers to rub through the skin and fascia, rather than sliding over the skin; systematically cover the entire sacrum.

3. Imagine stimulating the plexus of parasympathetic nerves that affects the pelvic organs and is bundled deep to the sacrum. Take care to avoid pointed sacral pressure that could possibly stimulate uterine contractions.

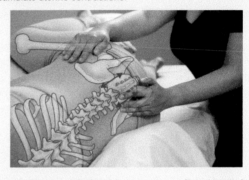

Figure 4.9 Autonomic Sedation Sequence 3–1–1 (Sacral Friction).

Rib Raking (Figure 4.10)

1. Stand behind the client's upper back, facing her feet. Using your outside hand (the opposite hand from the one you used above), spread your fingers into a rake-like formation. Place your hand just distal of her scapula on her lateral ribcage with a finger between each rib.

2. Beginning along the lateral midline, gently stroke lateral to medial, following the ribs and continuing to her spine.

3. Reposition and repeat at a frequency of approximately one-second intervals for one minute.

4. If you are able to comfortably reach beneath the table-side ribs, do the same rib raking there for another minute.

5. Imagine as you stroke her sides that you are collecting and solidifying her around her spinal core.

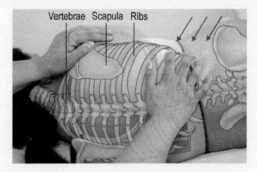

Vertebrae Scapula Ribs

Figure 4.10 Autonomic Sedation Sequence 3–1–1 (Rib Raking).

Hints

- Use a light application of lubricant to facilitate glide on Steps 1 and 3 of this sequence, or all three can be completed over clothing or sheets without oil or lotion.

- This technique is most effective if you perform all three procedures in the sequence described and for the length of time required.

- If you or your clients seem impatient with the repetition and simplicity of this technique, try adding a visualization of a peaceful spot or of brushing away their worries and tensions, or have them practice deep abdominal breathing to further encourage a relaxed state. You might also try shortening each step for a proportionate time, but be sure to include all three steps of the sequence.

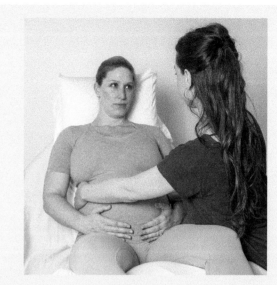

Figure 4.11   Breathing Enhancement.

Breathing Enhancement (Figure 4.11)

Intentions

To facilitate relaxation and increased kinesthetic awareness; to re-educate breathing toward complete diaphragmatic activation and maximum lateral and posterior ribcage excursion; to facilitate retraining those who breathe paradoxically to breathe diaphragmatically; to reduce overuse of upper chest and neck muscles that can contribute to headaches, neck and back pain, and thoracic outlet syndrome; to facilitate maximum maternal and fetal oxygenation; to prepare for the breathing demands of labor.

Procedure

May be performed in any position; without lubricant.

1. Place your hands on your client's lower lateral ribcage. Offer her the following visualization:

   - "Imagine your torso as a folded umbrella with the edge of the umbrella at your lower ribcage."

   - "As you inhale, see the umbrella opening."

   - "As you exhale, imagine it closing against the center pole."

   - "Continue to open and close the umbrella in your imagination as you breathe."

2. This visualization is especially useful to increase lateral and posterior costal breathing.

Hints

- Alternative Visualization

   1. Ask the client to place one hand on her lower abdomen and the other on the center of her chest.

   2. Instruct her to inhale through her nose and exhale through her mouth gently and deeply without strain.

   3. Offer her the following visualization: "See your baby nestled in your uterus, deep within your pelvis. Imagine that your inhaling breath gently touches her or him. As you exhale, imagine your caressing breath gently leaves her or him. Watch these waves of movement as you continue to breathe fully in this way for as long as desired."

- Observe any straining, especially chest over-inflation or activation of the scalenes and other neck muscles. Verbally encourage her to breathe effortlessly, without force.

- Enhance her awareness with your hands on the specific areas toward which you are guiding her breath.

- When a client has difficulty with visualizing, switch instead to kinesthetic cues. For example, with her hands on her abdomen, ask her to lift her hands away from her spine with her inhale and allow them to sink toward her spine with her exhale.

- Encourage frequent, daily breathing practice, particularly for those who breathe paradoxically (meaning their abdomens collapse on inhale and expand on exhale).

- See online resources for more on breathing guidance.

Cervical Transverse Rocking (Figure 4.12)

Intentions

To induce a sedative, calming effect by reducing compression on the parasympathetic nerves traversing here; to reduce strain and promote relaxation in surrounding soft tissue; to reduce headache; to evaluate the quality and quantity of joint motion and points of tenderness as a guide to where to apply deeper work.

Procedure

Best performed in sidelying or semireclining position (described for sidelying position); without lubricant.

1. Stand at the head of the table and facing the client. With your fingers pointing posteriorly, place the middle finger of your hand nearest her face on the transverse process of the highest reachable ceiling-side vertebra (maybe C2). Slide your other hand under her neck with your fingers pointing anteriorly. Use your middle finger on the table-side transverse process of the same vertebra. (Remember that the transverse processes of the cervical vertebrae are roughly in line with the ear, more anterior than many imagine them to be.)
2. Create a slow and fluid transverse rocking motion to C2 by rhythmically alternating pressure that lifts then depresses that vertebra for three to five repetitions.
3. Repeat to mobilize the entire cervical spine, working gradually down to C7 and repeating this focus one vertebra at a time.

Hints

- Visualize creating more space between vertebrae and re-establishing fluid cervical movement.
- Your movement should be small and slow, your rhythm steady; envision the frequency of a relaxed heartbeat.
- Create this movement by flexing and extending your knees, and keeping your hands soft, rather than by flexing and extending your fingers.
- If the client is nauseated, delay these procedures.

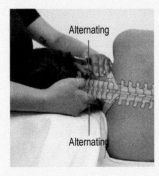
Alternating

Alternating

Figure 4.12 Cervical Transverse Rocking.

Foot Reflexive Zone Therapy (Figure 4.13)

Intentions

To promote normalization of function throughout the body and in specific areas, and to stimulate relaxation.

Procedure

May be performed in any position; with or without lubricant.

1. Use the side of your thumb and/or a finger or a knuckle to create bone-to-bone pressure into the foot. Travel with tiny, overlapping movements, compressing the skin and undifferentiated nerves of the foot against the foot bones.
2. Rhythmically inch along the entire foot. Press rather than rub to achieve the desired effect. Imagine that your finger or thumb moves like a tiny inchworm.
3. Repeat three times in each zone to specifically address areas of client complaint or observed tension.

Precautions

- Maintain a level of pressure that does not exceed slight pain. If the client perceives a high level of pain, move to another area, returning to the painful zone later.
- Prevent calf cramps by keeping the ankle joint in a neutral or dorsiflexed position.
- Avoid calcaneus reflex zones to ovaries and uterus, and avoid overstimulating the endocrine glands (see Chapter 2 for more on location and types of pressure to avoid).
- Avoid acupuncture points Liver 3, Kidney 3 and Urinary Bladder 60, which may stimulate uterine contractions under certain circumstances (see Chapter 2 for more on location and types of pressure to avoid).
- Exercise caution with substance abusers, if the pregnancy is tenuous or if this is the first session of zone therapy.

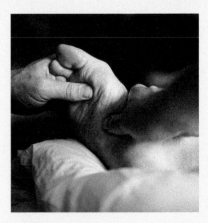

Figure 4.13 Foot Reflexive Zone Therapy.

Occiput Traction and Rocking (Figure 4.14)

Intentions

To induce a sedative, calming effect by reducing compression of the vagus nerve; to reduce strain and promote relaxation in soft tissues of the neck; to reduce headache; to evaluate the quality and quantity of joint motion and points of tenderness as a guide to where to apply deeper work.

Procedure

Best performed in sidelying or semireclining position (described for sidelying position); without lubricant.

1. Stand at the head of the table, facing the client's head.

2. Place the medial (pinky-side) edge of your hand nearest her face on her ceiling-side occipital ridge. Cup your hand so that her ear is not compressed. Use the lateral (pointer-side) edge of your other hand on the table-side occipital ridge. Let the sides of your fingers mold around the ridge of the occiput without digging in with the fingertips.

3. Exert gentle, gradual traction of her occiput away from the cervical vertebrae by leaning away from the table. Add gentle, slow, micro-rocking motions while maintaining a steady traction as you rock. Continue for a minimum of 30 seconds.

Hints

- Your movement should be small and slow, your rhythm steady; envision the frequency of a relaxed heartbeat.

- Aim to re-establish easy joint motion as you visualize the vagus nerve enjoying more space.

- If the client is nauseated, delay this procedure.

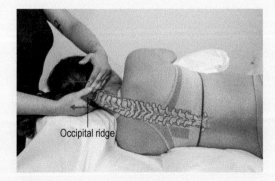

Figure 4.14 Occiput Traction and Rocking.

Structural Balancing Education

Intentions

To promote vertical head, spine and pelvic alignment, which can help reduce many musculoskeletal and physiological discomforts; to encourage more optimal alignment and functionality in everyday activities; to locate areas needing reduction of tension and those needing muscular toning.

Procedure

May be performed with the client clothed and either seated or standing (best performed and described for standing); without lubricant.

Occipital Lift (Figure 4.15)

1. Verbally guide your standing client to imagine the area immediately behind her ears lifting upward as it shifts more posterior.

2. After she imagines that movement three times, place your hand around her occiput. Lightly pull posteriorly and lift toward the ceiling to let your hand guide this movement as she does it.

3. Alternate image: Have her imagine that a string attached to crown of her head pulls skyward, lifting her head with it and allowing the cervical spine, ribcage and pelvis to follow.

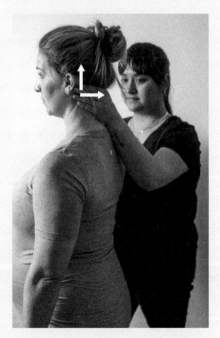

Figure 4.15 Structural Balancing Education (Occipital Lift).

Ribcage Alignment (Figure 4.16)

1. Ask your client to imagine that a string attached from the opposite wall to her sternum is pulling her upper body slightly forward.

2. From behind your standing client, spread your relaxed hands on the lateral, lower sides of her ribcage. After three imaginary movements, ask her to initiate this movement. As she does, use your fingers to direct her lower ribcage slightly more posterior. At the same time, lift her upper ribcage slightly forward with an anterior rotation of your thumbs.

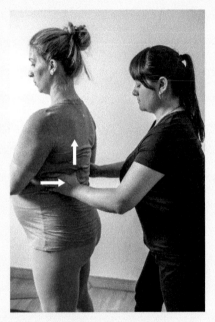

Figure 4.16   Structural Balancing Education (Ribcage).

Pelvic and Lumbar Alignment (Figure 4.17)

1. Verbally guide your standing client to imagine that an attached string lifts her pubic bone skyward. Have her imagine another string attached to her tailbone that is weighted and extends down toward the earth.

2. After three imaginary movements, ask her permission to put one hand on her sacrum and the other just superior of her pubic bone. As she initiates this imagined movement, guide her pelvis: press her sacrum, encouraging her to tuck her pelvis without engaging her buttock muscles, and gently lift her belly skyward.

Hints

- Due to proprioceptive habituation, many clients will feel as though they are falling forward with these realignments. Where possible, use a full-length mirror so that she may verify that she is indeed more vertical.

- Encourage her to realign herself throughout her day and whenever she feels pain, strain or fatigue.

- For other approaches to prenatal postural guidance, consult Bowman 2016; Simkin et al. 2018.

- Note that in Figures 4.15–4.17 the white arrows denote both client and therapist's movements.

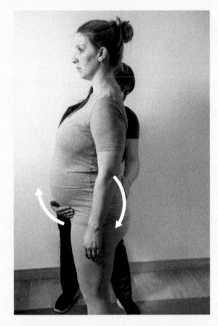

Figure 4.17   Structural Balancing Education (Pelvic and Lumbar).

Other Full-Body Integration Techniques

Choose from your own technique repertoire to promote relaxation and parasympathetic stimulation, integration, grounding and emotional support. That may include the following: gentle, full-body Swedish and Esalen-style massage; facial massage, especially to the temporalis, masseter and frontalis muscles, and other techniques for relieving headaches (tension, sinus or migraine); craniosacral therapy, focusing on still-point, occipital cranial base, transverse diaphragm releases, traction, and leverage release of L5–S1; polarity therapy; and jin shin jyutsu.

Torso Techniques

This grouping of techniques focuses on relieving pain throughout the trunk. They offer relief from prenatal changes to anterior, posterior and lateral structures. More specifically, these techniques treat shoulder and back stiffness and fatigue; ribcage pain; lumbar and pelvic pain, spasms and cramping; buttock pain, including piriformis syndrome, uterine broad ligament referral and/or sciatica; and the stabbing midline pain of symphysis pubis dysfunction.

These techniques may help create more space for the uterus and for other organs in the pelvic, abdominal and thoracic areas. They offer relief from tension, ligament strain, referred trigger points and other myofascial pain (see Chapter 1 for more on prenatal back and pelvic pain and other musculoskeletal complaints). Use these techniques generously in your sessions, particularly in your clients' second and third trimesters.

Precautions

- Observe all precautions in Chapter 2 regarding abdominal massage.

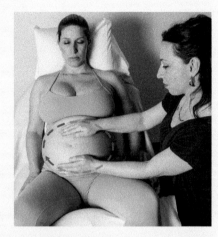

Figure 4.18 Abdominal Effleurage.

Abdominal Massage (Figure 4.18)

Intentions

To facilitate relaxation; to lubricate the abdominal skin, reducing dryness and itchiness; to gently mobilize torso joints; to facilitate connection with the baby; to reduce leg edema.

Procedure

May be performed in any position (described for supine or semi-reclining); with lubricant.

1. Use your flat, relaxed palms to apply oil with superficial effleurage strokes, circling around her abdomen. Complete a circle with one hand as the other makes a half circle.

2. Going no deeper than when spreading oil, make superficial thumb or finger fanning motions, moving medially from her sides toward her umbilicus.

3. To facilitate edema relief in the legs, use your flat fingers in small superficial circles concentrating in the lower abdominal region. Follow circling with long, superficial strokes from just superior of the inguinal ligament and pubis, moving toward the umbilicus. Then use superficial leg strokes as detailed in Figure 2.7A–D.

4. To more directly mobilize the torso joints, contact the lateral ribs with one hand and her ilium on the other side of her body with the other hand. Very slowly and gently alternate pressing and pulling on her sides to create a fluid and subtle undulation of her torso.

Laminar Groove Inching (Figure 4.19)

Intentions

To relax and reduce pain from the spinal ligaments and paravertebral musculature, especially the more intrinsic intertransversus, interspinalis, semispinalis, multifidi and rotators; to locate and extinguish trigger points in these muscles; to mobilize the spinal and rib joints.

Procedure

Best performed in and described for the sidelying position with lubricant.

1. Stand at pelvic level, facing the client's head. Spread oil over her back.

2. Place the middle and index fingers of your outside hand near the ceiling-side lumbosacral junction. Sink deeply into the laminar groove of the spine.

3. Maintaining your depth, rock your weight further toward the spine, and flex and rhythmically extend your distal phalangeal joints (the movement should resemble an inchworm). Slide up the groove parallel to the vertebral spinous processes, sinking into the spinal rotators and vertebral ligaments. Work from the lumbosacral junction to the seventh cervical vertebra.

4. Repeat on the table side of the spine.

Hints

- Extinguish trigger points as you locate them, or after completing the inching.
- Perform this procedure alternatively by using a knuckle or thumb.
- You can create inching variations by directing your pressure more medially or more anteriorly; also, by beginning at C7 and working caudally.

Precautions

- Inch immediately lateral to the spinous processes, but not directly over them.
- Support the client to maintain her securely on her side by using your inside hand and forearm along her torso.

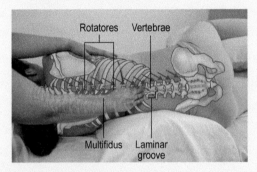

Rotatores   Vertebrae

Multifidus   Laminar groove

Figure 4.19 Laminar Groove Inching.

Lateral Pelvis Deep Tissue Sculpting (Figure 4.20)

(Adapted from Osborne 2002.)

Intentions

To relax chronic tension in the gluteals and femoral rotators; to reduce hip and other pelvic joint pain; to locate and eliminate trigger points; to assist in better pelvic and hip joint alignment; to reduce pain referred from the broad ligaments; to reduce compression of the sciatic nerve.

Procedure

Best performed in and described for the sidelying position; without lubricant.

Gluteus Medius

1. Stand posterior to the client's pelvis, facing her feet. Support the client using your inside hand and forearm along her torso to maintain her securely on her side. Using no lubricant, place the proximal forearm or the fist of your outside arm on the lateral side of her pelvis.

2. Sink gradually into the gluteus medius at its attachment inferior to the iliac crest until reaching tissue resistance. Confirm with your client that she is experiencing pleasure, on the borderline of pain, but not more. Hold for a minimum of 30 seconds, waiting for tissue changes that might move you along the gluteus medius fibers toward the insertion or that take you deeper into the gluteus minimus. Release your pressure as slowly and gradually as you applied it.

3. Continue performing a series of compressions for a minimum of 30 seconds each until reaching the insertion in the iliotibial tract. Limit any movement on the skin to elongation of fibers beneath.

Gluteus Maximus

1. Reposition yourself slightly while continuing to maintain the client securely on her side by using your inside hand at her ilium. Sink gradually into the gluteus maximus until reaching tissue resistance. Begin at its attachment on the sacrum and posterior iliac spine. Confirm with your client that she is experiencing pleasure, on the borderline of pain, but not more.

2. Hold for a minimum of 30 seconds, waiting for tissue changes that might move you along the gluteus maximus fibers toward the insertion or that take you deeper. Release your pressure as slowly and gradually as you applied it. Continue these melting compressions until you reach the superior aspect of the greater trochanter.

3. If there are no spider veins, reposition distal of the greater trochanter, and proceed similarly down the iliotibial tract.

Hip Rotators

1. Reposition yourself again to use the knuckles, forearm or elbow to sink gradually into the channel between the ischial tuberosity and the greater trochanter, until reaching tissue resistance. Confirm with your client that she is experiencing pleasure, on the borderline of pain, but not more. Hold for a minimum of 30 seconds, waiting for tissue changes that might take you deeper into the hip rotators and reduce compression on the sciatic nerve. Release your pressure as slowly and gradually as you applied it.

2. Carefully sculpt the attachments around the greater trochanter.

Trigger Points

(Adapted from Howard et al. 2000.)

1. As you sculpt, be alert to any points that elicit a jump response from the client or refer pain elsewhere. Extinguish these trigger points with a medium pressure on the point until the initial pain diminishes, and the client reports no pain remaining. Continue compressing for an additional 7 to 20 seconds. If possible, stretch the area around the trigger point for 30 to 60 seconds or perform localized strokes.

2. Work similarly with the many typical trigger points (indicated by red dots on Figures 4.20 and 1.5) in these muscles and in the iliotibial tract. They generally refer to the hip joint, thighs, pelvis and sacrum (particularly the sacroiliac joint).

3. Also, palpate the quadratus lumborum and leg muscles for tender points referring to the hip and lateral pelvis.

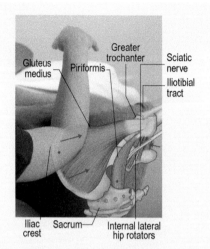

Figure 4.20 Lateral Pelvis Deep Tissue Sculpting.

Precautions

- The sciatic nerve is embedded beneath the gluteus maximus and within the lateral rotators, and it may be sensitive to deep compressions. Change position, direction or depth of pressure if the client experiences an electrical, burning, numbing or painful sensation down the posterior leg when you sink in.

- Avoid creating pain from excessive pressure into the supratrochanteric bursa.

- When extinguishing trigger points, adjust your pressure so that she experiences only a slight painful sensation. Take care to not defensively activate her sympathetic nervous system.

- Do not perform these techniques on areas where there are spider veins. Use mobilizations instead.

Lumbar Lengthening (Figure 4.21)

(Adapted pelvic lift technique from Maupin 2004.)

Intentions

To reduce lumbar pain by realigning the pelvis and spine, and by reducing strain to the sacrouterine ligament; to re-educate client movement; to improve iliopsoas strength through eccentric contraction.

Procedure

Must be performed in supine position with no pillows or bolsters on the table; without lubricant.

1. Ensure that any lubricant previously applied to the client's back has been removed before she lies supine on your table.

2. Stand at pelvic level facing the client's head, on the side of the table that allows your dominant hand to be closest to the table. Direct her to slide each foot toward her buttocks about halfway so that her feet are about 12 inches (30 cm) apart, resting comfortably, with knees bent and, if preferred, resting together.

3. Instruct her to turn her tailbone as though tucking a tail between her legs and lift first her pelvis, then her lumbar spine and, if possible, her thoracic spine from the table into a bridging movement. Then instruct her to do the reverse: slowly drop one vertebra at a time toward the table, so that her pelvis comes down last as her spine lengthens (see white arrows on Figure 4.21). Find phrases – like "Keep your bottom up, but let your waistline come down" – to aid lumbar lengthening.

4. Once the client has learned this movement, have her lift again. Place the palm of your dominant (inside) hand as high as possible on the spine, with your middle finger on one side and index finger on the other side of the spinous processes and raised perpendicular to the table. Let your forearm and back of the hand rest on the table. Place your other hand lightly on her upper chest.

5. Direct her verbally to set her torso back down, as above, starting at your fingers. Hook your fingers deeply into the fascia and draw them inferiorly, as shown with the dotted red line, while she gradually comes back to her resting position (end of Step 2). Encourage elongation through her thoracic, lumbar and sacral areas, both with your words and your hands. You may want to let your other hand lightly follow down the anterior of her torso at the level where your hand beneath is.

6. Repeat two more times.

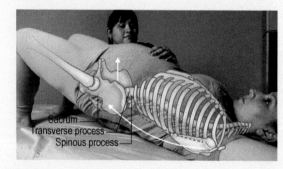

Figure 4.21 Lumbar Lengthening.

Hints

- Slide your hand between her back and the table from her side rather than going between her legs.

- Avoid trapping your hand under her by coordinating your stroke with her movement.

- Try the following verbal instructions: "Begin at the top of your spine to drop your vertebrae one at a time to the table. Very slowly continue while leaving your bottom up. Let your waistline come down, and now finally your bottom."

Precautions

- Do not press into her abdomen.
- Remove torso supports and bolsters from the table prior to performing. To prevent possible supine hypotensive syndrome, do not exceed three to five minutes of unsupported supine positioning as you do this technique.
- Eliminate this procedure for clients at high risk or those with complications, and if she has heartburn or hiatal hernia.

Lumbosacral Joint Decompression (Passive Pelvic Tilt) (Figure 4.22)

Intentions

To reduce lumbosacral joint pain; to reduce sacrouterine ligament referred pain in the sacrum and lower back; to reduce lumbar pain from the intervertebral joints and surrounding myofascial tissues; to facilitate maintaining pelvic/spinal alignment and flexibility.

Procedure

Best performed in and described for the sidelying position; without lubricant.

1. Stand behind the client's lower back, facing her feet. Cover her sacrum with the soft fist or palm of your outside hand. Place your other hand on her anterior superior iliac spine (ASIS).
2. Apply firm, anteriorly directed pressure to the sacrum that also turns her coccyx, as though tucking a tail. Allow your hand on her ASIS to remain relaxed but guiding a slight posterior movement.
3. Hold this tilted position for 30 seconds to one minute, creating stretch in the lumbosacral joint. Add rhythmic, small-amplitude rocking of the pelvis in the same direction while holding the tilt.

Hints

- This passive pelvic tilt can lead naturally into instruction in pelvic alignment (see Figure 4.32).
- If common tender points between the first/second and second/third sacral spines are present, use your whole hand to apply anterior directed pressure to the apex of the sacrum and hold for 90 seconds.
- Teach partners to perform this simple, effective comfort measure so that they may assist in daily relief of low back and hip pain, and for "back labor" (see Chapter 5 for more).

Precautions

- Avoid pointed, bone-to-bone pressure to the points that coincide with the sacral sulci – Urinary Bladder 31–34 (BL-31 to BL-34) – by applying generalized pressure with a broad tool such as the posterior flat of your fingers or the palm of your hand (see Chapter 2 for more on these precautions).
- Allow your hand on the ASIS to assist the primary movement of her pelvis that occurs by your tucking her sacrum and coccyx rather than forcefully pulling the ASIS or flexing your fingers into the pelvic bowl.
- Position your fingers to avoid inappropriate contact at the gluteal cleft.
- This technique requires considerable sustained pressure to be effective. Keep your wrist joint aligned in all planes to avoid straining your wrist.

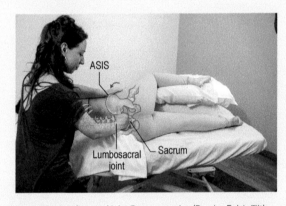

Figure 4.22   Lumbosacral Joint Decompression (Passive Pelvic Tilt).

Paravertebral Deep Tissue Sculpting (Figure 4.23)

(Adapted from Osborne 2002.)

Intentions

To relax chronic tension and reduce pain from shortened posterior myofascial structures, primarily the erector spinae group and lumbodorsal fascia; to eliminate pain from trigger points; to assist in pelvic and spinal realignment, easing strain and pain from the sacroiliac, lumbosacral and intervertebral joints; to facilitate fuller breathing by opening the posterior torso.

Procedure

Best performed in and described for the sidelying position; without lubricant.

1. From the head of the table, support the client using your inside hand and forearm along her torso to maintain her securely on her side.

2. Begin in an identified area of tension or near C7. With your outside fist, knuckles or fingertips, sink gradually into the paravertebral myofascial structures until tissue resistance. Confirm with your client that she is experiencing pleasure, on the borderline of pain, but not more. Hold for a minimum of 30 seconds, waiting for tissue changes that might move you along the paravertebral myofasciae toward their insertion or that take you deeper into the tissue layers. Release your pressure as slowly and gradually as you applied it.

3. Continue performing a series of compressions, for a minimum of 30 seconds each, all the way to the base of the sacrum. Limit any movement on the skin to elongation of fibers beneath. Change your tool (from elbow or fist or knuckles, to fingertips or thumbs) as the muscles narrow above and over the sacrum.

4. Work one side at a time or both sides simultaneously.

5. Extinguish any trigger points located during sculpting, especially in the longissimus thoracis (T8–T10), iliocostalis lumborum (L1), multifidus (S1) and quadratus lumborum (see red dots on Figure 4.23). Modify your pressure on an identified trigger point until the sensation is no more intense than pleasure on the borderline of pain. Request feedback from her about changes in pain intensity. Once her pain dissipates, continue to compress for 7 to 20 seconds.

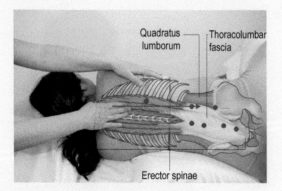

Figure 4.23 Paravertebral Deep Tissue Sculpting.

Quadratus lumborum

Thoracolumbar fascia

Erector spinae

Hints

- Perform all sculpting before applying oil. Do not force an unbroken stroke if the tissue is not elongating; a series of compressions is equally as effective. Remember to hold stationary for a minimum of 30 seconds or until myofascial change occurs. A combination of strokes and compressions is most likely.

- Change your position and tools as needed to avoid excessive leaning over the table or hand discomfort.

- As an alternative to sustained pressure on a trigger point, slowly move the client to a position that eliminates the pain and hold her there for 90 seconds. Gradually return her to her original position. (Adapted from strain–counterstrain technique in Jones 1981.)

Precautions

- Work in either the muscle bellies or along the lateral border of the erector spinae group. Do not sink directly over spinous processes.

- In the lumbar area, be sure to direct pressure more inferiorly than anteriorly to avoid excessive lordosis.

- Remember that low back pain can be a symptom of early labor or miscarriage, especially if unrelieved by a position change. Kidney infections can create lumbar pain, too. Severe, persistent mid-back pain, especially on the right side and shoulder and unaffected by positional changes, also can be referred pain from the liver and/or the kidneys during pre-eclampsia. Evaluate carefully for symptoms of complications and refer to the maternity healthcare provider for diagnosis and guidance.

Pectoral Girdle Mobilizations

Intentions

To create gentle joint mobilizations that reduce strain and promote relaxation of neck and upper pectoral girdle soft tissue; to reduce pressure on the vagus nerve and brachial plexus to induce a sedative, calming state and ease arm pain; to facilitate easier, fuller breathing; to evaluate the quality and quantity of motion as an indicator of tension and a guide to where to apply deeper work.

Procedure

Best performed in the sidelying and semireclining position (described for sidelying); without lubricant.

Stretching (Figure 4.24)

1. Stand at the head of the table. Place your hand that is closest to the client's back on her ceiling-side shoulder, between her neck and the acromioclavicular joint; place your other hand over that joint.

2. Gently press the pectoral girdle toward her feet. Maintain traction to stretch between her upper back and her neck.

3. Add rocking motions to the traction. Your movement should be small and slow, your rhythm steady; envision the frequency of a relaxed heartbeat. Do not release the traction as you rock. Maintain for a minimum of 30 seconds.

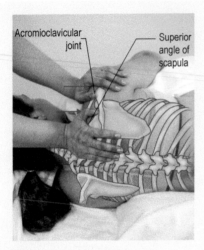

Figure 4.24 Pectoral Girdle Mobilizations (Stretching).

Circling (Figure 4.25)

1. Move to stand behind the client at her upper back and face her head. Slip your table-side arm under her ceiling-side arm so that her forearm is resting across your forearm. Gently bend her elbow to tuck it within your own flexed elbow; encircle her shoulder joint with that hand. Place your outside hand directly over her scapula or just medial to it.

2. Open her pectoral girdle horizontally with rhythmic, gentle lateral rocking of the scapula and humerus, and circular scapular movements. Emphasize quality of movement by using only very small-amplitude mobilizations, performed at the pace of a relaxed heartbeat. Include combinations of all scapulothoracic junction movements: elevation/depression, forward rotation/downward rotation, abduction (protraction)/adduction (retraction). Spend a minute or more slowly exploring each movement combination, stretching tight areas and/or shortening tense muscles to reset tension levels.

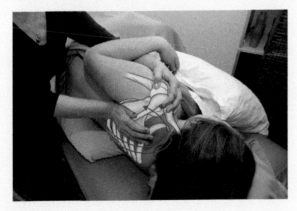

Figure 4.25 Pectoral Girdle Mobilizations (Circling).

Hints

- Once you feel confident with this movement, experiment with these variations. Move your other hand from the acromioclavicular joint to the ceiling-side occiput. Maintain the caudal direction of the hand on the shoulder; then create a counterstretch by leaning away with the other hand, tractioning the occiput. Do not release the traction as you gently rock. Maintain for a minimum of 30 seconds. Change her head angle to create a variety of stretches.

Precautions

- Rock gently to prevent the client tensing to keep herself securely on her side.
- Avoid extremes of range of motion.
- If the client is nauseated, eliminate these procedures.

Pectoral Girdle Deep Tissue Sculpting

(Adapted from Osborne 2002.)

Intentions

To create myofascial change that reduces chronic tension and pain in the pectoral girdle musculature; to reduce pain and improve breathing by assisting in realignment of the head, cervical and thoracic spine, and ribcage; to relieve pressure on the brachial plexus (that can be causing arm and hand pain) and on the vagus nerve; to reduce pain by locating and extinguishing trigger points.

Procedure

May be performed with the client in any position (described for supine or semireclining); without lubricant.

Upper Trapezius (Figure 4.26)

1. Stand at the head of the table. Use one or both fists to work either unilaterally or bilaterally on the shoulders.

2. Sink gradually into the upper trapezius, beginning near the base of the neck until tissue resistance. Confirm with your client that she is experiencing pleasure, on the borderline of pain, but not more.

3. Hold for a minimum of 30 seconds, waiting for tissue changes that might move you along the trapezius myofascia toward its insertion along the scapula or that take you deeper into the tissue layers. Release your pressure as slowly and gradually as you applied it.

4. Continue performing a series of compressions for a minimum of 30 seconds each until you reach the acromioclavicular joint.

5. Extinguish any trigger points discovered.

6. If performed unilaterally, repeat on other side.

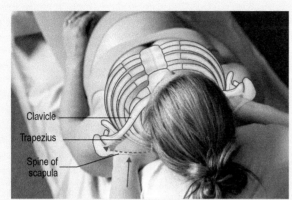

Figure 4.26 Pectoral Girdle Deep Tissue Sculpting (Upper Trapezius).

Levator Scapulae (Figure 4.27)

1. From the side or head of the table, use knuckles or fingertips to sink gradually into the levator scapulae attachment on the superior angle of the scapula until tissue resistance. Confirm with your client that she is experiencing pleasure, on the borderline of pain, but not more.

2. Hold for a minimum of 30 seconds, waiting for tissue changes that might take you deeper into the tissue layers. Release your pressure as slowly and gradually as you applied it.

3. Extinguish any trigger points discovered.

4. If performed unilaterally, repeat on other side.

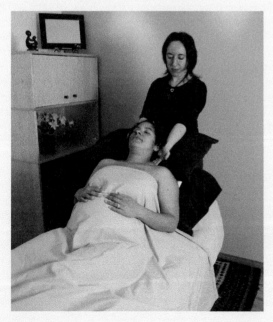

Figure 4.27 Pectoral Girdle Deep Tissue Sculpting (Levator Scapulae).

Scalenes (Figure 4.28)

1. From the side or head of the table, use fingertips to sink gradually toward the scalenes until tissue resistance. Apply unilateral pressure just posterior to the clavicle at a point just lateral to the sternocleidomastoid origins. Maintain a vector of pressure toward the client's feet. Confirm with your client that she is experiencing pleasure, on the borderline of pain, but not more, and no numbness or tingling in her arm.

2. Hold for a minimum of 30 seconds, waiting for tissue changes that might take you deeper into the tissue layers. Release your pressure as slowly and gradually as you applied it.

3. Extinguish any trigger points discovered.

4. Repeat on other side.

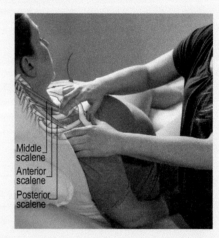

Figure 4.28 Pectoral Girdle Deep Tissue Sculpting (Scalenes).

Pectoralis Major (Figure 4.29)

1. Stand at the side of the table level with the client's abdomen and facing her opposite shoulder.

2. Using the fingertips of your hand closest to her feet, reach across her body to sink gradually into the upper pectoralis major fibers (clavicular section), just superior to breast tissue and just lateral to her sternum, until tissue resistance. Confirm with your client that she is experiencing pleasure, on the borderline of pain, but not more.

3. Hold for a minimum of 30 seconds, waiting for tissue changes that might take you deeper into the tissue layers or might move you along the myofascia toward the humeral insertions. Release your pressure as slowly and gradually as you applied it.

4. Continue performing a series of compressions for a minimum of 30 seconds each until you reach the humeral insertions.

5. Extinguish any trigger points discovered.

6. Move to the opposite side and repeat to work both sides.

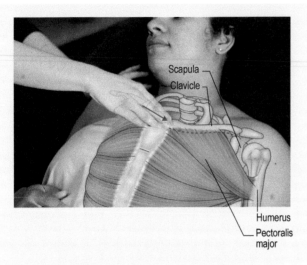

Figure 4.29 Pectoral Girdle Deep Tissue Sculpting (Pectoralis Major).

Pectoralis Minor (Figure 4.30)

1. Stand at the side of the table level with the client's abdomen, facing her head. Slightly abduct the arm closest to you, with her elbow flexed.

2. Use the posterior surface of your inside hand to medially displace her breast so that you may access her axilla without compressing into breast tissue. (Alternately, you may ask her to hold her breast away from her armpit.)

3. Place the fingertips of your outside hand at about the level of the fifth rib; sink gradually into the axillary fascia just deep to the pectoralis major until tissue resistance. Direct the vector of your pressure toward her sternal notch. Confirm with your client that she is experiencing pleasure, on the borderline of pain, but not more, and no numbness or tingling in her arm.

4. Shift your inside hand to the shoulder joint and forward-rotate the scapula to sink deeper. Alternately, downward-rotate the scapula to create stretch of the axillary fascia and pectoralis minor against your fingertips.

5. Hold for a minimum of 30 seconds, waiting for tissue changes that might take you deeper into the tissue layers. Maintaining some of your pressure, slightly release and redirect your vector of pressure to similarly contact attachments on rib four and then on rib three.

6. Extinguish any trigger points discovered.

7. Move to the other side of the table and repeat.

8. Perform similar work to any other tense pectoral girdle muscles.

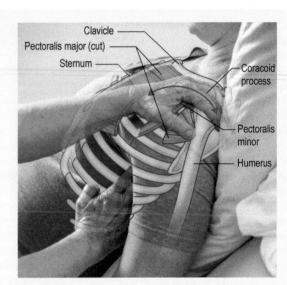

Figure 4.30 Pectoral Girdle Deep Tissue Sculpting (Pectoralis Minor).

Precautions

- Avoid painful and dangerous pressure into the brachial plexus. Redirect the vector if numbness or tingling occurs down the client's arm.

- Avoid pressure into the "careful triangle," bordered by the sternocleidomastoid, clavicle and anterior trapezius.

- Avoid painful pressure on the acromioclavicular joint.

- Use only broad pressure when sculpting the trapezius and be specific to the superior angle of the scapula when sculpting the levator scapulae insertion, to avoid stimulating Gall Bladder 21 point (GB-21, the apex of the shoulder).

- If your client has had surgery or radiation on the breast or axilla, including mastectomy, breast reduction or augmentation, multiple modifications are necessary. Do not perform pectoralis minor sculpting unless you are fully trained in relevant adaptations.

Pectoral Girdle Cross-Fiber Friction (Figure 4.31)

(Adapted from Cyriax and Cyriax 1996.)

Intentions

To reduce chronic tension and pain from adhesions in the pectoral girdle and neck, especially in the levator scapulae, supraspinatus, cervical soft tissues and rhomboids; to encourage realignment of the upper torso and neck; to reduce pain from trigger points in the pectoral girdle and neck.

Procedure

May be performed with the client in any position (described for side-lying); with lubricant.

1. Stand posterior to the client's torso and facing her head.

2. Use the fingertips or thumb of your outside hand to sink to the depth of the desired muscle.

3. Maintain depth of pressure to pin that tissue between your fingers and the underlying bone. Create the cross-fiber friction movement via rotation of your torso, rather than contraction of your fingers or wrist. Continue, without sliding over the skin, for two to five minutes.

4. Focus on the levator scapulae belly and insertion, the supraspinatus near its lateral musculotendinous junction, the insertion of the rhomboids, and the posterior cervical extensors.

5. Extinguish any trigger points discovered during friction.

Hint

- Create variations of friction: change the angle of the relevant joint, or rock the joint, in order to mobilize the affected tissue under your compressing thumb or fingers.

Precautions

- Use only broad pressure on the apex of the shoulder to avoid stimulating Gall Bladder 21.
- Maintain the client's alignment so that she does not roll forward onto her belly.

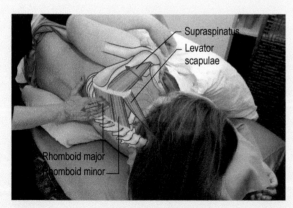

Figure 4.31   Pectoral Girdle Cross-Fiber Friction.

Intentions

To re-educate the client in efficient iliopsoas activation; to encourage proper lumbar and pelvic alignment with the legs; to tone the iliopsoas; to reduce pain around the lumbosacral joint and referred from the sacrouterine ligament; to reduce strain and pain in the lumbar spine and sacrum; to promote femoral circulatory flow by encouraging proper support of the uterus in the pelvic bowl.

Procedure

This is a client-activated exercise that you can teach before or after a session, in sidelying, sitting and/or standing position (described for sidelying).

1. Ask the client to imagine a long animal tail of her choice (a monkey tail is a useful image for many) attached to her tailbone and pulled between her legs, with the end at chest level where she can grasp it.

2. Verbally guide her to imagine pulling her tail up over her head – and to imagine feeling her tailbone curling under as she does so – then releasing it back to the beginning position at chest height. Ask her to imagine this movement two more times, coordinating the imagined movements with her breath: pulling the tail over her head on the exhale, returning to chest height on the inhale.

3. Standing at her lower back, facing toward her feet, place the palm of your outside hand over her sacrum; position your fingers to avoid contact with the gluteal cleft. Place your inside hand over her ilium, with your fingertips resting gently on her lateral abdomen just superior of her inguinal ligament.

4. Pay attention to which muscle groups she is using as you now instruct her to continue imagining pulling her tail and allowing the resulting pelvic movement (direction indicated by the white arrow on Figure 4.32). Encourage her to coordinate the imagery and the pelvic tilting with her breathing, as above.

5. Ask her to continue gently tilting and releasing the pelvis for up to one to two minutes; refine her muscle usage with each repetition.

6. Encourage her to repeat pelvic tilting periodically throughout her day, in lying, standing and seated positions, to help reduce pelvic congestion and lower back strain.

Hints

- Expect some clients to make tiny tilts, even when initially only visualizing the movement.

- The goal is to make this movement by contracting the iliopsoas muscles, with a slight activation of the lower rectus abdominis fibers. You should feel this underneath the fingertips of your inside hand. If you feel her gluteal muscles tightening, she may be using these or other extrinsic muscles (the hamstrings, rectus femoris or upper abdominals). That type of large-amplitude pelvic movement creates a pelvic thrust rather than a pelvic tilt, which is ineffective for bringing awareness to the iliopsoas. Request that she inhibits use of any extrinsic muscles. She may have to make her tilts smaller or limit herself to simply imagining this movement for several practice times before the psoas can activate in isolation.

- Remember that after 22 weeks, clients should not lie supine without adaptations for more than three to five minutes.

- For other approaches to appropriate pelvic alignment and pelvic tilting, consult Rizco 2020; Simkin et al. 2018; Bowman 2016; Noble 2003; Calais-Germain 2003; Franklin 2003.

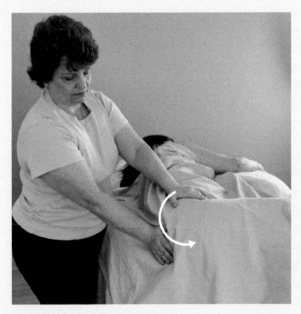

Figure 4.32 Pelvic Alignment Education.

Pelvic Girdle Decompressions (Figure 4.33)

Intentions

To maximize the available pelvic space and the space between the ribcage and ilium for uterine growth and optimal fetal position; to mobilize all the posterior pelvic ligaments, from the iliolumbar and sacroiliac joint ligaments through the long dorsal and sacrotuberous ligaments; to lengthen the oblique abdominals, quadratus lumborum and other lumbar paravertebral structures; to reduce possible pressure on the sciatic nerves as they traverse under the iliolumbar ligaments' fascial hoods.

Procedure

May be performed in supine, semireclining or sidelying (described for sidelying); without lubricant.

1. Stand behind the client, facing toward her ceiling-side knee. Place your hand closest to her head on her iliac crest and the other hand on her ceiling-side buttock between the lateral edge of her sacrum and her greater trochanter.

2. Using the hand on her buttock, distract and hold the ilium from the sacrum by leaning toward her knee and initiating rocking motions (see arrow on Figure 4.33). Maintain the traction on soft tissues for a minimum of 30 seconds. Your movement should be small and slow, your rhythm steady; envision the frequency of a relaxed heartbeat. Continue the rocking and the traction on soft tissues for a minimum of 30 seconds.

3. Stop the movement, release most of your pressure and turn slightly to face toward the foot end of the table. Use the heel of your inside hand just superior to her iliac crest and lean inferiorly, toward the foot of the table, tractioning the ilium away from the ribcage. Focus on mobilizing the most medial of this tissue around the iliolumbar ligament (see arrow on Figure 4.33). Maintain the traction on soft tissues for a minimum of 30 seconds. Your movement should be small and slow, your rhythm steady; envision the frequency of a relaxed heartbeat. After 30 seconds, stop the movement and slowly release your pressure.

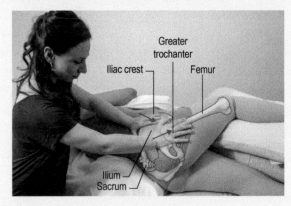

Figure 4.33 Pelvic Girdle Decompressions.

Hints

- Notice the quality and range of motion as you rock. Rigid, resistant areas are places where the soft tissues are most in need of further therapy.
- Once you are comfortable with each vector of decompression, combine them by putting pressure on both hands. This will simultaneously encourage more space between the ribs and the ilium, and between the sacrum and the ilium.
- Slightly adjust the vector and placement of your hand on the buttock to more specifically target other ligaments with similar movements.

Precautions

- In the sidelying position, maintain the client's horizontal alignment so that she does not roll forward onto her belly.
- Do not vigorously rock, and avoid extremes of range of motion.
- If the client is nauseated, eliminate these procedures.

Ribcage Deep Tissue Sculpting (Figure 4.34)

Intentions

To facilitate ribcage expansion to better accommodate the enlarging uterus; to facilitate deep abdominal breathing; to create myofascial change that reduces chronic ribcage tension and pain; to reduce pain from postural imbalances by assisting in ribcage realignment.

Procedure

May be performed in supine, semireclining or sidelying (described for sidelying); without lubricant.

1. Stand behind your client at her waist level, facing her head.
2. Create a drape that displaces the breasts sufficiently to allow modest access to the entire ceiling-side distal border of the ribcage (see Figure 3.8 for draping instructions).
3. With the flat of your fingertips of your inside hand, contact the distal costal cartilage border of the ribcage at xiphoid level on the ceiling side.
4. Lean away from the client to sink gradually into the attaching structures until tissue resistance. Confirm with your client that she is experiencing pleasure, on the borderline of pain, but not more. Remain on the distal costal cartilage, avoiding slipping inferiorly onto the abdomen.
5. Hold for a minimum of 30 seconds, waiting for tissue changes that might take you along the flat anterior surface of the distal costal cartilage. Limit any movement on the skin to elongation of fibers beneath. Release your pressure as slowly and gradually as you applied it.

6. Continue posteriorly, performing a series of compressions for a minimum of 30 seconds each, until reaching the floating eleventh rib.

Hint

- Encourage additional relief by directing the client to more lateral (costal) breathing during these procedures (see Breathing Enhancement, Figure 4.11). Use your outside hand on the lateral ribcage as a tactile cue for her breathing.

Precautions

- Do not curl your fingertips under the ribcage, and avoid any pressure into the abdomen.
- Do not press directly on the xiphoid process or into breast tissue.
- Use a breast drape or ask the client to shift her breast, if necessary.

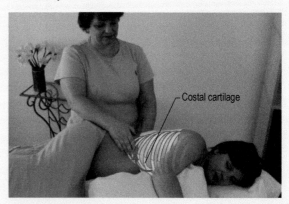

Costal cartilage

Figure 4.34   Ribcage Deep Tissue Sculpting.

Ribcage Trigger Points (Figure 4.35)

Intentions

To reduce pain by locating and extinguishing trigger points, particularly in the rectus abdominis, external obliques and intercostals; to deepen breathing.

Procedure

May be performed in supine, semireclining or sidelying (described for sidelying); with lubricant.

1. Stand behind your client at her waist level, facing her head.
2. Create a drape that displaces the breasts sufficiently to allow modest access to her lower ribs (see Figure 3.8 for draping instructions).
3. Spread a small amount of lubricant on her ceiling-side anterior and lateral ribs.

4. Place a finger or two of the inside hand on the rectus abdominis attachment near the xiphoid process. Create a stationary friction to check for tenderness and/or pain referral. Be alert for any areas eliciting a jump response from your client or any ribcage pain. Trigger points here may refer as far posterior as the mid-back.

5. Change your pressure on the point until the sensation is no more intense than pleasure on the borderline of pain.

6. Request client feedback on changes in pain intensity. Once her pain has dissipated, continue to compress for 7 to 20 seconds.

7. If possible, stretch the trigger area for 30 to 60 seconds, or perform localized fanning-type strokes over the point with your thumbs.

8. Relocate your fingertip lateral of the sternum to friction between the most superior two ribs that you can reach without touching the breasts. Begin creating a forward/back sawing motion that gradually works into the external oblique, serratus anterior and intercostals. As you make repeated passes in these tissues, friction between only two ribs with each pass, exploring between ribs 6 and 10 and from as near the sternum to as near the spine as possible. These trigger points are most prevalent in areas of soft tissue dysfunction and spasm.

9. Treat each trigger point as above for the rectus abdominis attachment.

Precautions

- Do not curl your fingertips under the ribcage.
- Avoid any pressure into the abdomen, directly on the xiphoid process or into breast tissue.
- Ask the client to hold their ceiling-side breast out of the way, if necessary.
- Do not create high levels of pain that would activate the sympathetic nervous system.

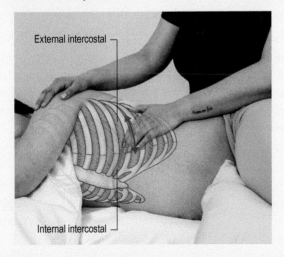

Figure 4.35   Ribcage Trigger Points.

Intentions

To create ligament and myofascial relaxation in and around the sacroiliac joint; to reduce sacroiliac joint immobility, compression and rotation; to assist in pelvic and lumbar repositioning that reduces lumbar strain and pain, and makes more room in the pelvis for the growing baby to be well positioned.

Procedure

Best performed in (and described for) the sidelying position; without lubricant.

This technique contains two different subtle movements of the sacroiliac joint, approximation and traction. When held for at least 30 seconds, each can reduce pain. The approximation will shorten joint structures and surrounding tissues to relax them; the traction distracts the ilium from the sacrum to create more space in the joint. Use either or both, depending on your client's needs.

Approximation (Figure 4.36)

1. Stand in front of the client at the level of her ceiling-side knee, facing her hip. Gently cup that knee and slowly lean into the patella, thus pressing her femur directly into the acetabulum and approximating the hip joint. Subtly lean further, pressing the ilium closer to the sacrum and approximating the sacroiliac joint (but not so far that you twist her lumbar spine).

2. Maintain that closing of the joint and add a rocking movement for a minimum of 30 seconds. Your movement should be small and slow, your rhythm steady; envision the frequency of a relaxed heartbeat.

3. If your other hand can reach the posterior iliac spine, you can confirm movement specificity and stabilize the client.

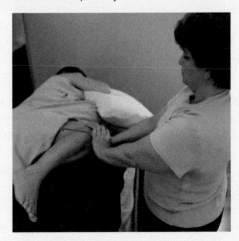

Figure 4.36   Sacroiliac Joint Decompression (Approximation).

Traction (Figure 4.37)

1. Stay in the same body position, standing in front of the client at the level of her ceiling-side knee, facing her hip, but adjust your hand position. Place one hand under her ceiling-side thigh, keeping palm and fingers soft so there is no focused pressure into the medial leg. Place the palm of the other hand over the lateral aspect of that same thigh.

2. Slowly lean away to distract the femur from the acetabulum. Lean slightly further to distract the ilium from the sacrum (sacroiliac joint) (but not so far that you twist her lumbar spine). Maintain your traction and add a rocking movement for a minimum of 30 seconds. Your movement should be small and slow, your rhythm steady; envision the frequency of a relaxed heartbeat.

3. If she prefers approximation or traction, perform only her preference, and show her how to recreate this at home.

Precautions

- Maintain the client's horizontal alignment so that she does not roll onto her belly.

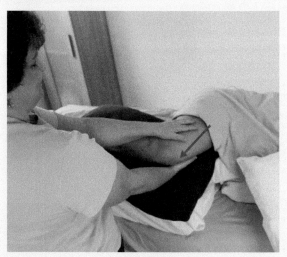

Figure 4.37 Sacroiliac Joint Decompression (Traction).

Sacroiliac Joint Rhythmic Deep Tissue

Intentions

To create ligament and myofascial relaxation in and around the sacroiliac joint; to reduce sacroiliac joint immobility, compression and rotation; to assist in pelvic and lumbar repositioning that reduces lumbar strain and pain, and compression on the sciatic nerve roots, and makes more room in the pelvis for the growing baby.

Procedure

Best performed in (and described for) the sidelying position; without lubricant.

This technique contains two different angles, or vectors, each affecting different ligamental combinations. Use either or both, depending on your client's needs.

Knee Vector (Figure 4.38)

1. Stand behind the client at lumbar level, facing her feet. Use fingertips or thumb of your inside hand. Sink gradually just medial to the ceiling-side posterior iliac spine, into the sacroiliac joint ligaments until reaching tissue resistance. Confirm with your client that she is experiencing pleasure, on the borderline of pain, but not more.

2. Place the palm of your outside hand between the sacrum and the greater trochanter. Initiate gentle traction toward the ceiling-side knee, shifting the ilium away from the sacrum. Then add a subtle rocking. Your movement should be small and slow, your rhythm steady; envision the frequency of a relaxed heartbeat. (This is the same movement shown in Figure 4.33 and described in Step 2 of that technique.)

3. Maintain this blend of pressure, traction and rocking for a minimum of 30 seconds for myofascial change.

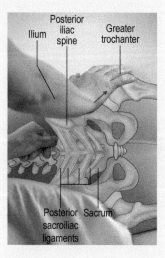

Figure 4.38 Sacroiliac Joint Rhythmic Deep Tissue (Knee Vector).

Foot Vector (Figure 4.39)

1. Stay in the same body position but change hand position. Now place fingertip or thumb of your outside hand between the posterior iliac spine and the lower lumbar transverse processes. Sink gradually into the client's iliolumbar ligament until reaching tissue resistance. Confirm with your client that she is experiencing pleasure, on the borderline of pain, but not more.

2. Place the palm of your inside hand immediately superior of the lateral iliac crest.

3. Initiate gentle traction toward her table-side foot, shifting the ilium longitudinally in relationship to the sacrum, while stretching the iliolumbar ligament. Then add a subtle rocking. Your movement should be small and slow, your rhythm steady; envision the frequency of a relaxed heartbeat. (This is the same movement shown in Figure 4.33 and described in Step 3 of that technique.)

4. Maintain this blend of pressure, traction and rocking for a minimum of 30 seconds for myofascial change.

Hints

- Maintain a steady, melting compression while you rock, going deeper only as the structures soften.

- As needed, create variations to address other combinations of the sacroiliac joint ligaments (especially the sacrospinous and the sacrotuberous ligaments) by relocating the rocking hand or the sculpting hand.

- Try other vector variations to the iliolumbar ligament work when client has sciatica symptoms. This is especially relevant for sciatic nerve compression caused by torsion in the pelvis.

Precautions

- Maintain the client's horizontal alignment so that she does not roll forward onto her belly.

- If she experiences any pain, numbness or tingling down the posterior leg (typical of sciatic nerve compression) or in the trochanteric bursa, reposition or reduce pressure.

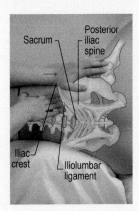

Figure 4.39 Sacroiliac Joint Rhythmic Deep Tissue (Foot Vector).

Spinal Rocking (Figure 4.40)

Intentions

To induce a sedative, calming state; to create gentle joint mobilizations that reduce strain and promote relaxation of the surrounding soft tissue; to evaluate the quality and quantity of joint motion as an indicator of tension and a guide to where to apply deeper work.

Procedure

Best performed in (and described for) the sidelying position; without lubricant.

1. Stand behind the client's head, facing the foot end of the table. Contact her spine with your outside hand. Gently mold either the posterior side of your flattened fingers or your flat palm against the spinous processes of the upper thoracic vertebrae.

2. Shift your weight slowly and gradually into the client's spine. The direction of your pressure should primarily be anterior and secondarily be caudal. Slowly release your pressure but remain in contact with the spinous processes to feel her torso spring back toward your soft hand.

3. After feeling the rebound of the torso back toward you, again slowly press anteriorly, and continue to create a gentle, undulating rocking motion of her spine, ribcage and pelvis. Your movement should be small and slow, your rhythm steady; envision the frequency of a relaxed heartbeat.

4. Rhythmically rock three to five times in that spinal segment, and then move inferiorly to the next segment, maintaining your rhythm and contact, to gently press on the next group of spinous processes.

5. Repeat this subtle undulating mobilization to rock the entire spinal column and pelvis.

6. Repeat several times, and/or reverse directions to rock from the sacrum up to the seventh cervical vertebra.

Hints

- More specific mobilizations of individual vertebrae are possible by using knuckles or fingertips to focus your pressure. Move up or down the spine, vertebra by vertebra, as above.

- Support the client to maintain her securely on her side by using your inside hand and forearm along her torso.

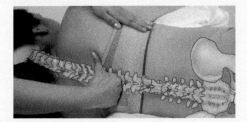

Figure 4.40 Spinal Rocking.

Symphysis Pubis Rebalancing

(Adapted from a muscle energy technique in Chaitow 2013.)

Intentions

To reduce the pain of symphysis pubis dysfunction; to improve motion and/or stability of the joint via resisted action of adductors and abductors.

Procedure

Best performed in supine or semireclining positions (described for semireclining with leg supports removed); without lubricant.

This technique consists of two different client movements. Use either or both, depending on your client's responses.

Abduction (Figure 4.41)

1. Stand at the client's pelvis, facing her head. Direct her to draw each leg up so that the soles of her feet are resting on the table about 12 inches (30 cm) apart. Ask her to rest her knees together.

2. Hold her knees together and ask her to try opening her knees (abduction movement) for five seconds, then relax.

3. If this resisted movement creates pain that does not subside within three to five seconds, discontinue the procedure and do not repeat. If her response is neutral or the procedure relieves pain (often with a clicking sound), then repeat three to five times.

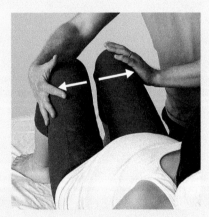

Figure 4.41   Symphysis Pubis Rebalancing (Abduction).

Adduction (Figure 4.42)

1. From the same client position as above, release your hold on her knees. Ask her to part her knees so that one or both of your forearms fits between them.

2. Ask her to try squeezing her knees together (adduction movement) against your forearms for five seconds, then relax.

3. If this resisted movement creates pain that does not subside within three to five seconds, discontinue the procedure and do not repeat. If her response is neutral or the procedure relieves pain (often with a clicking sound), then repeat three to five times.

Hints

- If in supine, in weeks 14 to 22, remove the torso support pillow prior to performing.

- In semireclining, you may need to remove knee and foot supports.

- Typically, one of these movements (and occasionally both) will relieve symphysis pubis pain. Teach the client to perform the effective one at home on her own or with her partner's help.

- Also offer her Structural Balancing Education (see Figures 4.15–4.17) and other procedures from the torso techniques group that may help reduce pressure on this joint by correcting excessive lumbar curvature.

Precautions

- To prevent possible supine hypotensive syndrome, do not exceed three to five minutes of unsupported supine positioning. Use the semireclining position with high-risk patients or those with complications.

- If one or both of these movements create pain that does not subside immediately, discontinue the procedure.

- Remember that anterior pelvic pain can be a symptom of early labor or miscarriage, especially if unrelieved by a position change. Evaluate carefully for other symptoms of complications and refer to the maternity healthcare provider for diagnosis.

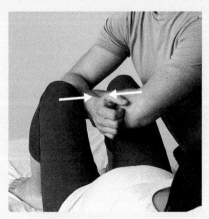

Figure 4.42   Symphysis Pubis Rebalancing (Adduction).

Other Technique Suggestions

For the upper torso, choose additional techniques from your own repertoire that relieve the strain of anterior weight load, alleviate neck and upper torso musculoskeletal pain and dysfunction, and rebalance structure and movement. These may include: craniosacral techniques, especially releases for the thoracic inlet and respiratory diaphragm, inducing still-point, dural tube rocking, and V-spread to painful sites; strain–counterstrain to the anterior and posterior spine, ribs and shoulder joint; stretching; structural integration; Swedish massage of the chest and upper back; trigger point therapy to the pectoralis major and minor, trapezius, rhomboids and rotator cuff.

See the previous section of this Technique Manual for details on neck work, and for zones on the foot for musculoskeletal strain in the pelvis, back, shoulders and ribs.

For the lower torso, choose techniques from your own repertoire that reduce stress on major joints (especially the intervertebral and facet joints, the lumbosacral junction, the sacroiliac joints and the symphysis pubis), relieve muscle tension (especially in the erector spinae, quadratus lumborum, rotators, multifidi, piriformis and gluteals), and that retrain appropriate abdominal strengthening, alignment and movement. These may include: assisted resisted stretches; craniosacral therapy, including traction or leverage release of L5–S1, medial compression of ASIS to release sacroiliac joints, V-spread to painful sites and dural tube rocking; strain–counterstrain technique for quadratus lumborum and anterior pelvic points, especially those on the pubic bone; Swedish massage of the back and posterior pelvic muscles; zones on the foot for musculoskeletal strain in the back, sacroiliac joint, symphysis pubis, coccyx and sacrum (avoiding reproductive organ reflexes); and other rhythmic passive movements.

Leg Techniques

Use this grouping of techniques to reduce leg pain from general muscle tension, varicose veins, restless leg syndrome and edema. They also address specific problematic areas: hip joint achiness, posterior thigh pain (piriformis syndrome or uterine broad ligament referral), medio-anterior upper thigh pain (uterine round ligament referral), numbness and pain on the anterolateral thigh (lateral femoral cutaneous nerve compression), leg weakness/numbness (femoral nerve compression), knee pain, calf cramps, or numbness (tarsal tunnel syndrome) and pain in the feet.

To fully treat these complaints, you will also need many of the torso techniques detailed in the grouping above. Remember that trunk muscles that cross to the extremities, trigger points referring distally, nerve entrapments and ligament referrals from the uterus are all possible sources of leg pain (see Chapter 1 for more on prenatal extremity complaints).

Anterior Hip Deep Tissue Sculpting (Figure 4.43)

(Adapted from Osborne 2002.)

Intentions

To reduce hip joint and surrounding myofascial tissue pain; to relieve tension contributing to excessive anterior pelvic rotation; to free blockages to fluid return from the legs; to reduce pressure on the symphysis pubis, linea alba, nerves and other inguinal structures, and strain to the uterine ligaments, particularly the broad and round ligaments.

Procedure

May be performed semireclining or sidelying (described for semireclining); without lubricant.

1. Stand at the client's pelvis, facing toward her feet, and use the fist or proximal forearm of either arm. Sink gradually into the rectus femoris and sartorius attachments at the ASIS until reaching tissue resistance. Confirm with your client that she is experiencing pleasure, on the borderline of pain, but not more.

2. Hold for a minimum of 30 seconds, waiting for tissue changes that might take you deeper into the tissue layers. Limit any movement on the skin to elongation of fibers beneath.

3. Release your pressure as slowly and gradually as you applied it but maintaining your feel of the ASIS. Reposition your fist or forearm slightly to sculpt the tensor fasciae latae, as you did with rectus femoris, by sinking gradually just lateral to the ASIS and aiming down toward the table.

Precautions

- Always work lateral of the femoral triangle, on the lateral side of the rectus femoris and sartorius. Use a soft fist or the side of your proximal forearm and avoid poking deeply into clot endangerment sites there and on the medial thigh.

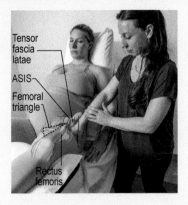

Figure 4.43 Anterior Hip Deep Tissue Sculpting.

Hip Joint Infinity Mobilization 🌐

Intentions

To alleviate compression and to reduce pain and restricted hip joint movement, particularly related to chronic lateral rotation; to alleviate fluid congestion in the leg by relaxing and lengthening myofascial structures directly associated with the inguinal ligament; to help allow for more upright alignment of the torso.

Procedure

May be performed in any position (described for sidelying); without lubricant.

1. Stand in front of the client, at the level of her ceiling-side knee and facing her hip in a horse-riding stance. With relaxed hands, lift the ceiling-side leg and remove any supports that would limit leg and hip movement. Secure the covering sheet around her thigh near the knee.

2. Slide your hand and forearm closest to her head outside the secured sheet and along her medial thigh to support the distal thigh and knee. Use the hand closest to her feet to medially support her calf.

3. As you cradle her leg in your arms, bring it as close as possible to your torso to better support the weight of the leg.

4. Subtly traction the hip, then slowly and meditatively move the leg through small-amplitude combinations of the hip joint's varied motions. Imagine the movements occurring in thick honey so that the pacing is extremely slow.

External Rotation (Figure 4.44)

5. Lift the knee while lowering the supported calf and foot toward the floor in an arcing motion.

6. Create that motion by sidebending and shifting your weight toward the foot end of the table.

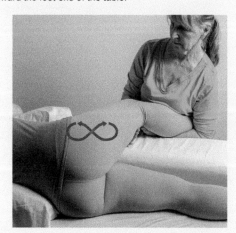

Figure 4.44   Hip Joint Infinity Mobilization (External Rotation).

Internal Rotation (Figure 4.45)

1. Lift the calf and foot while lowering the supported knee toward the floor in an arcing motion.

2. Create that motion by sidebending and shifting your weight toward the head end of the table.

3. Smoothly flow between external and internal rotation of her hip joint while at various degrees of hip flexion.

4. As shown by the red line in Figures 4.44 and 4.45, imagine the knee drawing an infinity sign (a sideways figure 8) as you move her, with the hip joint as the center of the infinity sign.

Hints

- Increase the range of motion as mobility increases.
- Combine these movements with passive and/or active stretching in various positions.
- Integrate positional release (holding in the direction of hip movement that has most ease for a minute or more).

Precautions

- Avoid torque on the client's knee and pointed pressure into her medial leg.
- Do not move her torso with these movements; instead, isolate movement at the hip joint itself.
- Do not perform these movements if the client is experiencing symphysis pubis dysfunction or has other pelvic instability.
- Stay within the normal joint range to avoid overstretching.

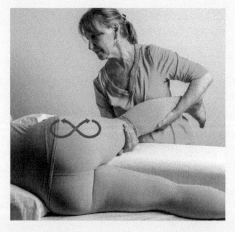

Figure 4.45   Hip Joint Infinity Mobilization (Internal Rotation).

Intentions

To alleviate compression of hip joint structures and reduce pain in surrounding myofascial tissue; to reduce sciatic nerve entrapment; to alleviate fluid congestion in the leg by relaxing and lengthening myofascial structures around the hip.

Procedure

May be performed with the client in any position (described for side-lying); without lubricant.

1. Stand behind the client at the level of the pelvis and facing the ceiling-side knee.
2. Lightly place your hand closest to her head on the ASIS to fix the pelvis and to stabilize her position.
3. Place the palm of your other hand superior to the greater trochanter. Distract the femur from the acetabulum by leaning your weight into your palm and directed toward her knee.
4. Maintain your pressure and add rocking motions to the traction. Your movement should be small and slow, your rhythm steady; envision the frequency of a relaxed heartbeat. Do not release the traction as you rock. Maintain for a minimum of 30 seconds, then release gradually.

Precautions

- Allow the hand on the ASIS to stabilize the pelvis so that you make the movement by gently leaning rather than forcefully pulling the ASIS. Do not flex your fingers into the pelvic bowl.
- Maintain the client's horizontal alignment so that she does not roll forward onto her belly.
- Keep your hand soft to avoid painful pressure on the supratrochanteric bursa.
- If the client is nauseated, delay this procedure.

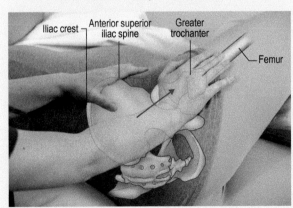

Figure 4.46 Hip Joint Decompression.

Intentions

To alleviate chronic external femoral rotation and resulting myofascial pain, especially in the femoral rotators and flexors, and the iliotibial tract; to reduce lateral femoral cutaneous, femoral and sciatic nerve compressions; to alleviate fluid congestion in the leg by relaxing and lengthening myofascial structures around the hip.

Procedure

Best performed in (and described for) supine or semireclining position; without lubricant.

1. Stand at the level of the client's knee, directly facing it, with your feet shoulder-width apart and weight evenly distributed. Place the fists or heels of both hands just superior of the knee and posterior of the iliotibial tract. Sink towards the midline and lift slightly to internally rotate the femur in the acetabulum.
2. Maintain rotation to stretch the posterior structures of the hip joint. Add rocking motions to the rotation. Your movement should be small and slow, your rhythm steady; envision the frequency of a relaxed heartbeat. Do not release the rotation as you rock. Maintain for a minimum of 30 seconds.
3. Maintaining internal rotation with one hand, move further proximally and posterior of the iliotibial tract to make similar motions at several points before stopping just distal of the hip joint.

Precautions

- Avoid point pressure into the medial side of the thigh.

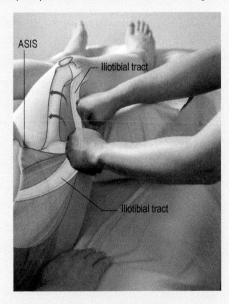

Figure 4.47 Hip Joint Internal Rotation and Rocking.

Wrist Passive Movements (Figure 4.50)

Intentions

To relieve pressure on the median nerve in the carpal tunnel; to relax chronic tension in the hand muscles; to mobilize the wrist and hand joints.

Procedure

May be performed in any position (described for sidelying); with or without lubricant.

1. Stand at the back of the table and extend the client's ceiling-side elbow with palm facing the table. Place both of your thumbs on her posterior wrist and wrap your fingers around to the anterior wrist.

2. Sink into the anterior wrist and gently spread apart the hamate/pisiform and tubercle of the trapezium. This will stretch the flexor retinaculum.

3. Hold this space between the bony borders of the carpal tunnel, then mobilize the carpal and wrist joints with small-amplitude, oscillating motions. Avoid extremes of range of motion.

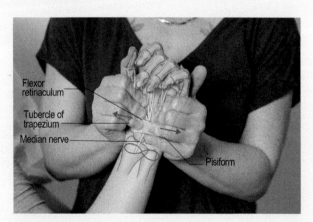

Figure 4.50 Wrist Passive Movements.

Wrist Retinaculum Cross-Fiber Friction (Figure 4.51)

Intentions

To relieve pressure on the median nerve in the carpal tunnel by reducing fibrous adhesions in the flexor retinaculum.

Procedure

May be performed in all appropriate positions (described for sidelying); without lubricant.

1. Stand at the head end of the table at the corner closest to the client's face. Flex the elbow and position the table-side forearm so the posterior side is fully supported by the table and any small wedges necessary.

2. Use your thumbs or several fingertips to compress firmly into a section of the flexor retinaculum. Maintain your pressure; move perpendicular to the ligament with a rapid friction motion.

3. Continue for three to five minutes of friction in that section, without sliding on the skin; then move to the next segment and repeat, until you have frictioned across the entire retinaculum.

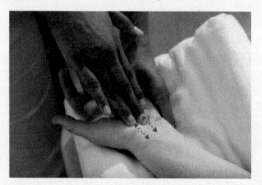

Figure 4.51 Wrist Retinaculum Cross-Fiber Friction.

Gastrointestinal and Urinary Tract Discomforts

Upset stomach, food cravings and constant urinating make for many pregnancy jokes. And then there is morning sickness and heartburn, constipation and hemorrhoids, urinary incontinence, and even the occasional hiatal hernia or uterine prolapse! The jokes are far less funny when you are experiencing any of these discomforts.

Lifestyle adaptations – mostly outside of our usual scope of practice to recommend – make the most impact on these common pregnancy complaints. There are a few techniques that may work reflexively to normalize and balance the involved organs.

Foot Reflexive Zone Therapy

Deep pressure to zones on the feet (see Figure 4.13) may reduce the discomfort of nausea, heartburn, constipation, hemorrhoids, bladder and kidney infection, and other common prenatal complaints (Lett 2000). Teach and encourage her to regularly work these zones:

- Nausea or hiatal hernia: plantar surface proximal to metatarsophalangeal joints.

- Constipation: plantar surface of left foot, moving across the midline of the foot and then toward the heel over the fourth metatarsal.

- Hemorrhoids: plantar surface of the foot, on the most distal edge of the calcaneus and along the Achilles tendon from its attachment on the calcaneus to approximately 2 inches (5 cm) proximal (avoid pinching the sciatic nerve).

- Bladder: in the "puffy" area of the medial arch just distal to the calcaneus.

- Kidneys: midline of the plantar surface of the foot.

Wrist Acupressure

Focused, rhythmic pressure to the Nei Guan (Pericardium 6, or PC-6) point, as shown in Figure 7.3, may help relieve nausea (Belluomini et al. 1994). Locate Pericardium 6 (PC-6) between the flexor carpi radialis and the palmaris longus muscle tendons on the anterior surface of the forearm, two client fingerwidths proximal of the wrist crease. Teach your client how to apply deep, rhythmic thumb or fingertip acupressure to this point on each forearm four times daily for 10 minutes each application. Studies suggest that this can help to reduce the severity and frequency of nausea (Ozgoli and Naz 2018).

Other Comfort Measures

Breathing Enhancement (see Figure 4.11) and other techniques from the Full-Body Integration section above may be helpful too. Choose other techniques from your own repertoire that promote gastrointestinal and urinary tract balance. These may include gentle, full-body Swedish and Esalen-style massage; craniosacral therapy; polarity therapy; and Asian bodywork therapies.

Chapter Summary

As a baby develops from two cells, its unique genetic imperatives unfold in generally predictable stages. The mother also adapts uniquely yet predictably. You now have both general goals and many individual techniques to increase your pregnant client's comfort and lessen her burdens. Use your understanding of what she is likely to be experiencing at each stage, along with any and all details she offers, to weave these clinically matured techniques from a broad range of modalities into your sessions. Always work with specificity, focused intention and respect for safety concerns.

With those guidelines, your sessions will move far beyond just general adaptations of a basic massage. Let each treatment respond to the uniqueness of your client and her baby. Do not forget to review the suggested session outlines available online, and the session design ideas in Chapter 8. Then, like a jazz musician improvising on a lyrical theme, let your intuition and creativity infuse the organic development of each session.

Think it through

To deepen your knowledge, go to our online resources, answer the test questions for this chapter and explore further.

References and Further Reading

ACOG (American College of Obstetricians and Gynecologists) (2015) Physical Activity and Exercise During Pregnancy and the Postpartum Period. Committee Opinion 650. December.

Aldabe D, Ribiero DC, Milosauljevic S et al. (2012) Pregnancy related pelvic girdle pain and its relationship with relaxin levels during pregnancy: a systematic review. Eur Spine J. 9(1):1769–1776.

Alexander DF (2017a) Vagus nerve outflow: essential to the healing process. Massage Magazine. 17(11):16–18.

Alexander DF (2017b) The jugular foramen: the cradle of autonomic stability. Massage Magazine. 17(8):21–24.

Alexander DF, Shea M (2017) Restoring vagal tone: improving your client's quality of life. Massage Magazine. 18(1):22–24.

Becker I, Woolley S, Stringer MD (2010) The adult human pubic symphysis: a systematic review. J Anat. 217(5):475–487.

Belluomini J, Litt RC, Lee KA et al. (1994) Acupressure for nausea and vomiting of pregnancy: a randomized, blinded study. Obstet Gynecol. 84(2):245–248.

Bowman K (2016) Diastasis recti. Seattle: Propriometrics Press.

Çakır Koçak Y, Sevil Ü, Ergenoğlu AM (2018) The Effect of Pregnancy Massage on the General Well-Being and Satisfaction Levels of Pregnant Women: A Randomized Controlled Trial, ISS2018 3rd International Science Symposium, "New Horizons in Science," Pristine, Kosova, September 5–8, pp. 97-102 (abstract submission/oral presentation).

Calais-Germain B (2003) The Female Pelvis: Anatomy and Exercises. Seattle: Eastland Press.

Chaitow L (2013) Muscle Energy Techniques, 4th edn. Philadelphia: Elsevier.

Cyriax J, Cyriax PJ (1996) Cyriax's Illustrated Manual of Orthopaedic Medicine, 2nd edn. Oxford: Butterworth–Heinemann.

Dalton E (2020) How Do Ligaments Cause Sciatica? Available at: https://erikdalton.com/blog/how-do-ligaments-cause-sciatica/ [accessed April 22, 2020].

DeCherney A, Roman A, Nathan L (eds) (2019) Current Diagnosis and Treatment: Obstetrics and Gynecology, 12th edn. New York: McGraw-Hill Education.

DeLoughery TG (2015) Bleeding and thrombosis: women's issues. In Hemostasis and Thrombosis. Cham: Springer International.

Devis P, Knuttinen MG (2017) Deep vein thrombosis in pregnancy: incidence, pathogenesis and endovascular management. Cardiovasc Diagn Ther. 7(Suppl 3):S309–S319.

Field T, Hernandez-Reif M, Hart S et al. (1999) Pregnant women benefit from massage therapy. J Psychos Obstet Gynecol. 20(1):31–38.

Franklin E (2003) Pelvic Power: Mind/Body Exercises for Strength, Flexibility, Posture and Balance. Hightstown, NJ: Elysian Editions, Princeton Book Co.

Gibbs R, Karlan B, Haney A et al. (eds) (2008) Danforth's Obstetrics and Gynecology, 10th edn. Philadelphia: Lippincott, Williams & Wilkins.

Hanlon P (2014) Pregnancy massage: provide relief for clients with varicose veins. Massage Magazine. Available at: https://www.massagemag.com/pregnancy-massage-may-provide-relief-for-varicose-veins-27827 [accessed December 22, 2014].

Hartman RE (ed.) (2013) Natural Childbirth Exercises for the Best Birth Ever. Aurora, CO: Mile High Press.

Hartman RE (2016) Natural Childbirth Exercise Essentials. Englewood, NJ: Parkland Press.

Health Direct (2018) Pelvic girdle pain in pregnancy. Available at: https://www.pregnancybirthbaby.org.au/pelvic-pain-during-pregnancy [accessed July 6, 2020].

Herman H (2004) Pregnancy and Postpartum: Clinical Highlights. San Diego: Prometheus Group. Seminar notes.

Howard F, Perry C, Carter J et al. (2000) Pelvic Pain: Diagnosis and Management. Philadelphia: Lippincott, Williams & Wilkins.

Howland RH (2014) Vagus nerve stimulation. Curr Behav Neurosci Rep. 1(2):64–73.

Jalalodini A, Nourian M, Saatchi K et al. (2016) The effectiveness of slow-stroke back massage on hospitalization anxiety and physiological parameters in school-age children: a randomized clinical trial study. Iran Red Crescent Med J. 18(11):1–10.

Jones L (1981) Strain Counterstrain. Indianapolis: American Academy of Osteopathy.

Keramati M, Sargolzaei I, Moghadasi A et al. (2019) Evaluating the effect of slow-stroke back massage on the anxiety of candidates for cataract surgery. Int J Ther Massage Bodywork. 12:2.

Klein A (2013) Peripheral nerve disease in pregnancy, in Clinical Obstetrics and Gynecology: An Overview. Philadelphia: Lippincott, Williams & Wilkins.

Kozhimannil D, Johnson P, Attanasio LB et al. (2013) Use of nonmedical methods of labor induction and pain management among U.S. women. Birth. 40(4):227–236.

Lett A (2000) Reflex Zone Therapy for Health Professionals. London: Churchill Livingstone.

Longworth JC (1982) Psychophysical effects of slow stroke back massage in normotensive females. ANS Adv Nurs Sci. 4:44–46.

Luchau T (2017) The sympathetic sacrum. Massage and Bodywork Magazine for the Visually Impaired. 32(2):97–99.

Maupin E (2004) A Dynamic Relation to Gravity, vol 2. San Diego: Dawn Eve Press.

Mayo Clinic (2014) Physical Medicine and Rehabilitation: Mayo Clinic Pelvic Floor Dysfunction Program in Minnesota. Available at: https://www.mayoclinic.org/departments-centers/pelvic-floor-dysfunction-program/overview/ovc-20467221 [accessed July 14, 2020].

Mayo Clinic (2019) Pregnancy and Exercise: Baby Let's Move! Available at: http://www.mayoclinic.com/health/pregnancy-and-exercise/pr00096. [accessed June 15, 2019].

Merck Manuals Consumer Version (2019) Available at: https://www.merckmanuals.com/home/women-s-health-issues/normal-pregnancy [accessed April 4, 2020].

Mukherjee B (2015) 10 potent acupressure points to treat swelling, water retention and edema. Modern Reflexology. Available at: https://www.modernreflexology.com/?s=edema [accessed July 14, 2020].

Myers T (2013) The pelvic lift: A Rolf-approved session finisher. Massage and Bodywork. 28(1):91–96.

Myers TW (2014) Anatomy Trains: Myofascial Meridians for Manual and Movement Therapists, 2nd edn. New York: Churchill Livingstone/Elsevier.

Nievenberg C (2015) Live science: Body changes during pregnancy. Available at: https://www.livescience.com/50877-regnancy-body-changes.html [accessed May 19, 2015].

Noble E (2003) Essential Exercises for the Childbearing Year, 5th edn. Harwich: New Life Images.

O'Hair C, Armstrong K, Rutherford H (2018) The potential utility for massage therapy during pregnancy to decrease stress and tobacco use. Int J Ther Massage Bodywork. 11(3):15–19.

Osborne C (2002) Deep Tissue Sculpting, 2nd edn. San Diego: Body Therapy Associates.

Osborne C (2009a) Pre-and Perinatal Massage Therapy: Survey of Massage Therapists. San Diego: Body Therapy Education. Available at: https://bodytherapyeducation.com/recommended-products-services-resources/graduates-survey/ [accessed January 1, 2020].

Osborne C (2009b) Ah, what relief! Deep tissue sculpting for lumbar pain, March 5. Available at: https://bodytherapyeducation.com/ah-relief-deep-tissue-sculpting-lumbar-pain/ [accessed July 14, 2020].

Osborne C (2010) Maternity massage therapy. Massage Magazine, October:58–63. Available at: https://bodytherapyeducation.com/wp-content/uploads/2015/12/MaternityMTspecialization.pdf [accessed July 15, 2020].

Osborne C (2016) The Pregnant Pelvis: An Introduction to Safe, Effective Prenatal Massage Therapy. March 3. Available at: https://bodytherapyeducation.com/the-pregnant-pelvis-an-introduction-to-safe-effective-prenatal-massage-therapy/ [accessed March 3, 2016].

Ozgoli G, Naz MS (2018) Effects of complementary medicine on nausea and vomiting in pregnancy: a systematic review. Int J Prev Med. 9:75.

Patijn J, Mekhail N, Hayek S et al. (2011) Meralgia paresthetica. Pain Practice. 11(3):302–308.

Rattray F, Ludwig L (2000) Clinical Massage Therapy: Understanding, Assessing and Treating over 70 Conditions. Ontario: Talus.

Ricci SS (2017) Essentials of Maternity, Newborn, and Women's Health Nursing, 4th edn. Philadelphia: Wolters Kluwer.

Riczo D (2020) Back and Pelvic Girdle Pain in Pregnancy & Postpartum. Minneapolis: OPTP.

Scheumann D (2007) The Balanced Body: A Guide to Deep Tissue and Neuromuscular Therapy, 3rd edn. Baltimore: Lippincott, Williams & Wilkins.

Simkin P, Klaus P (2011) When Survivors Give Birth, 2nd edn. Seattle: Classic Day.

Simkin P, Whalley J, Keppler A et al. (eds) (2018) Pregnancy, Childbirth and the Newborn: The Complete Guide, 5th edn. New York: Da Capo Press.

Soma-Pillay P, Nelson-Piercy C, Tolppanen H et al. (2016) Physiological changes in pregnancy. Cardiovasc J Africa. 27(2):89–94.

Stager L (2010) Nurturing Massage for Pregnancy. Baltimore: Lippincott, Williams & Wilkins.

Stillerman E (2008) Prenatal Massage: A Textbook of Pregnancy, Labor, and Postpartum Bodywork. Philadelphia: Mosby/Elsevier.

US Dept. HHS (US Department of Health and Human Services) (n.d.) Stages of Pregnancy. Available at: https://www.womenshealth.gov/pregnancy/youre-pregnant-now-what/stages-pregnancy [accessed July 14, 2020].

Werner R (2015) A Massage Therapist's Guide to Pathology, 6th edn. Baltimore: Lippincott, Williams & Wilkins.

Wick M, Limbeck P (eds) (2018) Mayo Clinic Guide to a Healthy Pregnancy. New York: Rosetta.

Yates S (2010) Pregnancy and Childbirth: A Holistic Approach to Massage and Bodywork. Edinburgh: Elsevier.

Zulak D (2018) Clinical Assessment in Massage Therapy. Edinburgh: Handspring.

Studying this chapter will prepare you to:

1. plan therapy sessions for your pregnant clients and/or teach their partners to help them prepare emotionally and physically for labor and birth

2. describe your role as a massage therapist in supporting women in labor and birth

3. identify key ethical, physical and emotional challenges involved in assisting at labors as a massage therapist

4. describe the four stages of physiological labor and birth, and the common accomplishments and challenges of the laboring mother, and how you can support each stage of labor

5. facilitate labor positions and apply massage techniques that support each stage of physiological labor and birth, as well as positively influence women's self-confidence.

Labor Techniques
Supporting a Positive Birth Experience

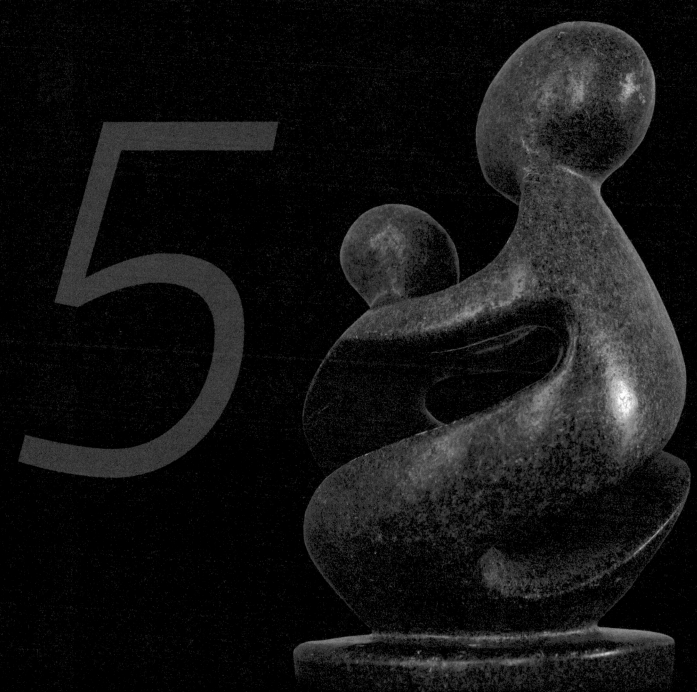

Chapter 5

Chapter Overview

Birthing a baby is perhaps one of life's most profound rites of passage. It can be a transformational journey of self-discovery, challenge and strength. As a knowledgeable, prepared massage therapist, you can accompany your client, offering her and her partner meaningful physical and emotional support during this sacred experience. This chapter explores your potential role in the preparation for and the process of labor and birth. It offers general guidelines for the typical progression through labor and birth's four stages (Box 5.1) and features a manual of labor and birth techniques to creatively meet your clients' needs.

As a massage therapist, you can offer touch and positional comfort measures in hospital, birth center and home birth settings. Your client may have a spontaneous vaginal birth with no medical intervention, or she may plan to choose – or later accept – medical intervention as detailed in this chapter. In all circumstances, you can have a positive impact on each client's experience. Your goal as a massage therapist who is supporting labor and birth is to help each client have a positive birth experience – as she defines it. Birth generates many emotional and ethical issues that uniquely impact you, the client and the client–therapist relationship. This chapter also initiates your exploration of your feelings and the realities of supporting births, so that you will know best how to integrate labor and birth support in your unique practice. As a result, you may decide to focus on preparations in prenatal sessions with clients, to teach mothers and their partners in a small group setting, and/or to commit to attending the labor and birth as a massage therapist. Our extensive experience with labor and birth will offer insights and tips to accomplish each.

This chapter will guide you in applying your massage therapy skills to the many facets of labor and birth. There is far more to know about labor and birth than this chapter can cover; therefore, we invite you to learn more about the many medical and non-medical options for childbirth (see online resources). We suggest you explore childbirth education classes, birth doula workshops and **networking** opportunities in your local community with other maternity, birth and parenting professionals. ⊕

Supporting Physiological Labor and Birth

Skilled, therapeutic touch nurtures **physiological labor and birth** – that is, the understanding that labor, just like pregnancy, is a natural process powered by the innate capacities of mother and baby. Studies suggest that birth is more likely to be both healthy and safe when labor's normal physiological processes are honored. That said, some women and babies may develop complications that need medical care to ensure healthy and safe outcomes (Buckley 2013). Even in the presence of complications, know that your work can still nurture these normal physiological processes. Alongside the client's chosen medical intervention, you can enhance the potential for her and her baby's best outcomes.

Physiological labor and birth have numerous positive short- and long-term health implications for both mother and baby. These include ideal neuroendocrine system function with enhanced release of oxytocin – the hormone of love and healing – and beneficial **catecholamines** – our stress hormones. These hormones facilitate both protective physiological responses and effective labor contraction patterns. Some examples include enhancing endorphin levels, baby's cardiorespiratory transition and body temperature regulation, successful **lactation,** and bonding behaviors between mother and baby. Along with a lack of high-quality relationships between a family and their medical care team, the absence of effective, nurturing labor support is one of the most common rea-

Box 5.1 Four stages of physiologic labor and birth						
Stages	First			Second	Third	Fourth
Phases	Early (latent)	Active	Transition	▪	▪	▪
Cervical dilation	0–6 cm	6–8 cm	8–10 cm	Pushing to birth of baby	Birth of placenta	Golden hour

sons for later dissatisfaction with childbirth. That lack is often associated with post-traumatic stress disorder (PTSD) after childbirth (Simkin et al. 2017). Regardless of when and to what extent you offer labor and birth support, your major contributions can include the following intentions.

Increasing Self-Confidence for Labor

The best predictor of how a person will experience labor sensations and pain is her self-confidence in her ability to cope with pain (Simkin et al. 2017). Your prenatal massage sessions can help prepare your client's body and mind to be confident about meeting labor and birth's opportunities and challenges. Your sessions can help her manage prenatal discomforts, improve her breathing capacity, and increase her inner attunement and body awareness – all building self-assurance for meeting labor and birth on her own terms.

Relaxing with Greater Breathing Awareness

Breathing contracts and relaxes the diaphragm, thereby stimulating the vagal nerve and providing the key to managing state of mind and stress levels. In labor, deeper breathing awareness allows the client to activate the nervous system's calming parasympathetic pathways on command. As early as possible in massage therapy sessions, observe her normal breathing patterns to help improve the quality of each breath. Improved breathing capacity not only benefits the pregnancy; it prepares her to trust her own access to a dominant parasympathetic state for the increased breathing demands of labor. This perpetual internal breathing ally aids your client in every labor and birth setting.

Guide her toward more multidirectional, deeper and diaphragmatic breathing, and suggest that she practices this, particularly in times of stress, tension or pain throughout the pregnancy. Include techniques for any restricted areas, paying particular attention to her ribcage, pectoral girdle and upper back muscles. During labor and birth, you can invite a return to this same familiar, deeper diaphragmatic breathing with a reminder to follow her breathing instincts as labor progresses (Chapter 4). Most laboring people use some kind of breathing as a coping strategy. They may receive a wide variety of information about breathing from childbirth education and the media. As a massage therapist, you are not teaching specific labor breathing patterns, but reminding your client to instinctively breathe for her different needs through each stage of labor.

Improving Movement and Flexibility

Women need ease of movement and flexibility to labor and birth most efficiently and comfortably. Ideally, they have the flexibility to move in and out of, as well as sustain, a variety of active and passive labor and birth positions (Figure 5.1). These include squatting, kneeling, lunging, and being on hands and knees – all of which require the hips, knees and ankles to fully flex and extend, as well as the thighs to fully abduct. For clients with pre-existing pregnancy-related pelvic girdle pain, try upright or forward-leaning positioning with bilateral pelvic symmetry and balance, while avoiding any movements that illicit pain (CPWHC 2014).

To provide your client with more of these options, you can include appropriate deep tissue massage, stretches, assisted–resisted exercise, and other passive movements and techniques for these areas in prenatal sessions. Seek particularly to reduce chronic tension and increase flexibility in the thigh adductors, quadriceps group, hamstring group, lateral and medial hip rotators, iliotibial tract, gastrocnemius–soleus and Achilles tendon, and lumbar spine (see Chapter 4). Tension in any of these muscles' pelvic attachments also limits expansion of the bony borders of the pelvic outlet, so focus on their origins and insertions as labor preparation. Remember and remind your client of the wisdom of pregnancy's hormonal effects, which will have beautifully increased her pelvic joints' flexibility to facilitate her baby's passage.

Freedom to move improves women's satisfaction with the birth experience (Simkin et al. 2017). When a laboring person feels safe and uninhibited, you can trust that she will spontaneously assume ideal positions that support the progress or naturally needed pauses or rest. Even with continuous electronic fetal monitoring, most hospitals offer telemetry options allowing free movement throughout her room and hallway as needed. Some medications

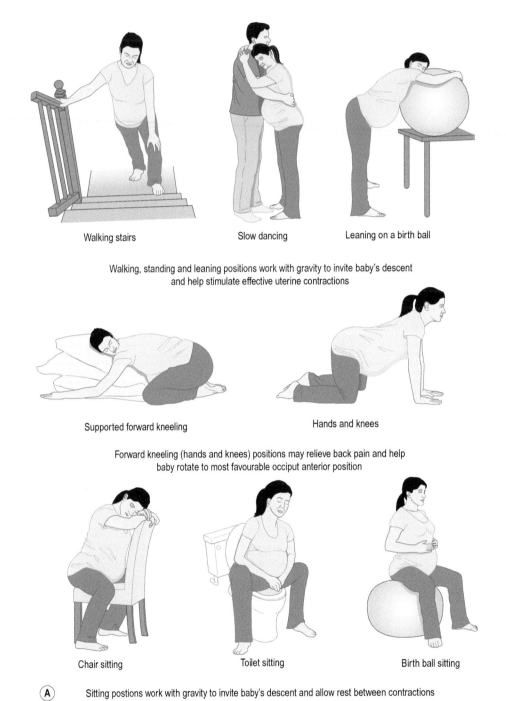

Walking stairs

Slow dancing

Leaning on a birth ball

Walking, standing and leaning positions work with gravity to invite baby's descent
and help stimulate effective uterine contractions

Supported forward kneeling

Hands and knees

Forward kneeling (hands and knees) positions may relieve back pain and help
baby rotate to most favourable occiput anterior position

Chair sitting

Toilet sitting

Birth ball sitting

(A) Sitting postions work with gravity to invite baby's descent and allow rest between contractions

Figure 5.1A–B
Labor and birth positions. Combine your expertise with muscle actions to help your client sustain and move in and out of these positions while recognizing normal joint range of motion that avoids muscle and joint strain. Some clients may find a single position that best suits their ease of movement and flexibility; other clients may prefer a variety of positions.

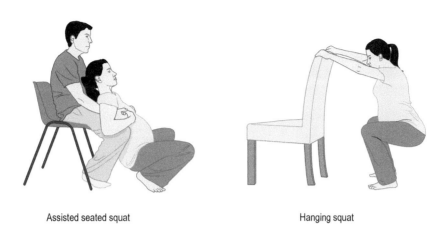

Assisted seated squat   Hanging squat

Squatting positions open the pelvis and use gravity to invite the baby's descent

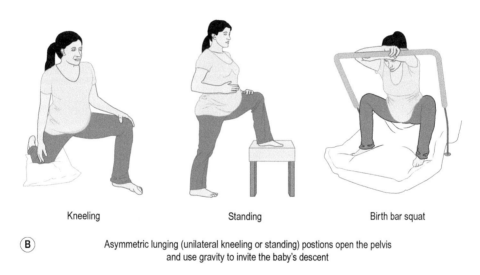

Kneeling   Standing   Birth bar squat

(B)   Asymmetric lunging (unilateral kneeling or standing) postions open the pelvis
and use gravity to invite the baby's descent

Figure 5.1A–B *(Continued)*
Used with permission by Ruth Ancheta, The Labor Progress Handbook, 4th edn. Oxford: Wiley-Blackwell, 2017.

administered via intravenous pump on a rolling IV pole stand can be easily moved with the hospital staff's guidance.

Be mindful of conserving your client's energy and follow her natural impulses to use resting positions. She will need to move in and out of passive, resting positions such as side position and resting forward-leaning or squatting positions. You can be helpful by using and setting up a variety of available supportive props – birth ball, pillows, bean bag, peanut ball, chair, stool, floor mat, bed, tub or household furniture – to assist these positions, movements and rest. If you are teaching expectant couples in their home or a group setting, it is fun and effective to have these props for realistic practice before the birth day.

Teaching Partners

Partners come in all shapes and sizes, and they help the laboring person in any number of ways. Most often, the birth partner is the baby's father, co-parent, husband, wife, life partner or lover. The birth partner may also be the pregnant person's mother, sister or friend (Simkin 2018). The last weeks and months of pregnancy provide a splendid opportunity to enhance partners' connection and relationship with the mother and baby. You can include your client's partner in an individual massage therapy session in the expectant couple's home (Figure 5.2), or offer a small group class to your clients and their partners. Teaching basic massage therapy techniques throughout pregnancy and in the last weeks of pregnancy – paying attention to both the mother's particular touch preferences and the ways that the partner also enjoys – is beneficial and increases their confidence as birth approaches. Again, the self-confidence of your client and her partner is one of the primary predictors for a positive birth experience. ⊕

Partners find it meaningful to have specific supportive touch techniques that they can contribute. One study found that the primary worry of partners was for any severe pain and suffering that their mates might experience (Bainbridge 2000). Another study concluded that the partner's labor massage can positively influence a laboring woman's perception of the quality of her birth experience. Eighty-seven percent of the massaged group in this study reported that partner massage was helpful in providing pain relief and psychological support (Chang et al. 2002).

Teach basic techniques such as long, slow effleurage strokes and petrissage kneading to relax tense muscles between contractions. Demonstrate on both your client and her partner, and then guide them as they practice the techniques and how to give feedback with "I prefer" and "I like when" statements. Avoid more complicated techniques that require advanced anatomical knowledge and depth sensitivity. Encourage the use of different labor positions, problem-solve with them, and invite them to continue practicing their new skills at home, refining their loving touch and enhancing their family's bonding. Specific techniques to teach partners include:

- Abdominal Effleurage (Chapter 5).

- Autonomic Sedation Sequence 3–1–1 (see Figures 4.8–4.10).

- Contraction Distraction (see Figure 5.10).

- Gluteal Double Squeeze or Double Hip Squeeze. ⊕

- Labor Stimulation Points (see Figure 5.12).

- Sacral Counterpressure (see Figure 5.13).

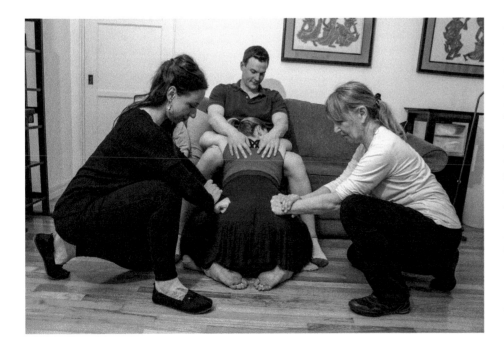

Figure 5.2
Teaching partners basic labor massage techniques.

Preparing the Pelvic Floor

As massage therapists, direct treatment to the pelvic floor is outside our scope of practice; however, you and your clients will benefit from an understanding of the critical role the pelvic floor plays in childbirth. Throughout a woman's life, layers of pelvic floor muscles act as a supportive sling for the pelvic organs and as sphincters at the urethra, vagina and anus. These muscles are essential to our daily rhythms of urination, defecation and sexuality. For birth, it is helpful to have an awareness of engaging their strength, relaxation and flexibility. A well-toned and flexible pelvic floor is more likely to remain intact through vaginal birth (Ricci 2017).

These pelvic floor muscles are perfectly designed to facilitate the baby's passage through the pelvis. During vaginal birth, they play a role in guiding and directing the baby into positioning for birth (Buckley 2013). The baby's head descends toward and passes against the deep and superficial transverse perineal muscles. The vaginal sphincter opens as the baby's head appears on the perineum, the most inferior aspect of the pelvic outlet, at "crowning." These perineal muscles also act as a tear-resistant body, supporting the posterior part of the vaginal wall against prolapse.

Pregnancy can present some challenges and opportunities for pelvic floor awareness and health. Some people do not have well-toned pelvic floor muscles before pregnancy, which can add further strain as the muscles adapt to changing posture, increasing fetal weight and movement. When the pelvic floor is tight, restricted by scar tissue or trigger points, or desensitized, a longer, more painful labor may ensue. Perineal trauma, from a surgical cut called an episiotomy or from a spontaneous perineal tear, occurs in more than 65 percent of vaginal births in the United States. Avoiding perineal trauma also means that a woman's postpartum healing will be quicker, and she is less likely to experience postpartum urinary stress incontinence (Ricci 2017). Fear of perineal damage is one of women's top concerns as they approach labor, and you may be able to help reduce this fear. If she is not learning pelvic floor exercises and perineal self-massage from other sources, you may offer to teach her these important preparations.

Points of view: Perineal massage

Self or partner perineal massage on a daily basis, beginning at 35 weeks of pregnancy, is associated with a decrease in perineal damage during birth. Women or their intimate partners can gently perform perineal massage without irritation or tissue damage, using a quality, water-soluble lubricant such as a food-based oil for 3 to 10 minutes each day. Within a few days or a week, the woman and partner may notice more elasticity in the perineal tissues with a reduction in any burning sensation during perineal massage. As her ability to relax increases, perineal massage pressure can gradually increase within her personal comfort level.

In a retrospective study of 368 women, prenatal perineal massage was found to be associated with reduced perineal trauma at birth, especially for women having first babies. In four controlled trials of digital perineal massage that included 2,497 women, prenatal perineal massage significantly reduced the incidence of perineal damage at birth that required suturing, as well as the incidence of episiotomy in first-time mothers. Mothers having a vaginal birth with their second or later child did not experience these same benefits. The meta-analysis also revealed that perineal massage did not significantly alter the depth of perineal tears when they did occur, or the incidence of assisted deliveries with vacuum or forceps. No significant differences were found in long-term postpartum pain, sexual satisfaction, or urinary and/or fecal incontinence in women who used perineal massage prenatally. In summary, prenatal perineal massage offers benefits to first-time mothers. The benefit from perineal massage may come from increasing the suppleness of the pelvic floor or likely from rehearsing conscious relaxation with crowning of the baby's head on the perineum (Simkin et al. 2017).

Older studies that sought to validate or invalidate the practice of perineal massage had conflicting results due to variables including the effectiveness of teaching techniques, timing and compliance with the practice by the participants (Hastings-Tolsma et al. 2007). Finally, the same term, "perineal massage," is also used to describe other, more aggressive, perineal techniques offered during the **second stage of labor** by medical providers, which have not been found to reduce perineal damage (Simkin et al. 2017).

Reminder

Internal perineal massage is outside of massage therapists' scope of practice. Some jurisdictions also legally limit external work on the pelvic floor and other pelvic structures due to their proximity to the genitals.

Enhancing Self-Awareness and Communication

Improving your client's self-awareness and her ability to communicate her needs and wishes can also contribute to a more positive birth experience. Specifically, her feeling of control through successful communication with those caring for her is more important to her short- and long-term satisfaction with her birth than whether or not she has an easy or a difficult birth (Simkin et al. 2017). You can help her to explore how she can fully express her needs and her desires to her partner, other family and friends, her healthcare team and you. To do so, she first needs self-awareness and communication with herself.

In prenatal sessions, you can ask her a question or request feedback that requires her to pay closer attention to her experience. Ask "Where do you feel the effects of my pressure?" or say "Describe the types of sensation you are experiencing." While gently rocking her spine, ask her to "Share where you feel the reverberations in your body beyond this movement."

These types of interaction can develop her attention to her internal experience and begin training her to express that verbally. You can further validate the benefits of hearing your client's needs and preferences by asking for them in prenatal sessions. For example: "Would you prefer to be sidelying or semireclining for today's session?"; "Silence today, or would you prefer soothing music?"; "What are the top three areas in your body needing attention with massage today?" If she has difficulty with turning her awareness inward and communicating her needs, you can ask for her feedback to potentially include more of this type of work in her prenatal sessions.

Getting Real about Attending Labor and Birth

Before committing to supporting your client's labor and birth, you should carefully reflect on your personal motivations, needs and feelings, as well as on the practicalities of being a reliable professional to a laboring person.

Exploring Motivations

Much of our understanding of the importance of the role of labor support comes both from birth doula research showing the benefits of continuous physical and emotional support, and from the work of professional doula organizations such as DONA International (DONA International 2019). The cornerstones of supporting a laboring person are understanding her birthing experience wishes and being of service in terms of her wishes. Our massage therapy scope of practice intersects physical comfort, pain reduction, autonomic sedation and emotional support with facilitating communication about her wishes. You must respect her choices and not direct her medical care in any way. It is critical to examine your own motivation and intentions before embarking on this commitment. Motivations such as resentment from your own or someone else's birth experiences, any of your beliefs about how birth "should" be, or a conviction that pharmaceutical interventions are "bad," "preferable" and so on are your own feelings, and it is essential to put them aside when supporting a client's birth, her beliefs and her choices.

Labor Techniques: Supporting a Positive Birth Experience

What would you do?

You may aspire to assist birthing clients in response to the increasing rates of birth medical intervention. The very nature of your work may lead you to be a natural birth supporter. What if your client chooses a hospital birth with pharmaceutical pain relief as soon as it is possible, and she is open to any and all medical interventions? Can you objectively and non-judgmentally support her during her birth? Before pursuing this work, take time to explore your feelings about birth and to become clear in your intention. This protects you, your clients and our profession from compromised positions and unethical actions.

Considering Practical Implications

You must consider the practicalities and implications of offering labor support, which mean always being on call throughout your client's 37th to 42nd weeks of pregnancy. Before committing, carefully examine positive and negative impacts on your lifestyle and your practice. What personal and professional support needs to be in place so that you can depart for a birth – at any time of the day or night and for an undetermined length of time? If you attend a birth overnight or for more than one day, what rest and recovery time will you need after the birth? Are the potential impacts of this commitment understood and supported by your family, friends, clients and professional colleagues? After careful consideration, you may decide that you cannot make the commitment to continuous labor support. Instead, perhaps, you will offer your invaluable ongoing prenatal massage preparations and then plan for postnatal massage sessions. Maybe you will organize a group class for expectant couples interested in more hands-on labor support education. You may want to develop a referral list of other local labor massage therapists and birth doulas who can commit to attending births.

Committing to Supporting Labor and Birth

If you decide that you have the requisite flexibility and support to make this sacred commitment, we recommend pulling your support system close when you are on call. We also suggest that, one month before your client's due date, you write a contract with your client that includes important details. Open communication to clarify her wishes for her birth experience, as well as your mutual expectations, is essential to maintaining professional client–therapist relationships during and after the intimate, oxytocin-rich experience of birth. In your contract, you can clarify:

- Who will be at the birth?

- What are her birth preferences or **birth plan** (Box 5.2), including her expectation of your massage therapy support?

- What are her feelings and any prior experiences that help you to understand her joys and fears relating to labor and birth?

- How will she communicate with you at her first signs of labor?

- Where will she labor and birth? At what stage of labor are you agreeing to join her for support, where (including addresses), and for what duration after the birth?

- What post-birth meeting or ritual will you offer her for closure?

- What compensation and payment have you agreed to?

- What is your backup plan if there is an unforeseen circumstance – an illness or emergency – that prevents you from attending the birth? Will you provide a backup or a refund?

- What work is and is not in your scope of practice? Have you clarified that you do not provide medical advice or speak on her behalf to her healthcare providers?

- What other details do you both want to confirm in writing?

By her 37th week of pregnancy, have your birth bag packed and ready in your car, containing two sets of comfortable, professional clothes with pockets, shoes, food, drink, toiletries, mobile phone and charger. Ensure that

Box 5.2
Benefits of a birth plan

A birth plan is a document written prenatally by a woman and her partner to introduce themselves and to present their priorities for and concerns about the upcoming birth. Parents discuss these priorities and concerns with their maternity healthcare provider, childbirth educator and others, with the final birth plan being placed in the medical chart during the last weeks of pregnancy. In labor, the woman and her partner can also present a copy, with the intention that all those involved will review and honor it.

Benefits of a written birth plan include:

- The client and her partner can better prepare to make informed decisions, and their preferences are more likely to be honored when there is a birth plan. This collaborative communication tool promotes satisfaction in the birth experience.

- All involved in the client's care can consult it as a shared decision-making tool. This allows the client and her partner to focus on labor, instead of explaining their preferences and decisions to the many different providers caring for them throughout labor and birth.

- Non-medical care support people, including the massage therapist, can refer to it to clarify her medical intervention choices, instead of speaking for the client to maternity healthcare providers, thereby avoiding the perception of directing her medical care.

Flexibility in the birth plan is essential for flowing easily with changes in her wishes and as circumstance requires. When there is a change in plan, and parents are informed of why the change in plan is deemed necessary and participate in decisions, they are more likely to be satisfied with their care (Simkin et al. 2017). Ideally, your client understands the protocols of her chosen birth setting and makes requests that her healthcare providers can realistically honor within that setting's protocols.

your mobile phone is always on and charged, and have a plan for contacting other clients whose appointments you need to cancel and reschedule. ⊕

After the birth and in the early weeks, honor the client's need to rest; check in periodically by text. Two to four weeks after attending the birth, plan for a short closure meeting or ritual at your client's home and bring a thank-you letter to the baby and family. Give the new mother and her partner time to talk about the birth, validating her and her partner's feelings and feedback about your role as the massage therapist. As you close the visit, again express your gratitude for the opportunity to be of service to them during this special time. If she has postpartum needs that are beyond your agreed contract or outside of your scope of practice, provide necessary referrals. Before you leave, ask to schedule her next postnatal massage appointment with you to resume your massage client–therapist relationship in your professional setting. With this closure ritual, you will find it easier to resume your prior relationship without taking time in her massage sessions to process her birth experience with you. A continued therapeutic relationship is beneficial for your client as you work with her through postpartum and perhaps further into motherhood. The experience of being with her in labor and birth has the potential to bring you more understanding of and insight into her needs in your ongoing massage therapy work.

Ethical Considerations

Labor and birth's emotional landscape can include feelings of vulnerability for your client. Through your presence, behaviors and words, you can validate those feelings and empower her too. In the most vulnerable moments, she may not initially know what she wants or needs, and instead she may ask your advice. If and when you need to talk, do so between contractions, when she can more easily concentrate on your words. Share information and repeat instructions as needed. Remind and invite her to look inside to find and communicate her wishes, rather than offering advice or making decisions for her. Your role also extends to her partner, who may also feel vulnerable at times; remember to facilitate, not take over, their involvement in the birth experience.

When working with expectant clients, particularly around the vulnerability and sensitivity of labor and birth, **transference** dynamics are very common. Transference occurs if a client displaces her thoughts, feelings or behaviors about a significant other onto you. She may then relate to you as though you were someone important from the past, often a parent. Whether the feelings are positive or negative, this dynamic can create other dilemmas that can compromise your care of her. Be aware of this tendency and do your best not to build or intensify the transference. Also remember your own vulnerability to **countertransference**, seeing your client as an important someone from your past or projecting your feelings onto her. You lose objectivity and your connection with her when this occurs, or when you project your own feelings onto her or identify with her (Greene and Goodrich-Dunn 2004).

Before supporting a birth, consider watching a variety of labor and birth videos to become more familiar with what birth can look like. Giving birth can have an inherent sexual and sensual element. As a massage therapist adhering to professional boundaries, this can be unsettling; nevertheless, it is essential to understand that the same brain centers activated during labor and birth are also energized in sexual activity. Respected home-birth midwife and author Ina May Gaskin reminds us, "What gets the baby in, gets the baby out!" During labor and birth, when a woman feels safe and uninhibited expressing herself, her deep, low sounds can be very similar to those of lovemaking. This helps the jaw and throat to relax, encourages deep breaths, and has a reflexive relaxation effect on the diaphragm, cervix and abdominal wall (Gaskin 2019). Her rocking movements and open leg positions may also appear sexual. These are all positive signs of physiological birth and invite effective uterine contractions that support labor's progress.

Develop your comfort in witnessing and encouraging these common labor and birth behaviors. Also explore how to use your body, eye contact and draping expertise in service to her wishes to be touched, fully or partially clothed in her personal clothes or hospital gown, or completely unclothed. Remember that she may need more or different physical contact than your accustomed use of your arms and hands, and she also may be wearing less or no clothing, so consider how you will maintain a professional stance. Examples include making your eye contact with her face and eyes, instead of uncovered parts of her body; using your own clothing barrier and perhaps sheets or pillows between you when you are touching and holding her; and, whenever possible, having her partner, rather than you, offer her a close embrace. In your next postnatal session after the birth, be sure to re-establish your normal professional draping and physical contact boundaries.

Caring for all

Diverse family structures are not new. When we open our eyes, we find a growing number of these families in our communities. Consider how you might support diverse family structures and celebrate what they uniquely bring to pregnancy, birth and parenthood. Women have long created families without partners – either by choice or because the biological father is not involved (DeParle and Tavernise 2012). People who identify as lesbian, gay, bisexual, transgender, queer, intersex and asexual (LGBTQIA) have been quietly having and raising children for generations. There are an estimated 1 million LGBTQIA parents in the United States, raising an estimated 2 million children (Family Equality Council 2012). With inclusive language and workplace practices, we can support all families on their paths to parenthood. Be aware of your biases and blind spots. And if you like, find these diverse families in your community and show up with a loving intention to listen, learn and serve.

Another ethical consideration is that the client–therapist relationship can deepen during and after a shared birth experience, with feelings akin to the closest personal relationships in your respective lives. Be aware of maintaining your professional role and boundaries to avoid becoming intertwined in an unhealthy, dual relationship. One example of blurred personal boundaries is accepting her personal invitations to her baby shower or the baby's future birthday parties alongside family and friends.

Another would be her requesting additional personal time with you beyond that contractually agreed to for her birth support. You may also feel deep gratitude for her inviting you into her birth circle and be tempted to offer her more than you contractually agreed to by bringing meals, additional gifts or offers of additional support time.

Reminder

Within the extraordinary and intimate process of labor and birth, continue to find ways to maintain professional boundaries with your clients.

Witnessing a woman giving birth can be a powerful experience for you too. Another ethical consideration is that you may need a confidential, professional place to reflect on what happened and your role in the birth experience. This is especially true if it was challenging for you, a difficult birth for the family, a traumatic birth or one with an unexpected outcome (see Chapter 7). Be prepared to discuss the birth with a trusted professional colleague in a private, confidential setting to honor any processing that you may need. Be mindful to not process your feelings and experiences with the family. The only exceptions to this would be expressing your gratitude and validating her and her partner's feelings about the birth.

From the treatment room

It's a personal and professional juggling act to balance being on call to attend births as a birth doula and massage therapist. To begin, I got my support team in place. I asked my family if they would be willing to be my "doula support angels" with the understanding that I would sometimes be on the phone with a client in early labor or be at a birth during family meals or my son's basketball games or in the middle of the night. After a birth, my family fed me a protein-rich meal before tucking me in to sleep for the rest of the day ... or next day. My other "doula support angels" were my amazing birth doula group, who provided backup doula support. I didn't miss any family birthdays and holidays, except for one Mother's Day when I attended a repeat client's glorious vaginal birth after Cesarean (VBAC)! I planned out-of-town vacations and commitments months in advance to avoid my clients' due date windows. My wonderful massage therapy clients also had to flex with me when I was called to a birth or still sleeping afterwards. They were gracious, kind, understanding. We managed disappointments as best we could with rescheduling their appointments. I thank my clients and "doula support angels" for the many blessings of attending approximately 200 births and also for supporting me in the challenging edges of balancing it all.

– **Michele Kolakowski,** therapist

Attending Labors and Births

Most women want and need supportive people around them during labor and birth. Their labor progress depends on emotional, interpersonal, physical and physiological factors, all of which we can positively influence as an attending massage therapist. Progress is facilitated when your client feels safe, respected and cared for; when she can remain active, mobile and upright; and when her pain is adequately and safely managed. Her sense of well-being is enhanced by a caring, attentive partner or loved ones, as well as competent, confident and compassionate maternity healthcare providers and a calm, comfortable and well-equipped birth setting (Simkin et al. 2017).

Like any labor assistant, a massage therapist provides consistent, responsive physical and emotional care throughout her client's labor. Your refined skill in touch therapies and in pain and stress reduction, and as a practiced listener to the nuances of the body and mind, is extremely valuable and somewhat unique on most birthing teams. As such, your most direct intentions include the following:

- supporting the normal progression of labor and birth
- helping to conserve and regenerate physical and emotional energy

- facilitating breathing and comfort with massage therapy, stretching and visualizations

- assisting in relief of muscle cramping, exhaustion and pain, especially in the back, abdomen, pelvis, legs and arms

- enhancing the partners' relationship, allowing space for and encouragement of the partner's involvement and care.

A summary of 15 Cochrane reviews and three non-Cochrane reviews of pharmacologic and non-pharmacologic methods of labor pain relief found benefits with relaxation, massage, acupressure, and immersion in water (hydrotherapy): these four improve mother's satisfaction with pain relief and the birth experience, have possible efficacy in managing labor pain, are non-invasive and appear to be safe (Simkin et al. 2017). A recent study specific to lower back massage in labor found that it has a significant effect on both reducing labor pain and increasing birth satisfaction. Positive feedback from women about massage and their requests for massage in labor corroborate the value of our work – not only for easing pain, but also for cultivating feelings of greater self-confidence and developing positive interactions with those attending the birth (Erdogan et al. 2017). Massage therapy and other natural coping strategies – movement, position changes, relaxation, breathing and emotional support – offer non-pharmacologic pain relief that is effective with few negative side effects (Ricci 2017). All of these methods of pain relief are well within a massage therapist's scope of practice.

Reminder

Remember that your scope of practice is nurturing the mother through labor and birth. As a massage therapist, you do not offer any medical advice, assess and determine labor progress, or make decisions for your client. You also support the active role of partners or family members unless you are asked to step in as a substitute.

Collaborating with Physicians, Midwives and Nurses

The majority of American women birth in a hospital or medical center under the care of a physician or a certified nurse midwife (Box 5.3). This reality affords you a wonderful opportunity to represent our profession in a medical setting. In hospitals, nurses provide most of the bedside care during labor and birth. They have a primary responsibility to support, monitor and record a patient's labor progress and the well-being of her and her baby. The nurse maintains close communication with the physician or midwife, who initially visit periodically and then more consistently when their patient enters labor's second stage. Your massage therapist role and the nurse's role can blend well together, especially when you respect their knowledge and actively support their medical monitoring and charting responsibilities. When you are both present with the mother, the two of you bring expertise. Remember to communicate and

---

Box 5.3
Best-performing maternity care hospitals

As healthcare consumers during pregnancy, many expectant families research their options and choose which hospital they will birth at. Their choice may be influenced by several factors: the hospital where their preferred maternity care providers have medical privileges; convenience and proximity to home and/or work; and the quality of the hospital's maternity care. Expectant families can review the annual maternity care statistics of hospitals at Leapfrog Hospital Survey (www.leapfroggroup.org/compare-hospitals). Leapfrog is currently the only publicly available source for this data. Most, but not all hospitals, are willing to make their data public. The Leapfrog Hospital Survey includes measures that are endorsed by the National Quality Forum and aligned with other healthcare data collection entities, including the Centers for Medicare and Medicaid Services and the Joint Commission for Accreditation of Healthcare Organizations.

collaborate positively in service to the family. In fact, by you taking the primary role of calming and supporting their patients, you support nurses in their other essential responsibilities and can perhaps bring more ease and joy to their demanding jobs. Don't forget to leave any judgments and agenda about medical personnel and procedures outside your client's birthing room or space. Work with the partner, nurse, midwife and physician to rotate your continuous support and breaks, so that everyone is nourished and rested. Keep their rotating shift changes in mind, and welcome the new, incoming medical staff with your positive, collaborative spirit.

Attending a birth at home or at a free-standing birth center is an opportunity for the labor massage therapist to fully bear witness to the power of physiological labor and birth while working alongside certified nurse midwives, direct entry midwives and nurses. Again, be prepared for them to welcome your presence and your work as a non-pharmacologic form of support.

In all these settings, once the second stage of labor is underway and pushing begins, the physician, midwife and nurses will remain with the patient or stay nearby to support her active pushing efforts. As they assist delivery of the baby and the placenta, your hands-on skills again can complement their medical expertise as you focus on the mother's comfort and energy.

There can be uncertain moments for the mother, her partner and perhaps even you, when medical professionals are present and medical intervention is being considered. A common time that this may occur is when a woman wants to know her labor progress and asks her medical professional to check for cervical **effacement** and **dilation** – a snapshot of the current labor picture. Hearing lower numbers than expected can be disappointing and discouraging. It can be helpful to remember that these numbers are not a crystal ball nor a reliable indicator of labor's future timeline. Stay true to your role by validating her feelings. Encourage your client to trust that her labor and birth are unique for her and her baby. Offer a different comfort measure and position, but often the best intervention is patience and time. If a medical intervention is necessary or chosen, strong emotions can sometimes arise for the mother and her partner. Validate

her instincts and choices without any sign of disappointment or judgment of her or her maternity healthcare provider. By adapting and thinking quickly on your feet in these emotional moments, you can continue to calmly and confidently support your client.

Some massage therapists who offer labor and birth support want to learn more, improve their collaboration with medical professionals and take on the birth doula's advocacy role in discussing medical interventions and other available options. As a massage therapist, you already have a thorough understanding and experience of how the body and mind respond to touch; however, you may want to pursue birth doula training as part of your continuing education. This also can broaden your other non-touch support skills, expand your understanding about physiological labor and birth, and familiarize you with interventions, as well as the art of birth doula advocacy. 🌐

Understanding Hormonal Influences

Next, we will present an overview of the complex cocktail of hormones that intimately impact your interactions and techniques used during labor and birth.

Shifting from Gestation to Birth

During pregnancy while the baby is growing, high levels of progesterone prevent uterine contractions; therefore, labor's first hormonal step is to decrease progesterone. This process is initiated by the baby as the uterus stretches during the last few days and weeks of gestation, bringing corticotropin-releasing hormone and cortisol. In turn, this triggers a rise in the steroid hormone estriol, a form of estrogen that is predominant during birth. As estriol rises, it inhibits progesterone synthesis by the placenta and prepares the smooth muscles of the uterus for labor. Estriol and other estrogens increase the sensitivity of the uterus's smooth muscles to the forthcoming hormones that will stimulate uterine contractions. As estrogen begins to stimulate uterine contractions, the uterus also produces **prostaglandins**. These further contribute to a decrease in progesterone levels. Relaxin relaxes the cervix, as well as pelvic ligaments, for added flexibility in labor and birth as the baby passes through the pelvis.

Oxytocin, endorphins and catecholamines are other important labor hormones with a specific function that either facilitates or inhibits the effects of the others. It is their hormonal balance that determines the overall effect on labor progress. Nowhere is this more apparent than in the coordination of the uterine muscle layers' action. The uterus is composed of beautiful, interconnected layers of smooth muscle, each in a different orientation for coordinated uterine contractions. The vertical layer is responsible for effacement and dilation, which it brings about by pulling on the lower uterine segment, thereby thinning and opening the cervix and facilitating labor's progress. When the horizontal and circular uterine fibers contract, this further facilitates effective labor progress and the baby's descent. Uterine muscle actions are governed hormonally by oxytocin – the hormone of love, calm, connection and closeness. The number of oxytocin uterine receptors multiply at the end of pregnancy, and oxytocin levels gradually increase throughout labor, peaking around the time of birth (Buckley 2015).

Oxytocin also reduces both pain perception and memory of aversive experiences (Simkin et al. 2017). Oxytocin is not only a hormone; it is also a signaling substance in the brain that, when released during birth, skin-to-skin contact and breastfeeding, induces key physiological and psychological adaptations in both mother and baby. Oxytocin stimulates their ability for social interaction, decreases anxiety and stress, and stimulates functions related to growth, restoration and health (Uvnäs-Moberg 2014).

Endorphins are the body's naturally occurring opiates, secreted from the pituitary gland in the presence of pain. They help to reduce stressful feelings and to induce feelings of pleasure. During labor, endorphins create an altered, dreamy, trance-like state where the woman turns inward, following instinctual behaviors (Simkin et al. 2017). These powerful endorphins in labor are responsible for the "other consciousness" or right-brain orientation that is characteristic of laboring women who are well supported and undisturbed in their labor. Massage therapy may increase the production of endorphins, as well (Ricci 2017).

Stress Hormones

Catecholamines, the stress hormones – including **epinephrine** and **norepinephrine**, cortisol and others – counteract the effects of oxytocin and endorphins during

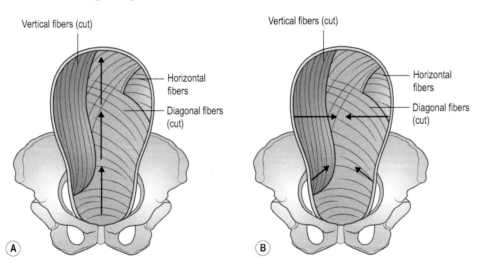

Vertical fibers (cut)
Horizontal fibers
Diagonal fibers (cut)

Vertical fibers (cut)
Horizontal fibers
Diagonal fibers (cut)

(A)   (B)

Figure 5.3A–B
Effects of stress hormones on progress in the first stage of labor. **(A)** When a woman relaxes and feels safe, vertical uterine fibers produce effective cervical dilation and effacement; **(B)** under stress, both horizontal and vertical fibers contract, creating a less productive, more painful first stage.

labor. They prompt a sympathetic nervous system fight, flight or freeze response to the fear and distress caused by a real or perceived threat, and to severe pain and exhaustion. When a laboring person is in this fight- or flight-dominant state, the counteracting effects of catecholamines have a protective wisdom in that they slow down or stop uterine contractions until the real or perceived threat hopefully passes. Under stress, synchronized uterine muscle contractions are interrupted but the layer of horizontal, circular uterine fibers continues to contract. As a result, labor's progress, measured by cervical change, can stall or stop (Figure 5.3).

Also under stress, contractions then become more painful and can reduce blood flow to the uterus by as much as 65 percent (Buckley 2015). Fear or anxiety may cause the laboring person to perceive labor events or caregivers' words as threatening or dangerous, and she may remain vigilant or hyperalert. Fear and anxiety may also interfere with her ability to absorb and retain information that is being provided to her. High levels of catecholamines also suppress the usual endorphin effects that would otherwise alter her state of consciousness, and help her enter an instinctual, trance-like state. Note that, even in this "labor land" zone, a woman is aware that she is allowing herself to be in this state. She is also fully capable of becoming alert and making decisions when needed (Simkin et al. 2017). A laboring woman is more open to mental suggestion in this state and will respond positively to appropriate encouragement, images and visualizations. Creative, active imagery, positive statements (affirmations), prayer and your touch are usually dynamically effective during labor (Ricci 2017).

Understanding Sensation and Pain for Labor and Birth

Pain is a perception influenced by many factors, and fear and stress tend to further increase physical pain. Women are often culturally conditioned through the media and stories to expect and fear birth as painful, so it tends to be. Without exposure to a wider variety of potential birthing experiences, some women never consider the possibility that labor and birth could be an ecstatic, sensation filled, peak experience. To help her prepare mentally, invite her to explore her beliefs about pain in labor and birth.

Invite her to consider these new sensations as valuable, intelligent information that will guide her in labor and birth (Figure 5.4). Studies suggest a critical relationship between maternal confidence and the perception of pain during labor. More than half of the variance in early labor pain and approximately one-third of the variance in active labor pain is explained by one variable – the woman's confidence in her ability to cope with pain (Fulton 2015).

Pain and Suffering

Exploring the distinction between pain and suffering is also critical to our understanding of our laboring client's well-being. Labor pain is an intensely unpleasant bodily

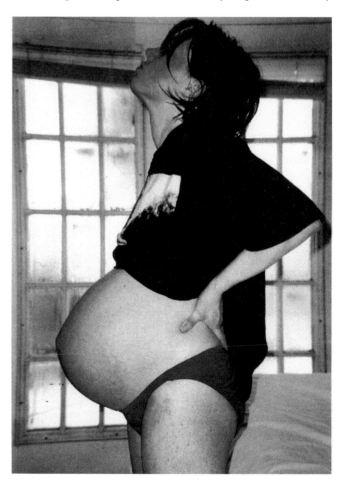

Figure 5.4
Labor and birth sensations.

sensation associated with contractions that she wants to relieve or avoid. Suffering, however, is a distressing psychological state that includes feelings of helplessness, fear, panic, loss of control and aloneness (Dekker 2018). Simkin and her colleagues postulate that it is not pain, but a fear of suffering – an inability to cope with pain – that is of concern. The woman fears how pain will affect her behavior – including "losing control, crying, writhing, struggling, showing weakness, behaving shamefully, feeling helpless, isolated, and not knowing how long the pain may continue and being unable to do anything to reduce it." Suffering is similar in definition to trauma. It can lead to emotional distress and even the post-traumatic stress disorder that sometimes continues long after the birth (Chapter 7). No woman should remain in a state of suffering in her labor and birth (Simkin et al. 2017). Your prenatal and labor care has the potential to help her avoid this suffering state.

In addition to your communication about how she is coping, also ask about and give her the chance to change the words that she prefers to use and hear during labor – for example, her personal name, "mama," "birthing goddess" or "woman warrior," and "uterine contraction," "pressure wave," "love squeeze," "rush" or "sensation." Also in many hospitals, laboring patients are asked periodically to assess their "pain" using a visual analog scale of 0 (no pain) to 10 (worst pain). The patient indicates her pain level, and, if it reaches a particular level, pain medications may be offered unless she indicates otherwise in her birth plan (see Box 5.2). Some women ask that their maternity healthcare providers use specific sensation language that resonates with them, thereby avoiding any mention of "pain."

In the *Labor Progress Handbook*, Simkin and her colleagues suggest two main approaches to managing pain with the primary goal of preventing suffering:

1. accepting the use of non-pharmacological methods to keep sensation manageable, rather than attempting to remove sensations of pain

2. avoiding pain by using medication to modify or remove sensations of pain.

As experts in the first approach, you can explore how you can help your client have both realistic expectations and strong coping skills, as well as the flexibility to accept both approaches if suffering presents and lingers.

Effects of Touch

Labor and birth sensations are big because the uterus's strong smooth muscles contract to thin and open the inferior opening at the cervix and move the baby through the pelvis and pelvic floor. Muscles, ligaments and their fascial attachments move and stretch in new ways as well. Massage therapy and other types of labor comfort measures to relieve these new, sometimes painful, sensations are based on the gate theory of pain. This concept suggests that local stimulation – pressure, stroking, friction, heat or cold – can fill the brain's sensory receptor sites before pain sensations arrive. This is because painful stimuli travel most slowly of all sensations to the brain. A hypothetical gate in the spinal cord will close the brain to painful sensation so that less pain is perceived (Ricci 2017). Pain management with touch stimuli is commonly most effective when you deliver continuous, tactile experiences just prior to and throughout contractions using slow, rhythmic and predictable movements and/or stationary compressions.

Consider the benefits of simultaneous touch stimuli that more effectively close the pain gate – for example, combining a firm sacral counterpressure with a cool washcloth over her forehead. Observe how your client uniquely responds to your labor massage therapy techniques. Know that one client might enjoy touch during contractions, and another enjoys it only between contractions. One client might require constant skin stimulation, while another wants only certain types of strokes, pressure or rhythm. Another client might respond best to massage of specific areas only. And sometimes you find one technique that your client loves throughout her labor and birth. With another client, her preferences might wax and wane through the hours – what was effective an hour ago no longer is, and what she discarded 10 hours ago is again her new favorite comfort measure. Use your intuition, understanding and experience-based wisdom to guide you and be willing to explore with and learn from your client. Track her constant or changing needs for physical closeness, as well as privacy. Know that your continuous, calm and reassuring presence may be more useful than any hands-on techniques, especially for the client who surprises herself because the touch she enjoyed in her prenatal massages is now overstimulating during labor.

Other Considerations

Because labor and birth may last a few hours or span a few days, you must have great endurance. Remember to eat, stay hydrated, and take mini-breaks for stretching and tension relief when possible. Efficient body mechanics help to conserve energy and reduce overuse injuries, especially to your hands, wrist and back. Reduce back strain from leaning over low, wide hospital beds by adjusting the bed height and having your client close to the bedsides. Use a rolling stool or chair when possible. When using deep, sustained pressure, as for back labor, align your hand, wrist and shoulder joints. Use your elbows, knuckles, knees and legs whenever possible.

Also, expect the unexpected at births. For example, a fearful person can burst with confidence when she enters labor. On the other hand, a healthy, positive woman who appears to have prepared extremely well for birth can have a challenging, complicated labor and birth that unfold very differently than her birth plan. Develop your concentration and regrouping skills to be more prepared for the unexpected, as well as for new people, equipment and procedures.

Points of view: Induction and augmentation of labor

As your client approaches full-term pregnancy, she may be exploring and discussing with her maternity healthcare provider the natural and medical options for labor induction or labor augmentation. She may turn to you for more information on natural methods, including acupressure and **reflexology** techniques, and/or requesting "let's get this show on the road!" As discussed in Chapter 4 and detailed in Chapter 2

(see Figures 2.8 and 2.9), before full-term pregnancy at 37 weeks, we respect the potential potency of labor-stimulating points by avoiding bone-to-bone pressure.

Accurate dating of the pregnancy is essential before cervical ripening and induction begin to prevent a preterm birth (Ricci 2017). Recent research reveals varying results and indicates that further study is needed to validate the efficacy of labor stimulation points (see Figures 2.8, 2.9 and 5.12) for cervical ripening, initiation of contractions and their augmenting effects on labor. A number of variables cloud the current research findings – optimal point selection from a variety of points, techniques (that is, acupuncture or acupressure), length of time for point stimulation, and the research subjects' unique **Bishop score** and parity (Schlaeger et al. 2017).

Acupuncture and acupressure have been used for more than two millennia in China to augment labor and reduce labor pain. Acupressure is digital pressure applied over acupuncture points. Suzanne Yates aptly describes the use of labor-related points for birth as "labor initiation or focus points" to distinguish these bodywork techniques from medical induction methods (Yates 2010). A Cochrane review of 13 trials of acupuncture and acupressure during labor found they reduced labor pain intensity (Simkin et al. 2017). Studies of acupuncture have demonstrated that acupuncture may reduce labor pain, the use of pain medications, forceps and vacuum-assisted births, and the length of labor. However, studies that examined the effect of acupuncture on labor that is induced or augmented for **premature rupture of membranes** found that acupuncture may increase the degree of cervical ripening, but did not reduce the amount of pitocin, a synthetic oxytocin, or epidural analgesia; nor does it shorten the length of induced labor. More relevant for our work, certain studies found acupressure may reduce labor pain and labor duration; however, others found acupressure did not increase cervical ripening or induce labor (Schlaeger et al. 2017). Studies with more specific acupressure protocols show it may help promote cervical ripening – using Spleen 6 (SP-6) for 20 minutes, repeated every 24 hours in the morning until labor. Another study using Shiatsu showed that it may result in less use of pitocin to induce labor – using Spleen 6 (SP-6), Gall Bladder 21 (GB-21) and Large Intestine 4 (LI-4) for 15 minutes (Dekker 2017).

Reflexology is the application of pressure to areas on the feet based on the theory that reflexive areas (zones) on the foot correspond to organs and systems of the body. Reflexology may reduce the duration of the second stage of labor for primiparous women with low back and/or pelvic girdle pain (McCullough et al. 2017).

With deference to the historical use of acupressure and reflexology to invite labor and stimulate its progress, we suggest that you present this information to clients with this caveat – her body will reveal its wisdom and readiness to begin and progress through labor. Acupressure and reflexology cannot trump Mother Nature. Wherever she is at in her physical and emotional readiness for labor, integrating the labor stimulation points after 37 weeks of pregnancy (see Figures 2.8, 2.9 and 5.12) is safe and may support her next steps to begin labor and/or continue its progress while providing welcome pain relief. Her body and her baby will decide.

Pre-Labor

Let us first review the signs of pre-labor, to distinguish pre-labor from the four stages of labor and birth (see Box 5.1).

Uterine Contractions

Pre-labor is characterized by uterine contractions that ripen, begin to efface and move the cervix anteriorly. These are all positive signs and necessary precursors to the cervical dilation to come in true labor. Ideally, between the 37th and 42nd weeks of pregnancy, many physical, neuroendocrine and psychological elements coalesce and signal the baby's readiness to be born. The placenta, as well as the mother's and baby's brains, signal readiness for labor, which initiates the production of prostaglandins that soften or ripen the cervix (Simkin et al. 2017). Practice labor contractions called **Braxton Hicks contractions**, which have occurred earlier in pregnancy, now increase in number, frequency and strength under the influence of increasing oxytocin levels. As the cervix becomes softer, the **cervical mucus plug** that filled the cervical opening begins to release. As the cervical capillaries open, they release **bloody show**. Both discharges are evidence of this internal pre-labor process and a sign of pending labor in a few hours, days or weeks.

Other Signs

Often the baby drops lower into the pelvis, also known as lightening, bringing a noticeable increase in pelvic pressure and more ease in breathing. Heartburn and other digestive discomforts sometimes improve too. The spontaneous "breaking of waters" – a trickle or gush of amniotic fluid from a small rupture in the amniotic membrane and sac around the baby – occurs in pre-labor in only 10 percent of cases. More often, the amniotic sac ruptures after **active labor** begins and is well established. Vaginal secretions may increase, another result of shifting hormones preparing for birth, and the mother's breasts may leak **colostrum**, the thicker "golden milk" that contains essential nutrition and boosts immunity for the baby's first days. Women often greet this time with a mixture of anticipation, relief, and perhaps some anxiety about the labor and birth ahead.

General Guidelines

During pre-labor, you can include more specific breath awareness and techniques to improve your client's breathing capacity and rhythm. If she has Braxton Hicks contractions during your prenatal sessions, help her to identify where she tends to tense up and guide her toward relaxing. Maximize her relaxation and help to minimize any discomforts, as you have throughout the pregnancy. When discussing your client's self-care routine, this is also a good time to mirror it with your own early bedtime, daytime naps, light exercise, great nutrition and hydration as you await her call that labor has begun.

Specific Techniques

- A full-body relaxation or Swedish massage, reminding your client about breathing and relaxing her muscles while her uterus begins its work.

- Observing her body in a contraction, addressing areas of tensing with awareness and prenatal massage techniques (see Chapter 4).

- Auditioning a variety of massage techniques – long, slow effleurage during a contraction or static firm pressure at her neck, shoulders or sacrum. Determine what she feels most comfortable with, and establish a predictable ritual to return to in labor.

- Using deep tissue sculpting of tense muscles to help achieve deep muscle relaxation, especially to muscles attaching to the pelvis (see Chapter 4).

- Reminding or teaching the partner about basic massage techniques as a ritual.

- Grounding Hold (see Figure 5.11).

First Stage of Labor

Labor is distinguished from pre-labor because uterine contractions now change and progress the cervix's dilation. The onset of the **first stage of labor** is defined simply as that time at which the mother first perceived regular uterine contractions. It is not possible to distinguish first stage of labor from pre-labor, except by hindsight when the contractions cease or when active dilation begins (Simkin et al. 2017). First stage of labor is divided into three phases – early (latent), active and **transition** (see Box 5.1).

Early (Latent) Phase – First Stage of Labor

When contractions become more rhythmic and occur without respect to your client changing positions, this signals that the early first stage of labor is likely underway. The uterus gains momentum, with a trend toward stronger contractions that can vary from subtle to strong, and sometimes can be erratic in rhythm too. For your client and her partner, this time is often marked by growing excitement, anticipation and energy. Penny Simkin refers to the work of labor and birth, particularly in this first stage, as the three Rs – relaxation, rhythm and ritual – and as "personally meaningful rhythmic activities repeated with every contraction" (Simkin et al. 2017). This is an ideal time to establish this pattern, as well as the healthy, sustaining ritual of sips of hydration after every contraction and periodic snacks or small meals. To conserve energy through early first-stage contractions, "ignoring it until you can't ignore it" is also an effective early labor coping technique. Your client may want to call to talk with her physician, midwife or nurse in early labor.

Reminder

Remember Penny Simkin's three Rs – relaxation, rhythm and ritual – and incorporate each in your labor and birth massage techniques.

General Guidelines

During early labor, you may want to check in by phone with your client and her partner to offer reminders from any prenatal instruction, including the three Rs. Remind her of the wisdom of alternating rest, naps and sleep (Figure 5.5) with light activity and gravity positions (see Figure 5.1), especially when this early (latent) phase occurs at night. When early labor is slow and painful, your presence and hands-on techniques can be very helpful. Focus on reducing sympathetic nervous system arousal with relaxing, centering touch employing rhythmic, soothing strokes and holding. Try a variety of gravity-assisted positions and walking with alternating rest times that conserve her energy. Unless she requests otherwise, work with her partner to maintain close, supportive physical contact while she continues to hydrate and enjoy snacks between each contraction.

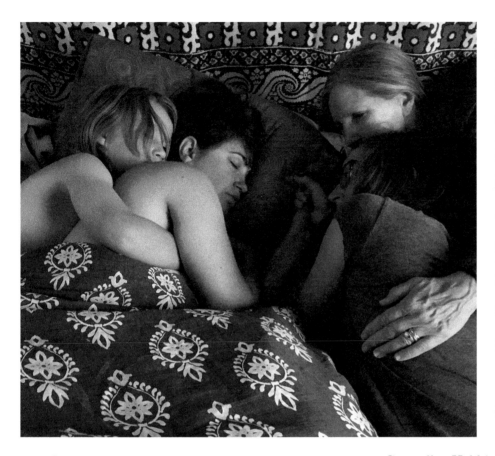

Figure 5.5
Resting in early labor.

Specific Techniques

Keep the three Rs in mind as you experiment with the effects of:

- Observing your client's body in a contraction, addressing areas of tensing with awareness and prenatal massage techniques (see Chapter 4).

- Experimenting with a variety of massage techniques – long, slow effleurage during a contraction or static, firm pressure at her neck, shoulders or sacrum. Determine what she feels most comfortable with and establish a predictable pattern.

- Using deep tissue sculpting of tense muscles to help achieve deep muscle relaxation (see Chapter 4).

- Reminding or teaching the partner about basic massage techniques as a ritual.

- Autonomic Sedation Sequence 3–1–1 (see Figures 4.8–4.10).

- Grounding Hold (see Figure 5.11).
- Labor Stimulation Points (see Figure 5.12).
- Localized Massage (see Chapter 5).

From the treatment room

I believe that if it wasn't for my pregnancy massage during my labor with my daughter, it wouldn't have gone as smoothly as it did. I was in active labor, but the massage helped me to be in such a relaxed state that I could get some rest and complete my labor without any drugs. My first was a Cesarean section, but this time was a "stop and drop" delivery, and vaginally. Just a few good pushes and my daughter was born. I mention my labor massage experience to every woman I meet who is expecting.

– Jessica, client

Active Phase – First Stage of Labor

At some point, a new plateau of regular longer and stronger contractions emerges. With each contraction, your client stops her usual activity, focuses inward and instinctively concentrates on her breathing and movement. The uterus contracts rhythmically in a more predictable and frequent pattern, pulling the cervix open and moving the baby's head down against it and through the pelvis, as measured by **pelvic station** – the relationship of the crown of the baby's head to the pelvic landmarks of the ischial spines.

In 2014, the American College of Obstetricians and Gynecologists (ACOG) changed the definition of the active phase from 4 centimeters of cervical dilation to 6 centimeters. With "six is the new four," it is easier to honor the wide variations in the normal first stage of physiological labor and allow the process to unfold at its own pace (Simkin et al. 2017). Physicians and midwives encourage a person in active labor to make her way to the hospital or birth center. If the woman is birthing at home, this is usually when the midwife comes to her home. If you have not already begun your labor support, this is an ideal time to join the new family before or during a change to a new environment with new people that might be stressful. If it is unclear to your client that active labor is underway, encourage her to follow her wise instincts of when it is time to contact her physician or midwife. Note that some women may feel safest being in their chosen birth setting earlier in labor to settle in, while others prefer to make any change of setting much later in labor.

General Guidelines

This is also the more active part of labor for you as the massage therapist. As the pace of labor increases, it is helpful for you to anticipate the next contraction, ready for a new or "tried and true" touch or position that your client enjoys. Stay mindful of your body mechanics as you support her there. Quietly observe and listen for the onset of the contraction with a hands-on comfort measure that begins and ends in sync with her work. Help her cope with the new stimuli with continuous contact – slow, steady, predictable, stationary or rhythmic – just prior to and throughout uterine contractions. Match the intensity of your contact to the increase, peak and decrease of each contraction.

Again, consider the effectiveness of combining multiple pleasant sensations that close the pain gate. For example, try stroking pressure on the erector spinae muscles with a nearby warm washcloth. Integrate your static or very

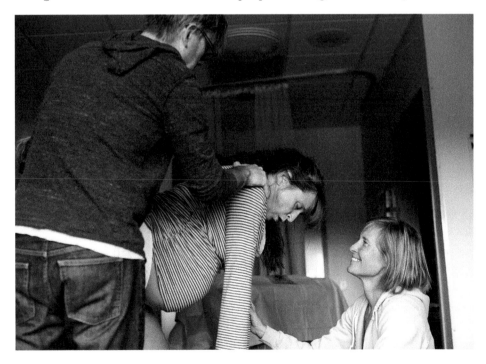

Figure 5.6
Inviting movement and validating strength.

slow-moving strokes during the contractions with slow and steady mobilizations matched to her instinctive rocking or swaying movements. If she is not moving through her contractions, invite movement through your hands. Initiate the movement and guide her in its rhythm, perhaps in sync with a slow breathing pattern. In standing positions, your hands can be on her shoulder, back and sacrum; in kneeling, your hands can be on her hips to gently rock her. For example, she may be leaning over pillows on the dining-room table or the hospital bed, with you or her partner applying counterpressure on the sacrum while inviting slow, deep breathing in sync with rhythmic swaying (Figure 5.6).

As soon as a contraction has passed, invite a complete exhale to release any remaining tension. Refresh and refuel with hydration and rest in between contractions. It may be helpful to remind your client that the rest times between contractions, when all added together, far exceed the total time her uterus contracts in labor and birth. Words of encouragement in trusting in the pace of active labor's work are helpful. Between contractions, use cleansing, faster and sometimes more energetic strokes to her back, shoulders, neck and limbs to encourage relaxation. Communicate a steady, sure, calm presence with your hands and movements, as well as your words, to help set the tone. Consider the possibility that no touch may also be an appropriate response, especially for some people who might experience touch as overstimulating or invasive in the vulnerability of birth.

When she experiences a new and higher plateau of longer and stronger contractions, validate that she is strong (see Figure 5.6). If and when she has a moment of doubt, validate her feelings, regroup by offering encouragement, or try a new position and comfort measure. When this stage of labor is painful and long due to physical factors, including baby in occiput posterior (OP) or asynclytic positions, offer your client positions and techniques that invite the baby's spontaneous movement to a more favorable position.

Note that a person in active labor should empty her bladder at least every two hours. This allows maximum space for the baby to pass through the pelvis and by the bladder, so integrate this regular ritual into her resting positions on the toilet. With intermittent or continuous electronic fetal monitoring, remain focused on her and avoid watching the monitors. Observe her response to the fetal heart tone monitor's volume. Some clients may find it reassuring while others find it distracting. Ask for the nursing staff's assistance to adjust the volume to the laboring person's preferences.

Keep an eye on the partner too and engage him or her in the relaxation, rhythm and ritual. Facilitate the partner's birthing experience with involvement that is personally meaningful and physically safe. Support the partner in taking meal and bathroom breaks, alternating continuous support of the mother with you. When your client has chosen to have others at her birth – a close friend, a parent or perhaps siblings – also attend to their involvement and how your client and her partner are responding to their support. Most laboring women prefer privacy, and it can be a balancing act to include the positive energy of many support people. Look for changes in her wishes and needs for privacy in active labor. With your client and her partner's permission, you may need to be directive in protecting her birthing space by modeling and diplomatically ensuring that she is surrounded by people who believe in her and support her birth plan.

Specific Techniques

- Abdominal Effleurage (Chapter 5).
- Cervix and Pelvic Floor Relaxation (Chapter 5).
- Contraction Distraction (see Figure 5.10).
- Cramp Relief. ⊕
- Heat and Cold Therapy (Chapter 5).
- Labor Stimulation Points (see Figure 5.12).
- Localized Massage (Chapter 5).
- Muscular Tension and Joint Pain Relief (Chapter 5).
- Sacral Counterpressure (see Figure 5.13).
- Sacroiliac Joint Decompression (see Figures 4.36 and 4.37).
- Sacroiliac Joint Rhythmic Deep Tissue (see Figures 4.38 and 4.39).
- Support Between Contractions (Chapter 5).
- Thigh Adductors Passive Relaxation (see Figure 5.14).

Hydrotherapy

Active labor is a wonderful time for a woman to consider using hydrotherapy in a **birthing tub**, **birthing pool** or shower if available. Laboring in a birthing tub or pool provides buoyancy, hydrostatic pressure, warmth and skin stimulation that induce relaxation. It can temporarily reduce pain awareness, may lower catecholamine production and may speed active labor progress (Figure 5.7). Timing of the bath may be important, as using it in early labor may slow the contractions for helpful rest periods; using it in the active phase often speeds cervical dilation. Controlling the water temperature to match the laboring woman's body temperature is safest. Her neck, shoulders and head are accessible for your relaxation work while her partner can join her in the tub to comfort and hold her. Women may enjoy water immersion through both first and second stages of labor, and sometimes the babies are born in the birthing pool or tub.

Professional midwifery organizations from various countries have extensive literature offering safety guidelines and reviews on water birth, including positive findings on pain relief and labor progress. There is less consensus on water birth among American physicians, so it is not currently offered in most hospitals (Simkin et al. 2017). Showers are readily available in almost all birth settings, and sitting on a birth ball while using an available hand-held shower spray on the back, sacrum and belly can provide great comfort during active labor.

From the treatment room

I have had the opportunity to accompany laboring women in many different environments. One memorable time was spent walking throughout a frigid Canadian winter night. I was bundled for the cold while Kathy had her coat wide open and pajamas on underneath! We slowly ambled along the quiet, dark streets, chatting, breathing together, arm in arm. At each contraction, every four minutes or so, she would take a deep breath and say, "Here we go." Then she'd wrap her arms around my neck, bend her knees, and we would breathe and sway back and forth for as long as the contraction took, then continue on our way. I remember we shared the night with the deer

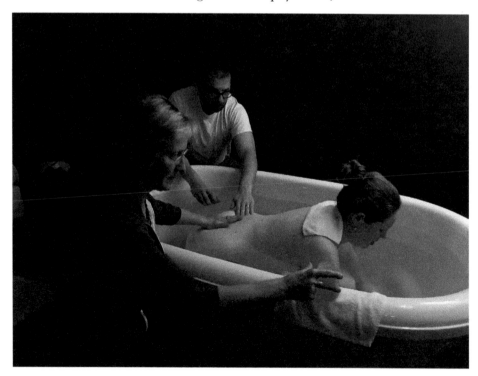

Figure 5.7
Hydrotherapy in active labor.

that had gathered in her wooded neighborhood to snack from the bird feeders there. They were comfortable with our presence, as we were with them. As the sky started to lighten, contractions were closer together and longer, so we made our way home. Kathy woke her partner and then climbed into the tub I was preparing. Dan called the midwives, who soon arrived and determined she was at 8 centimeters, and her baby was near.

– Linda Hickey, therapist

Back Labor

Back pain is common in pregnancy, as well as in labor, when sensations of the contracting uterus can radiate into the back; however, severely painful "back labor" often occurs when the baby is in a persistent occiput posterior (OP) position – the baby's head pressing on the laboring woman's sacrum and sacral nerve plexus. OP position is more common in first-time mothers. The good news is that even though the incidence of OP position is approximately 30 percent at the onset of all labors, most babies rotate to a more ideal occiput anterior (OA) position before birth.

Obstetricians, midwives, acupuncturists and chiropractors have effective techniques for turning babies from OP, as well as from the variety of breech presentations. Refer to these professionals when appropriate, remembering that "turning a baby" is outside your scope of practice. In addition, there are self-care practices, midwifery and birth doula techniques for helping babies shift their own uterine position. Although they are not massage therapy techniques, understanding their principles sheds light on some massage techniques in this chapter. Some labor attendants use a long scarf or rebozo to lift and jiggle the uterus and baby (Tully 2019). Positional changes that can work include a standing lunge, leaning into the raised hip and pelvis. These help with some uterine or joint ligament imbalances that might be restricting a fetal shift. Other labor attendants have the mother lie semi-prone or roll over in a sequential pattern to help reposition her baby. These protocols utilize gravity and any fetal inclination to move toward either the left or the right side.

Intradermal or intracutaneous sterile water injected into four specific points on the woman's back can be used as a non-pharmacologic approach for relief of back labor, as well as other back pain in labor (Simkin et al. 2017).

General Guidelines

As a massage therapist, you may be able to alleviate the pain of back labor with specific labor positions, movements and techniques. The hands and knees position often gives most relief. Couple it with the techniques below to help your client cope. Use heat and/or ice on the sacrum, and try sanitizable massage tools such as firm rubber balls or an ice-filled bottle for sacral pressure or rolling. Gentle abdominal massage and/or the baby lift technique can invite the uterus and baby to relax and spontaneously move to a more favorable position.

Specific Techniques

- Abdominal Massage (Chapter 5).
- Baby Lift. 🌐
- Gluteal Double Squeeze (see Figure 5.2) or Double Hip Squeeze. 🌐
- Labor TENS (Transcutaneous Electrical Nerve Stimulation) Unit. 🌐
- Lumbosacral Joint Decompression (see Figure 4.22).
- Paravertebral (see Figure 4.23) and Lateral Pelvis Deep Tissue Sculpting (see Figure 4.20).
- Passive and active pelvis tilt with rocking (Chapter 5).
- Pelvic Alignment Education (see Figure 4.32).
- Sacral Counterpressure (see Figure 5.13).
- Sacroiliac Joint Decompressions (see Figures 4.36 and 4.37).
- Sacroiliac Joint Rhythmic Deep Tissue (see Figures 4.38 and 4.39).

Epidurals and Other Pharmaceutical Pain Management

Recognizing the top priority of a safe birth for both mother and baby, new parents and their medical care team commonly treat pain management as the next priority. In industrialized countries around the world, more than half of all birthing women choose an epidural and other pharmaceutical pain management. While pain is sometimes a natural part of physiological labor and birth, the suffering of a long or difficult labor is now optional with pharmaceutical pain relief. While debates continue about safety and side effects, it is beyond this book's scope to address these topics; therefore, we will focus on realistic, practical ways that you as a massage therapist can continue to non-judgmentally support your clients who choose any pharmaceutical pain relief options. While there are various types of pharmacological means of managing labor pain, epidural anesthesia is the most commonly used during labor's active first stage and in hospital settings. This is true for women who plan to birth there, as well as those birthing at home or a birth center who choose to transfer to a hospital for access to available pharmaceutical pain relief options.

An epidural is an injection of a local anesthetic combined with a narcotic or opioid into the space around the dura, the tough membrane protecting the spinal cord. Those medications are continuously administered into the epidural space via a flexible catheter tube secured up the patient's spine. This tube is attached to a bedside rolling stand with a connected IV pump automatically adjusting to the desired, continuous dosage of medication throughout the remainder of the birth. Epidurals block the sensory and motor nerves as they exit from the spinal cord, usually providing very effective relief from the sensation of the uterus contracting. When an epidural is administered in an effective dose, the physician or nurse anesthetist still wants the laboring woman to be able to move her legs, with some assistance if needed. It is also ideal for your client to coordinate her second-stage active pushing efforts with the feelings of pressure arising from her ongoing rhythmic uterine contractions and the descent of her baby through her pelvis.

When a woman chooses an epidural, she remains in bed for her safety since her lower abdomen, pelvis and legs are affected. Epidural medications are gravity-sensitive; therefore, once the initial dose is evenly and effectively perfused, a nurse will periodically assist the laboring woman's turn from side to side, to direct the medication evenly through her lower body. The client who chooses an epidural will also have an IV fluid port in her hand or arm, a blood pressure cuff on her upper arm, and an oxygen pulse oximeter on her finger or toe, as well as a urinary catheter to empty her bladder. She will have access to a hand-held self-administering bolus button to make small increases in her dosage as needed, with a maximum lockout. Her nurses and physicians can return at her request to turn the epidural medication up, down and off as she wishes. When your client chooses other pharmaceutical pain management, such as IV medications or nitrous oxide inhalations, she remains in bed for her safety as well.

General Guidelines

Your supportive role continues and simply adapts when your client chooses an epidural or other pharmaceutical pain options. While the physician or nurse anesthetist administers, your client's partner and/or you can make a request to remain in the room. Your presence can help her manage her pain and reassure her, while staying in touch and talking with her baby as the painful sensations fade. During an epidural, it is advisable for the partner and you to be sitting in a bedside chair, facing her, while she leans forward as her physician or nurse guide her to do.

Once your client is in sidelying position, use your expertise with this position to ensure her comfort. Supply a pillow to be placed under her belly to support it, with her ceiling-side leg high and horizontally supported for comfort and safety (see Chapter 3). Peanut-shaped inflated birth balls are also readily available in more hospitals now. These provide support for positioning the laboring woman's ceiling-side leg in greater hip abduction without another person continuously supporting it (Simkin et al. 2017). Once the epidural has taken effect, she may immediately fall asleep, so pause your touch techniques during her rest and use these quiet moments for your own self-care. When she is awake, be ready at her bedside – standing or sitting on a stool – to integrate upper body massage techniques, being mindful to avoid her arm IV port, blood pressure cuff and other medical equipment. Invite her or her partner to keep in contact with their baby with abdominal effleurage, or offer to do that for her. They can also hold her belly, using words and visualizations of her baby moving down, the cervix opening, and the uterus strongly "hugging" the baby down and out. Be mindful of working around the electronic fetal monitoring equipment on her abdomen.

With lower body pain management no longer so relevant for you, your gentle passive movements of her hips and legs can be tremendously helpful. Perform those within normal range of motion, before and after position changes, in between her restful sleeps and during the pushing stage of labor. These movements not only are beneficial for keeping the pelvic joints mobile and pelvic muscles relaxed, but they also stimulate lymph drainage and relief from increased edema in her legs with the additional IV fluids. With an epidural, be mindful that she can perceive the pressure of contractions and your touch in her lower body, so keep working with her through those sensations. Continue to observe the medial leg contraindications, along with your body mechanics, as you perform these techniques and support her legs during the changes in positions and movements. Be mindful of avoiding pressure on medical equipment on her lower body, such as a urinary catheter attached to her inner thigh and a pulse oximeter sometimes attached to a toe instead of a finger.

If any breakthrough pain occurs, let her doctor or nurse know immediately and continue to work in that area, in the same ways as without pain medication, until it can be adjusted. If pain medication was not in her birth plan, validate her and her partner's possible feelings of relief and/or disappointment, as well as applauding their flexibility to be present to what is needed in the moment. Involve and also allow rest for partners and other support people. With the mother's awareness and permission, consider taking a short break or nap to nourish yourself while she and her partner rest too.

Specific Techniques

- Abdominal Effleurage (Chapter 5).
- All available upper body techniques (see Chapter 4).
- Grounding Hold (see Figure 5.11).
- Hip Infinity Mobilization (see Figures 4.44 and 4.45).
- Labor Stimulation Points (see Figure 5.12).

Reminder

When you massage during labor, continue to observe all precautions for blood clots in the legs.

Transition Phase – First Stage of Labor

In this last, relatively short phase of the first stage of labor, uterine contractions are at their strongest and longest, with only short breaks in between. As her cervix approaches full dilation to 10 centimeters open, all layers of her uterine muscles work simultaneously and intensely toward that goal. The rituals and techniques that you and her partner used in the early (latent) and active phases may not work now. Your client may appear fearful and unsure of what is happening and of her strength to cope with this last, relatively short, intense burst of uterine contractions. Nausea, vomiting and temperature fluctuations, as well as arm and leg trembling, are common during transition, with significant hormonal shifts occurring as the first stage of labor completes. Transition is often a time of surrender and "digging deep" for the laboring person.

General Guidelines

As a massage therapist, fully utilize your skills in autonomic sedation. Be solid ground for her so she can yield to the intensity of transition. This usually involves firm holding and communicating, perhaps taking a stronger role in directing her breath, keeping eye contact with you, or assisting her to a different position or movement. She might have wildly varying needs that change from moment to moment, including her desire for touch, assurance, warmth, cold and position changes. During transition, offer a firm, still hand on a tense area and avoid touch that overstimulates her senses. In the short rests between contractions, she may welcome slow, rhythmic massage or zone therapy on her feet to ground her. Back and pelvic pain is common, even with an OA presentation baby, so concentrate on firm, deep pressure on her sacrum, sacroiliac joints and paravertebral muscles. Rhythmic soft effleurage, moving proximal to distal on her inner thighs, may help calm her trembling legs.

Focus on providing positions that allow her to have her desired amount of physical support, as well as respecting her potential need for space with her partner and you. When she asks for space, be sure that you are still energetically and verbally close with her in this time of vulnerability and surrender.

It is usually a short time until she feels an urge to bear down and push. Often you can recognize this by a grunting or guttural noise made during a contraction's peak. A nurse or doctor may offer to check for full 10-centimeter cervical dilation, with the baby's head ready to descend through the vaginal birth canal. On occasion, a remaining cervical lip is present in front of the baby's head that needs to dilate a bit more to avoid cervical swelling or, very rarely, a tear. Her physician, midwife or nurse will suggest positions and ask her to pant through her remaining first-stage contractions to avoid bearing down on this cervical lip. This can be very challenging when she feels an overwhelming pushing urge, so provide extra attention and support for her to finish labor's first stage.

Specific Techniques

- Cervix and Pelvic Floor Relaxation (Chapter 5).
- Contraction Distraction (see Figure 5.10).
- Cramp Relief. ⊕
- Heat and Cold Therapy (Chapter 5).
- Hydrotherapy (Chapter 5).
- Labor Stimulation Points (see Figure 5.12).
- Localized Massage (Chapter 5).
- Muscular Tension and Joint Pain Relief (Chapter 5).
- Sacral Counterpressure (see Figure 5.13).
- Sacroiliac Joint Rhythmic Deep Tissue (see Figures 4.38 and 4.39).
- Support Between Contractions (Chapter 5).

Second Stage of Labor

Although this pushing stage of labor requires alertness and great physical effort, in some labors a woman's body does not feel an immediate urge to push as she completes labor's first stage. Instead, she may experience a restful 10- to 30-minute pause as milder uterine contractions continue. By "laboring down" and delaying the onset of active pushing, the laboring woman has a chance to regroup before her spontaneous, active urge to push emerges. An outpouring of catecholamines normally occurs during active pushing and has the beneficial effect of speeding the baby's descent through the birth canal by causing the "fetal ejection reflex." Many women also briefly exhibit fear, anger or even euphoria – typical catecholamine responses – just before and just after the birth. The second stage of labor ends when the baby is born (see Box 5.1) (Simkin et al. 2017).

General Guidelines

As her massage therapist, you can assist your client in changing positions every 20 to 30 minutes to explore and find the most effective positions and breathing that facilitate the baby's steady descent through the birth canal. It is vital to continue comforting and nourishing her through this athletic stage of labor. In addition to her own positional and breathing instincts, her physician, midwife or nurse may offer their direction and feedback. In a hospital setting, a birthing bed with the addition of a birth bar allows her to squat in gravity to open the pelvic outlet. She may prefer to sidelie, with hips and knees flexed and legs abducted in bed. With her partner's preference also in mind, choose your locations – at her head, at her side near her ear or at her back. Talk quietly with her or assist her by holding her leg during each push. In other birth settings, beds are also available, as well as squat stools. Birth slings dangling from the ceiling or a doorway jam may be available as other options to let gravity complement the mother's efforts. In birth centers and home births, some women may choose to enjoy their pushing and birthing in a birthing tub.

In whatever positions she chooses, stay attuned to her joints' integrity with pushing positions and movements. Partners and other support people often hold a laboring woman's legs for her during pushing, with knees and hips flexed, abducted and externally rotated, thereby opening the pelvic outlet. Remember that her ligaments are more lax in preparation for this very moment of pelvic flexibility as the baby passes through her pelvis; however, this also may make her more vulnerable to overstretching, especially with an epidural, when she cannot feel the movement, or if she has a pre-existing pelvic injury or instability. When caught up in the excitement of the baby's arrival, there is the potential to lose focus on how well-meaning, caring hands are actually compromising her spine and pelvic and knee joints.

Between contractions, help reduce the strain of those positions with your massage techniques. Offer reminders to take slow, calming diaphragmatic breaths, "kissing the baby's bottom on the way out." Offer her sips of an energizing hydration drink. Accentuate these relaxation moments with the relief of a cooling washcloth at her head or neck and the gentle breeze of a handheld fan. You can continue to use both touch and firm holding to ground her energetically and physically.

For breathing during her contractions, evidence suggests that her spontaneous bearing down efforts are more likely to have better outcomes for her perineum and baby, compared to outcomes when being directed to use Valsalva closed-glottis bearing down or "purple pushing." You can replace the use of outdated, loud cheerleading directions – such as "count to 10" – instead with your natural speaking voice. Offer positive encouragement, such as "Let yourself push naturally. Your body knows just what to do" and "That's the way, just like that" (Simkin et al. 2017). As the baby's head appears and crowns on her perineum, she may instinctively slow and steady her breath with panting. These can invite the pelvic floor muscles to fully relax and the perineum to stretch through the "ring of fire."

Also keep your eyes on her face, ready to make supportive eye contact as needed while others may be excitedly focused on watching the baby emerge. Keep a cooperative working relationship with her maternity healthcare providers. Remember that at least one additional midwife or nurse will join the team during pushing to care for the newborn. Be prepared to yield your position, as needed, to provide space for the physician, midwives and nurses to assist the mother in the birthing of her baby.

Specific Techniques

- Cervix and Pelvic Floor Relaxation (Chapter 5).
- Cramp Relief. ⊕

- Heat and Cold Therapy (Chapter 5).
- Labor Stimulation Points (see Figure 5.12).
- Lumbosacral Joint Decompression (see Figure 4.22).
- Pelvic Girdle Decompressions (see Figure 4.33).
- Support Between Contractions (Chapter 5).

What would you do?

Having flexible thigh adductor muscles that can relax while experiencing labor's intensity and possible pain often facilitates labor's normal progress. Given the concern about possible thrombi in the medial veins of the leg, how can you safely and effectively work in this area? What types of technique can you use and what do you need to modify or eliminate? ⊕

Labor Dystocia

The term **labor dystocia** refers to **protracted labor** or **arrested labor** progress in cervical dilation during the first stage of labor's active phase, or protracted or arrested descent during the second stage of labor (see Chapter 7).

Third Stage of Labor

In physiological birth with no complications, as the baby emerges, a woman reaches down to welcome and lift her baby to her chest. Alternately, her physician or midwife places the baby directly to the mother's abdomen or chest, skin to skin, with the umbilical cord still pulsating with its vital circulation for a few more minutes between mother and baby as baby takes its first breaths. With her new baby in arms, a new mother and her partner are usually singly focused on their new wonder of the world; however, her uterus still strongly contracts to completely release the placenta off its uterine attachment site, usually within 30 minutes of the birth. This wise adaption of continued uterine contractions after the baby and placenta are born reduces the risk of hemorrhage from the multitude of blood vessels traversing uterine fibers at this attachment site. As the birth day party begins, physician, midwives and nurses may give active, sometimes painful uterine fundal massage to encourage the uterus to contract more, to expel the placenta completely and to keep the uterus strongly toned. In hospital settings, it is routine protocol to administer pitocin by IV or intramuscular injection to keep the uterus well toned and firm, unless your client declines it. The **third stage of labor** ends when the placenta is born (see Box 5.1).

General Guidelines

During third stage, give the new family time and space to enjoy their new baby. Provide continued verbal encouragements and congratulations. Remind her to take slow, deep breaths through continued uterine contractions, uterine fundal massage and any needed local perineal numbing and repair. Sometimes, as your client holds her baby in one arm, she will reach out with the other hand to her partner or you for gentle, firm hand squeezes and caring eye contact. Offer this as she requests, and be prepared to yield your bedside position as needed to provide space for the physician, midwives and nurses to complete their care and assessment of mother and baby. If there is a delay in the placenta's release, you can offer acupressure techniques within your reach that stimulate stronger uterine contractions.

Specific Techniques

- Abdominal Effleurage (Chapter 5).
- Cervix and Pelvic Floor Relaxation (Chapter 5).
- Labor Stimulation Points (see Figure 5.12).
- Support Between Contractions (Chapter 5).

Fourth Stage of Labor

This final **fourth stage** – also known as the "golden hour" – consists of the first one or two postpartum hours (see Box 5.1). Prior definitions focused on the mother – stabilizing her vital signs, controlling her bleeding, beginning uterine **involution** and repairing any perineal tears. More contemporary definitions include family integration with mother and baby together,

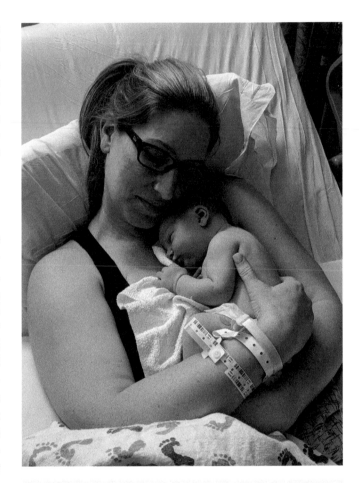

Figure 5.8
Fourth stage of labor: "golden hour."

preferably skin to skin and breastfeeding (Figure 5.8). American physicians Marshall Klaus and John Kennell first suggested in the 1970s that mothers and their babies benefit from being together during the first hour after birth. They asserted that both are hormonally primed to form crucial bonds as a survival technique. Over several decades, they developed their concept of the "sensitive period," lasting about one hour after birth. Their work was pivotal in highlighting the third and fourth stages of labor as times when feelings of love and attachment can flourish.

Many hospitals encourage early mother–baby contact immediately and for hours afterward. A large 2013 survey of new American mothers found that

58 percent reported having their babies in their arms during the first hour after birth. Sixty percent said the baby "roomed in" with them during the hospital stay (Simkin et al. 2017). With her baby hopefully skin to skin on the mother's chest, everyone can marvel at the baby's innate crawling reflexes, with little feet pushing and massaging her uterus. The baby also gives feeding cues and inches toward the mother's breast for a taste of colostrum, the first breast milk. Note if your client wants this family-centered "golden hour" and her hospital does not yet support these practices. In that case, encourage her to talk to her physician prenatally about integrating these evidence-based practice preferences into her birth plan.

General Guidelines

As in the prior third stage, continue to give the new family time and space to enjoy their new baby. Provide continued verbal encouragements, as well as reminders to take slow, deep breaths through her healthcare providers' continued uterine fundal massages every 15 to 30 minutes in the early postpartum hours. Uterine contractions also can be quite strong during breastfeeding's oxytocin release and especially in **multigravidas**. If you agreed to take photos or videos, keep in mind her stated preference about shots including her breasts and perineum. Continue to offer sips of hydrating drinks and one-handed nourishing snacks for both new parents while they enjoy their new baby – and remember to also nourish yourself. It is essential for her to feel completion in her birth experience with you. Take a quiet moment to express your gratitude for the honor of supporting her birth before you depart. After a good rest, describe your client's labor and birth in your records.

Specific Techniques

- Abdominal Effleurage (Chapter 5).
- Cervix and Pelvic Floor Relaxation (Chapter 5).
- Labor Stimulation Points (see Figure 5.12).
- Localized Massage (Chapter 5).
- Uterine Fundal Massage (see Figure 6.16).

What would you do?

Your 34-week pregnant client is distraught that her baby is in a breech presentation, rather than head down. A Cesarean birth terrifies her, and she asks you to help turn her baby from the breech presentation. How can you best support her in this difficult situation while staying within your own scope of practice? 🌐

Cesarean Births

A Cesarean section is abdominal surgery to birth the baby and placenta. With the proper support, it can be a positive experience for the mother and her family. Under epidural, spinal or, less frequently, general anesthesia, the physician team makes several surgical abdominal incisions through the multiple layers of skin, adipose and connective tissues, muscle layer and finally through the uterine wall (Figure 5.9). The physicians move and lift the baby's **presenting part** (head, pelvis or feet) through the incisions, followed by the entire body and the placenta. Dissolvable sutures close each layer's incision. The skin is closed with staples or sutures, and bandaged for the early days and weeks to prevent infection as the area heals. Increasingly, hospitals are integrating **family-centered Cesarean birth practices**, including a clear, sterile drape for the mother to view her baby's birth, as well as skin-to-skin placement and breastfeeding in the operating room. Newer surgical techniques on the lower segment of the uterus reduce the risk of **uterine rupture** in subsequent births (see Figure 5.9).

Supporting Cesarean Birth

Currently in the United States, one in three women birth by Cesarean. Labor dystocia is the most common reason for first-time Cesarean births. Dystocia also indirectly contributes to the number of repeat Cesarean births, especially in areas where the rates of vaginal birth after previous Cesareans (VBAC) are low. In fact, the ACOG estimates that 60 percent of all primary and repeat

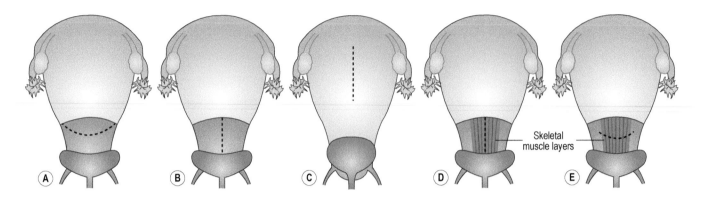

Figure 5.9A–E
Cesarean birth incision. Understanding the different possible incisions in the skin and through each layer of tissue can make your postpartum Cesarean Scar Massage (see Figure 6.13) more effective. **(A)** is the most common horizontal incision on both the skin and uterine layers. **(B)** is the most common vertical incision. **(C)** is the less common "classical" incision made through skin, the linea alba and the uterus. At the skeletal muscle layer, **(D)** is the most likely vertical incision and, in some cases, a horizontal incision **(E)** is required. The surgeon lifts the baby through all incisions and then sutures each layer, finishing with the skin. *Adapted from Gibbs et al (2008) Danforth's Obstetrics and Gynecology, 10th edn. Philadelphia: Wolters Kluwer.*

Cesareans are attributable to labor dystocia. Other situations for which a Cesarean birth may be indicated include certain maternal medical conditions, breech presentation of the baby, a **large-for-gestational-age** baby, and pregnancies of twins or **high-order multiples** of three or more babies (Simkin et al. 2017). Cesarean births are performed in hospital operating rooms and can be planned with a scheduled birth date that may change with an earlier onset of spontaneous labor or a medical complication for mother or baby. Cesarean births can also be unplanned when labor dystocia or other complications are present (Chapter 7).

General Guidelines

Like all childbearing decisions, the choice for Cesarean birth occurs after a caring, informed discussion between a woman and her physician or midwife. It also presents an opportunity to explore your beliefs and practice non-judgmental, **active listening** and support of her choice. Hospital policy, sterile operating room procedures, space requirements and the wishes of your client and physicians will determine which and how many support people are allowed in the operating room and in the adjacent recovery room after the birth. If you are welcomed into the operating room, you will be dressed in sterile surgical scrub attire. Freely cooperate with all medical staff and facilitate a great experience for the family. Sitting by her head near the anesthesiologist, keep your attention on her with unwavering eye contact and

From the treatment room

One of the teaching hospitals in Calgary has a viewing area attached to the obstetrical surgical suite. On the occasions the labor I was attending ended with a Cesarean birth, I have waited in the viewing area and stayed energetically with my client, keeping eye contact with her throughout the procedure. At each of these births, the midwife or doctor has acknowledged my participation in the event for the mother by bringing the baby over to the window to say hello and show me that all is well. Smiles of joy were all round – even those behind a mask.

– Linda Hickey, therapist

invite her breath, relaxation, and connection with her baby and partner. You often can touch her head, neck, shoulders and chest or hold her hand above the drape that defines the sterile abdominal surgical area below. Your client will experience sensations of pressure and movement in her lower body as her physicians help birth her baby. As with all births, avoid your own distractions by the sights, sounds and smells of medical equipment and procedures around you. If the family requests photos or videos by you, be clear on and follow the hospital's policy in the operating room.

When you are with a client in labor and a concern for her or baby's health prompts a Cesarean birth, the transition to the operating room may be either steady and slow, or happen quickly, leaving you in the labor room. Stay in contact with the nursing staff and the family. If allowed and requested, resume your support for her and her partner in the recovery room. Reconnecting with your client and her partner when you can and before you depart from the hospital is essential for a feeling of completion in the birth experience for everyone. Chapter 7 provides more guidance for difficult and traumatic births.

Technique Manual of Labor and Birth Massage Therapy

This section includes detailed instruction on how to perform selected techniques for labor and birth. Techniques are alphabetized, rather than organized according to the stage of labor and birth, so that you can be creatively flexible and responsive to your client. Some will be helpful throughout labor. Others may seem ineffectual, and then they may become invaluable. Labor massage therapy is truly an adventure of spontaneity, careful observation, trial, error and success. You will need to modify for client position and medical needs and equipment.

Each of the techniques is described as follows:

[Name of Technique]

Intentions

The outcome or purpose of the procedure. Understanding this underlying rationale will enable you to more precisely and effectively meet your client's evolving labor needs. It will also help you to modify for different labor positions and to share relevant information and improve communication with your client, her family and healthcare staff.

Procedure

Precise written instructions for accomplishing the technique (written with a specified client position in mind, if relevant), usually accompanied by a photo of a client and a therapist correctly performing the technique. (Note that, for clarity's sake, the client is usually clothed, rather than professionally draped as shown in Chapter 3.) Most figures have some of the following to convey further details:

- an overlay with the anatomical structures involved
- solid red arrows indicating the vector or direction of your pressure
- dashed red arrows marking the total area to apply the technique
- white arrows showing movement you request of your client
- red dots identifying typical trigger points to locate and extinguish
- an indication of whether to use a professional massage therapy lubricant.

These instructions may use the following terms:

- Outside hand = your hand farthest from the table when you are standing beside it. Which hand is "outside" depends on if you are facing the head or the foot end.
- Inside hand = your hand between your torso and the table when you are standing beside it. Which hand is "inside" depends on if you are facing the head or the foot end.
- Ceiling side = the side of your client's body that is highest from the table and usually most available to work with when she is sidelying.
- Table side = the side your client is lying on.

Hints

Tips for ease, variety or effectiveness. These are pointers for your own body use and ways to adapt the technique, including suggested alternatives for creating the same effect.

Precautions

Safety adaptations and guidelines. Certain techniques require specific guidance – in addition to that in Chapter 2 – so that they are not only effective but also safe.

Abdominal Effleurage

Intentions

To facilitate relaxation, especially of the abdominal muscles and uterus; to facilitate connection with the baby; to create space for the baby to spontaneously reposition; to facilitate cervical dilation.

Procedure

1. From a position beside the abdomen, use the flat, relaxed palms of your hands to apply the preferred lubricant with superficial effleurage strokes circling around the client's abdomen. Complete a circle with one hand as the other makes a half-circle to spread the oil, to make connection with the mother and the baby, and to warm the tissue (see Figure 4.18).

2. Use your flat fingers in small, superficial circles around her abdomen, concentrating on the lower abdominal region.

3. Hold gently at the edge of the baby's back with flat, relaxed hands, and gently rock and undulate the abdomen.

4. Reinforce the uterine muscles' action on the cervix with your effleurage strokes on the abdominal muscles. During the first stage, stroke gently from the pubic area upward toward the umbilicus to simulate the lifting force of the uterus's longitudinal smooth muscles fibers. Amplify this effect by suggesting that she visualizes each contraction gathering the cervix into the uterine walls to open it. In the second stage, let your strokes flow downward from the ribcage toward the pubic bone while she visualizes the baby moving down.

5. If a fetal position change is desired, deepen your pressure to the abdominal muscles but no deeper, making superficial thumb or finger fanning motions. Concentrate your strokes on the area to invite relaxation, space and the possible opportunity for the baby to spontaneously shift on its own to a more favorable fetal position. For example, to encourage a rotation from OP to OA, work on the lower segment of the abdomen superior to the pubic bone and on the side opposite the baby's face. Create long, superficial strokes laterally across her abdomen, moving in the direction of a desired fetal movement – left to right or right to left.

Hints

- If a fetal position change is desired, try the above procedures with the mother on all fours or on knees and elbows, so that gravity might shift the baby's head slightly out of the pelvic inlet. This will give a bit more space for the baby to rotate in response to the suggestion in your abdominal massage.

- In one of the above positions, wrap a folded sheet or rebozo around the mother's abdomen. Stand behind her, holding both ends of the sheet. Gently rock her abdomen back and forth as an alternate version of the rocking movement above.

- Wrap the folded sheet around the mother's hips and rock her pelvis instead.

- Encourage visualization and conversation between the mother and the baby to suggest the desired effect of the massage.

Precautions

- Secure her permission before touching her abdomen.

- Maintain pressure so that you are not penetrating deeply into the uterus. Be sure to use a flat, soft surface of your hand. Avoid tense fingers that poke or press beneath the ribcage, into the pelvic bowl, or in the inguinal or solar plexus region.

- If the client is nauseated, do not perform the rocking.

- When electronic fetal monitoring equipment restricts long strokes, shorten your strokes, and emphasize rhythm and the stroke's purpose.

- If a fetal position change is desired, work with the nurse, midwife or physician after they determine the baby's present position and the optimal preferred position, and as they monitor the baby's response to changes in positions, movements and techniques.

- Do not forcibly or aggressively attempt to make a baby move.

Cervix and Pelvic Floor Relaxation

Intentions

To relax the cervix, making it more responsive to dilation and effacement; to relax the pelvic floor so that the client will more readily yield to the power of contractions rather than resist them; to relax the pelvic floor through relaxation of the jaw and mouth.

Procedure

1. Encourage open-mouth exhalations to prevent the client from clenching her jaws in response to the pain.

2. Validate and support any low-pitched, guttural vocalizations she makes, such as groaning, moaning and repeated sounds. If her vocalizations become high-pitched and strident, she may be expressing fear, and she will be tighter in her upper body. Use your own voice to lead her to lower sounds that will calm her, bring her awareness deeper into her belly, relax her throat, and help to keep the masseter and temporalis muscles relaxed.

3. Grasp the three medial toes of both feet simultaneously. Press the three toes firmly together. Hold, or rhythmically release and hold at two- to four-second intervals during contractions to create a relaxation of the pelvic floor and/or the adductors.

4. Use imagery and visualizations to assist in opening of the cervix and relaxation of the pelvic floor muscles. For example, ask her to imagine that her cervix is the bud of her favorite flower. As each contraction begins and peaks, encourage her to imagine the bud slowly and easily opening into a large beautiful blossom, adding as much sensorial detail as possible.

Hints

- The toe grasp may work by stimulating meridians or medial fascial planes. If you are familiar with these systems, use visualization and energetic intention to supplement your pressure. This technique is more effective when the client's legs are completely supported.

- Keep in mind the concepts of Sphincter Law, described by Ina May Gaskin, as you work with these procedures: sphincters function best in an atmosphere of intimacy and privacy; sphincters cannot be opened at will; sphincters can close down when a person is upset, frightened, humiliated or self-conscious; and relaxation of the mouth and jaw is directly correlated to the ability of the cervix, vagina and anus to open fully (Gaskin 2019).

Contraction Distraction (Figure 5.10)

Intentions

To flood the brain with pressure and pleasurable sensations that distract from the pain of the cervix stretching, uterine ligament strain and other anteriorly felt pain; to relax the lower back.

Procedure

1. Use fingertips, thumbs, knuckles or elbows to compress firmly and directly perpendicular to the paravertebral muscles at the level of T10–L2. Apply this stationary, deep pressure to the lateral borders of the erector spinae and also at the lumbosacral junction during contractions to compete with uterine sensations.

2. Perform rhythmic effleurage, kneading, thumb fanning and/or nerve strokes to the area and to the entire sacrum during contractions.

3. Encourage rhythmic pelvic tilting during contractions.

4. Provide more general distraction with gentle abdominal effleurage; long, delicate strokes down the arms or legs; or soft, soothing fanning motions across the brow.

5. Address pain by stimulating Chinese acupuncture point Urinary Bladder 67 (BL-67). During contractions, apply firm pressure bilaterally with a fingernail into the flesh at the lateral, proximal corner of the nails of the fifth toes.

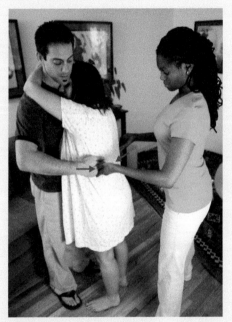

Figure 5.10   Contraction Distraction.

2. Use open, soft hands, making maximum contact. Slide your top hand under her neck, gently cupping her occiput. Slide your other hand down to hold her sacrum in your palm. Your hands stay in this position throughout the push and rest cycle. Guide the subtle movement of the spine – do not position and immobilize her.

3. In the resting minutes between contractions, promote parasympathetic stimulation by circling your sacral hand. With your superior hand, gently knead the cervical muscles and occipital attachments.

4. As the contraction begins, stop the movement of your hands and hold in place. Gently spread them apart, encouraging her head and upper chest into flexion and her sacrum into a pelvic tilt.

5. Hold this lengthening and gentle spinal flexion throughout the contraction and pushing. A subtle rocking between your hands for mobilization may also feel supportive.

Precautions

- Avoid the epidural site.

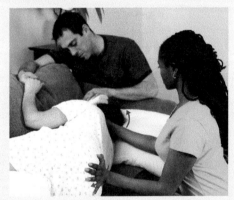

Figure 5.11   Grounding Hold.

Grounding Hold (Figure 5.11) 🌐

Intentions

To gently curve and encourage the spine into flexion for guiding the baby out, counteracting the client's natural tendency to pull away from the painful sensations of pushing; to promote the parasympathetic nervous system response; to relax tense muscles at the occiput and sacrum.

Procedure

Described in the sidelying position; modify for other labor positions.

1. Position yourself at the bedside at the client's shoulder height.

Heat and Cold Therapy

Intentions

To add this hands-on therapy as its own technique or in combination with other techniques to reduce pain sensation by sending a competing stimulus to the brain; to relax tense muscles; to comfort and soothe.

Procedure

1. Place a heat source on the lower abdomen, back or groin to ease pain. Use a warm blanket, washcloth, heating pad, water bottle or heated rice- or husk-filled sock.

2. Place an ice bag, cold wrap, frozen washcloth, or package of frozen peas or corn on the sacrum or low back to ease pain. Use a can of frozen drink or other object to roll firmly over her lower back.

3. Try other local applications of heat or cold that can soothe and relieve, including warm blankets or towels to reduce trembling; or cool washcloths for wiping her face, neck and anywhere it feels good to her. Her nurse, midwife or physician can also offer warm compresses on the perineal area to help relax the vagina and perineum.

Precautions

• Test the temperature to be sure that you can easily hold any hot or cold object in your hand. Put fabric between the object and the client's skin.

• Never apply heat or cold to an area affected by an epidural, as it lacks sensation and so she will not be able to give accurate feedback.

• Most hospitals will not allow microwaveable items to be placed on a laboring patient because of the risk of burn from uneven heating within the item.

Labor Stimulation Points (Figure 5.12)

Intentions

To strengthen uterine contractions and support labor progress by activating specific Chinese acupuncture points and reflexive points (see Figures 2.8 and 2.9 and "Points of view: Induction and augmentation of labor"); to reduce pain (Urinary Bladder 67 (BL-67)). The same points can have different effects with each client at her unique stage of pre-labor, labor and birth, and as each client will respond differently, based on their unique needs (Yates 2010).

Procedure

1. Press firmly with thumb tip or fingertip bilaterally into each of the acupuncture points (see Figures 2.8 and 2.9) after her 37th week of pregnancy and during labor and birth. On the foot and leg: Liver 3 (L-3) (as demonstrated by the female therapist in Figure 5.12), Kidney 3 (K-3), Urinary Bladder 60 (BL-60), Urinary Bladder 67 (BL-67) and Spleen 6 (SL-6). On the hand: Large Intestine 4 (LI-4). On the torso: Gall Bladder 21 (GB-21) and Urinary Bladder 31 to 34 (BL-31–34). Reflexive zone on the medial calcaneus includes the uterus.

2. Work on each point consecutively in six cycles of 10 seconds of pressure on and 10 seconds off. If this is not effective, extend your pressure to as long as one minute on and one minute off.

3. Work bilaterally, if possible, through all the points, followed by 15 to 30 minutes of rest, and then start again at the feet, if desired.

4. You are not required to use all the points. Notice when your client relaxes or reports that certain points feel "right." Also note when contractions and/or the baby's movements arise with specific points, and stimulate according to her wishes (Yates 2010).

Hints

• Use a marker or pen to mark each point on your client so that you can teach others to work these points too.

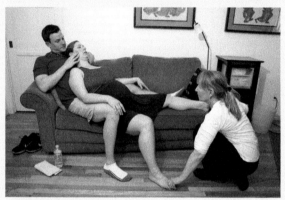

Figure 5.12　Labor Stimulation Points.

Localized Massage

Some women relax best to massage therapy in only one or two areas, particularly their head, hands or feet.

Intentions

To stimulate parasympathetic arousal that increases relaxation.

Procedure

1. Experiment with gentle, soothing facial massage, especially to the scalp, forehead and jaw. Hair stroking is very nurturing for many. Include her neck and upper shoulders. Gently undulate her cervical spine and traction and rock at the occiput (see Figures 4.12 and 4.14).

2. Thoroughly massage both of her hands, especially if she has been clenching them during contractions. Firm, midline palmar pressure simultaneous with friction on the dorsal surface of her hand simulates a traditional labor technique of clenching a comb or other object without generating maternal forearm tension. Try Wrist Passive Movements (see Figure 4.50).

3. Use Swedish, passive movements, or reflexive work on her feet. Use firm, rhythmic, inching pressure to create bone-to-bone contact at the zones reflexive to areas of tension and pain. Concentrate on the pelvis, perineal and back reflexes. To potentially encourage contractions, press the uterine points on the medial calcaneus. ⊕

4. Craniosacral therapy fosters relaxation and balance in all body systems, particularly maintaining physiological equilibrium (homeostasis). Use the biodynamic craniosacral approach (Shea 2008). Alternatively, induce the still point of the craniosacral fluid rhythms by holding and then releasing the ebbing and flowing fluid with light pressure against the mastoid area of the temporal bones, through holding the legs, or at the sacrum. Follow with release of the occipital cranial base, the thoracic inlet, and the pelvic and respiratory diaphragms. Relieve pelvic pain with sacral compression/decompression techniques. Consult craniosacral references for the V-spread technique to focus healing energy.

4. Other prenatal techniques from Chapter 4's Technique Manual that may be especially effective for muscle tension include: Laminar Groove Inching, Autonomic Sedation Sequence 3–1–1, Occiput Traction and Rocking, and Spinal Rocking.

5. Other prenatal techniques from Chapter 4's Technique Manual that may be effective for joint strain include: Sacroiliac Joint Rhythmic Deep Tissue, Sacroiliac Joint Decompressions, Lumbosacral Joint Decompression, Pelvic Girdle Decompressions, Hip Joint Infinity Mobilization and Symphysis Pubis Rebalancing.

Hints

- Use visual imagery to enhance the effectiveness of your massage techniques.

Precautions

- Avoid clot endangerment sites as blood clotting factors reach their highest levels at birth to prevent hemorrhaging.

Muscular Tension and Joint Pain Relief ⊕

Intentions

To relax generalized tension and specific muscles tensed in response to pain and to ease strain on pelvic joints as the baby descends and exits the pelvis. The most commonly tensed muscles during labor are: the masseter and temporalis; trapezius, levator scapulae, and other upper back muscles; hand and finger flexors; hamstrings and quadriceps; adductor longus, brevis and magnus; erector spinae, quadratus lumborum and other lumbar muscles; levator ani, transverse perineal and other pelvic floor muscles; and gastrocnemius, soleus and toe flexors. The most strained joints are: sacroiliac, symphysis pubis, lumbosacral, intervertebral and hip.

Procedure

1. Dissipate unproductive tension in these muscles by molding your hand to the area and asking her to focus on relaxing there.

2. During contractions, apply firm, stationary, deep tissue sculpting compressions with knuckles, fist, fingers or elbow. Cause no pain and maintain consistency of touch. Review Chapter 4's Technique Manual for general instructions and deep tissue sculpting principles that are applicable to any area.

3. Kneading, effleurage and other Swedish strokes help to relax chronically tightened muscles and prevent cramping. Perform rhythmic, firm strokes during or between contractions, as she prefers. Between contractions also use passive stretches, assisted–resisted stretches and/or shortening of tensed muscles to relax these areas by eliciting proprioceptive adjustments in muscle length.

Sacral Counterpressure (Figure 5.13) ⊕

(Adapted from Simkin et al. 2017.)

Intentions

To relieve pain in the sacrum and lower back, especially for those who have more extreme "back labor" due to the baby being in the OP position; to stimulate uterine contractions through activating the Urinary Bladder 31 to 34 (BL-31–34) points that correspond to the sacral sulci.

Procedure

1. From a position behind the client, use your elbow, knee or knuckle to apply very deep compressions on the sacrum. Protect her lumbar spine by simultaneously directing your pressure inferiorly toward her coccyx, creating a passive pelvic tilt.

2. Search for one or two "sweet spots" – specific points that, when firmly pressed, afford relief. Maintain firm pressure continuously during each contraction. You may need to support her pelvis with your other hand to keep her pelvis more aligned under your pressure.

3. Relocate further distally or switch to the other side of her sacrum to find a new "sweet spot" when relief begins to diminish because the baby has moved.

Hints

- Encourage her to try positioning herself on her hands or forearms and knees or sitting on a birth ball to facilitate a better fetal position. She might try pelvic tilting and rocking of her body forward and backward. These movements, especially in combination with the sacral counterpressure or cold packs, are often effective in reducing or eliminating back labor.

- If you have sufficient balance and control, you can use other bony body parts such as your heel, knee or ischium rather than your arms or hands.

- A massage tool, such as a knobble or T-bar, or a household item, such as a spoon or hairbrush handle, might be a good tool for achieving sufficiently deep and pointed pressure.

- Heat or cold, shower water or a vibrator applied to the sacrum also may be effective in sending competing stimuli to the brain.

Precautions

- Do not press the lumbar spine anteriorly with your pressure. Be sure that you or whomever you teach to do this is on the sacrum, not on the lumbar spine.

- If she has carpal tunnel or other wrist or hand pain, guide her to rest on her forearms or her fisted hand rather than on the palms.

- Because very deep pressure is necessary to create sufficient counterpressure, use efficient structural alignment as you apply your body weight to avoid injuring yourself.

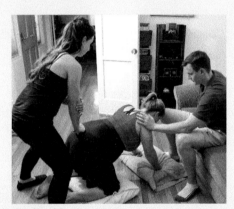

Figure 5.13 Sacral Counterpressure.

Intentions

To ease accumulating tension in ankles, knees or hips, and wrists, elbows or hands during labor positions and movements; to bring the laboring person's attention to these areas for conscious relaxation; to bring energy to the limbs in preparation for the next contraction.

Procedure for Legs

- Use your cupped, soft hands to quickly stroke up from knee to hip 5 to 10 times, covering the circumference of the upper leg. If the client's leg is in a position you can access, vibrate for 30 seconds, with featherlight pressure behind the knee, and then repeat the cupped hand light strokes 5 to 10 times on the lower leg, working your hands around the circumference of the leg again. Gently squeeze around the ankle and the top of the foot. End on the leg with a few upward full-leg strokes, beginning at the ankle and ending at the hip. Repeat for the other leg.

- If kneeling, your client may choose to rest between contractions by sitting back on her lower legs. Perform quick, superficial, upward strokes on the lower legs, and do gentle ankle and foot squeezes as she moves forward to hands and knees position, readying herself for the oncoming contraction.

Procedure for Arms

- At any time when your client is holding a bar, has hands clasped, or is leaning forward on bent wrist or forearms, use cupped hands and light touch to quickly stroke from wrist to shoulder. Cover the circumference of her arm with your hands.

- Grasp and circle her wrist with your palms, strip upward toward her shoulder several times and massage her hands before the next contraction begins to build.

Hints

- Movements between contractions, depending on her position, that also can help include: knee-high slow marching in place; arms above head or out to sides and shaking; rotating shoulders; walking.

- Encourage a change of position every 20 to 30 minutes, and suggest she attempts to urinate every two hours.

- If she is sitting on a ball, take care not to destabilize her balance with your strokes.

Precautions

- Suggest a change of position to a standing forward-leaning position if your client experiences numb or tingling sensations in her legs from the weighted flexion of her knees when kneeling or on hands and knees. Place pillows for space and padding behind or under her knees too.

- Observe precautions concerning no deep, pointed pressure on the medial aspect of the leg in pregnancy. During labor, light, fluid strokes are appropriate.

- When your client has an epidural or is limited in movement, use featherlight drainage techniques as above to lateral, anterior and posterior aspects of the leg only. Avoid the medial leg entirely because of the increased risk of clots due to inactivity.

Thigh Adductors Passive Relaxation (Figure 5.14)

Intentions

As labor preparation, to promote flexibility; to prepare emotionally for the exposure and vulnerability inherent in birthing; to assist in resolving issues related to prior births, medical procedures, sexual abuse or other experiences that may negatively impact the birth.

During labor, to induce relaxation and passive stretching of the thigh adductors; to promote the ability to squat and abduct the thighs during labor.

Procedure

Described in semireclining position.

1. Stand facing the client. Slide any leg bolster out from under her closest leg, and flex that knee to place her foot flat on the table or laboring bed near her other knee. Support this foot with your hand closest to the table or bed to prevent it from sliding, but allow it to evert with the following movements.

2. Place your other hand or forearm on the lateral side of her bent knee. Ask her to give over her leg weight to you by relaxing her inner thigh. Receive and distribute the entire weight of her leg into your legs to provide stable support.

3. Induce adductor relaxation by initiating very small-amplitude, rhythmic adduction and abduction movements while gradually externally rotating her hip. Initiate movement from your own legs rather than with just your arms.

4. Continue the small rocking movements as you gradually take the knee from her midline to maximum hip range of motion, without creating pain.

5. Allow the weight of the leg to further stretch the adductors for 30 seconds to one minute and/or perform assisted–resisted stretches.

6. Return the leg to the midline with similar rocking movements.

7. Relocate the bolster, extend this leg and then repeat on the other leg.

Hints

- If the client has difficulty releasing her leg to your movements, ask her to imagine your hand as a powerful magnet and her leg as metal. Have her imagine that the attractive force of the magnet makes it impossible for her to hold the weight of her leg.

- Whenever the muscles contract to regain control of the movement (the leg will feel lighter to you), reverse your movement to return to an angle where she was passive with adductors relaxed. Repeat your rocking movements through the resistant area until she is able to relax again.

- With expressed client consent, improve acceptance of the exposure inherent in birthing by repeated performance of this technique to her level of comfort following this progression in subsequent sessions: fully clothed and draped, fully clothed, with underwear and draped, without underwear and draped (when performed as preparation for labor).

Precautions

- Do not perform when she experiences symphysis pubis pain.
- If pain occurs in sacroiliac joints or other pelvic areas, provide pillow support under the lateral thigh to reduce maximum range of motion.
- Avoid overstretching ligaments.

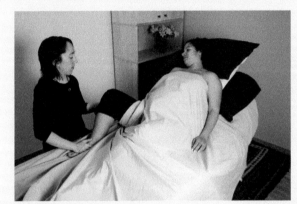

Figure 5.14 Thigh Adductors Passive Relaxation.

Chapter Summary

Accompanying a woman through labor and birth as a member of her birthing team is an honor you should consider experiencing. A massage therapist functions as a facilitator of relaxation, mind–body awareness, pain reduction, and physical and emotional nurturance. You can enhance your client's experience, her family's development, and, indirectly, the world. Performed by practitioners who are sensitive and attentive by nature, massage therapy lends itself beautifully to the emotional, energetic and physical support that is necessary for a woman to calmly and confidently labor and birth her baby. It is an incredible opportunity to fully experience the power of touch for humanity.

Think it through

To deepen your knowledge, go to our online resources, answer the test questions for this chapter and explore further.

References and Further Reading

ACOG (American College of Obstetricians and Gynecologists) (2019). Approaches to Limit Interventions During Labor and Birth. Available at: https://www.acog.org/Clinical-Guidance-and-Publications/Committee-Opinions/Committee-on-Obstetric-Practice/Approaches-to-Limit-Intervention-During-Labor-and-Birth [accessed July 1, 2019].

Bainbridge D (2000) Making Babies: The Science of Pregnancy. Cambridge, MA: Harvard University Press.

Buckley S (2013) Gentle Birth, Gentle Mothering: A Doctor's Guide to Natural Childbirth and Gentle Early Parenting Choices. Berkeley: Celestial Arts.

Buckley S (2015) Hormonal Physiology of Childbearing. Available at http://www.nationalpartnership.org/our-work/resources/health-care/maternity/hormonal-physiology-of-childbearing.pdf [accessed July 1, 2019].

Chang M, Wang S, Chen C (2002) Effects of massage on pain and anxiety during labour: a randomized controlled trial in Taiwan. J Adv Nurs. 38(1):68–73.

CPWHC (Chartered Physiotherapists in Women's Health and Continence and Directorate of Strategy and Clinical Programmes; Health Service Executive) (2014) Clinical Practice Guideline: Management of Pelvic Girdle Pain in Pregnancy and Post-Partum. Guideline no. 16; revised August.

Dekker R (2017) Natural Labor Induction Series: Acupuncture. Available at https://evidencebasedbirth.com/category/series/natural-labor-induction-series/ [accessed October 29, 2019].

Dekker R (2018) Pain Management During Labor. Available at: https://evidencebasedbirth.com/overview-pain-management-during-labor-birth [accessed January 24, 2018].

DeParle J, Tavernise S (2012) For women under 30, most births occur outside marriage. New York Times, February 17.

DONA International (2019) Benefits of a Doula. Available at: https://www.dona.org/what-is-a-doula/benefits-of-a-doula/ [accessed July 1, 2019].

Erdogan SU, Yanikkerem E, Goker A (2017) Effects of low back massage on perceived birth pain and satisfaction. Complement Ther Clin Pract. 28:169–175.

Center for American Progress (2012) All Children Matter: How Legal and Social Inequalities Hurt LGBT Families. Available at: https://www.americanprogress.org/events/2011/10/25/17153/all-children-matter-how-legal-and-social-inequalities-hurt-lgbt-families/ [accessed June 26, 2020].

Fulton B (2015) The Placebo Effect in Manual Therapy. Edinburgh: Handspring.

Gaskin I (2019) Ina May's Guide to Childbirth. New York: Bantam Dell.

Goldberg AE (2015) Cervical ripening. Available at http://emedicine.medscape.com/article/263311-overview [accessed January 30, 2020].

Greene E, Goodrich-Dunn B (2004) The Psychology of the Body. Baltimore: Lippincott, Williams & Wilkins.

Hastings-Tolsma M, Vincent D, Emeis C et al. (2007) Getting through the birth in one piece: protecting the perineum. Am J Matern Child Nurs. 32(3):158–164.

McCullough J, Close C, Liddle D et al. (2017) A pilot randomised controlled trial exploring the effects of antenatal reflexology on labour outcomes. Midwifery. 55:137–144.

Muza S (2012) Series: Welcoming All Families: An LCCE Shares Tips & Resources for Your Childbirth Practice. Available at: https://www.lamaze.org/Connecting-the-Dots/Post/series-welcoming-all-families-an-lcce-shares-tips-resources-for-your-childbirth-practice [accessed January 30, 2020].

Ricci S (2017) Essentials of Maternity, Newborn, and Women's Health Nursing, 4th edn. Baltimore: Wolters Kluwer.

Schlaeger JM, Gabzdyl EM, Bussell JL et al. (2017) Acupuncture and acupressure in labor. J Midwifery Women's Health. 62(1):12–28.

Shea M (2008) Biodynamic Craniosacral Therapy, vols 1 and 2. Berkeley: North Atlantic Books.

Simkin P (2018) The Birth Partner, 5th edn. Boston: Harvard Common Press.

Simkin P, Bolding A (2004) Update on pharmacological approaches to relieve labor pain and prevent suffering. J Midwifery Women's Health. 49(6):489–504.

Simkin P, Hanson L, Ancheta R (2017) The Labor Progress Handbook, 4th edn. Oxford: Wiley–Blackwell.

Supporting Healthy and Normal Physiologic Childbirth: A Consensus Statement by ACNM, MANA, and NACPM (2013) J Perinat Educ. 22(1):14–18.

Tully G (2019) Easier Childbirth with Fetal Positioning. Available at: https://www.spinningbabies.com [accessed July 1, 2019].

Upledger J, Vredevoogd J (1983) Craniosacral Therapy. Seattle: Eastland Press.

Uvnäs-Moberg K (2014) Oxytocin: The Biological Guide to Motherhood. Amarillo: Praeclarus Press.

Yates S (2010) Pregnancy and Childbirth: A Holistic Approach to Massage and Bodywork. Edinburgh: Elsevier.

Studying this chapter will prepare you to:

1. plan postpartum therapy sessions featuring safe and effective techniques and positions after vaginal and Cesarean births for both immediate postpartum recovery and long-term healing

2. identify common structural, physiological and emotional adjustments of the early postpartum period

3. discuss the benefits and goals of postpartum massage therapy after giving birth and throughout the postpartum time

4. describe the possible long-term effects of postpartum musculoskeletal concerns and address them in sessions

5. recognize signs of postpartum complications and make safe adaptations for postpartum massage therapy.

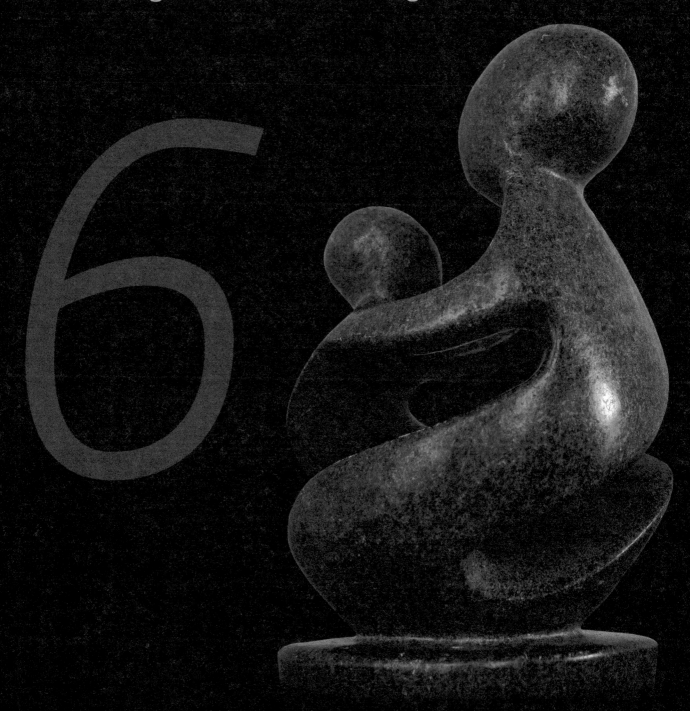

Postpartum Techniques:
Facilitating Restorative Healing

6

Chapter Overview

Every second, worldwide, five babies are born (Population Reference Bureau 2014). With each of these little miracles, a new mother is also born. With her newborn warmly snuggled against her, she transitions into the joys and challenges of motherhood. The newborn's early cues for comfort, nourishment and sleep are a curious new language for parents to learn. Each day, week and month brings changes and new developmental milestones for mother and baby. Caring for an infant can be both exhilarating and exhausting. Ideally, a new mother smoothly adapts and transforms – physiologically, structurally and emotionally – after her pregnancy and the baby's birth. To do so, she needs care, support and time to heal. This chapter is all about how massage therapy can help (Figure 6.1).

The meaning of the word postpartum is literally "bringing forth" and "after birth" (Johnson 2017). Medically defined, the postpartum period or **puerperium** is the six weeks following the birth of the placenta or completion of pregnancy through uterine involution – contractions that reduce the remarkable watermelon-size abdominal organ back to a pear-size pelvic organ. Many mothers, and the professionals who care for them, define this

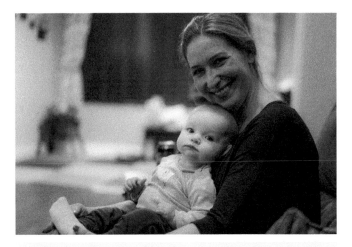

Figure 6.1
Motherhood can be exhilarating and exhausting. People need care, support and time to heal while caring for their infant and expanding family.

"fourth trimester" more holistically, noting the myriad of changes that can last well into the first year or beyond. From a massage therapy perspective, we also consider how new mothers hold and carry their babies outside the womb until they begin crawling, and ultimately walking, between 9 and 17 months of age (Simkin et al. 2018). Johnson (2017) insists that the very definition of postpartum drives home the point that, after birth, women are permanently postpartum!

In the hands of a skilled postpartum massage therapist, new mothers can enjoy a massage immediately after birth. This might be in the hospital, 48 or 72 hours before discharge, in a birth center, or at home, and may continue into the early weeks, months and years of motherhood (Kolakowski 2018). You can enhance a client's comfort and healing during this remarkable transition. This chapter provides an overview of your role in addressing the common concerns of the early postpartum period after vaginal and Cesarean births. And for your clients with older children, you can recognize the legacies of the pregnancy and birth, and how to help resolve residual postpartum issues.

No part of a woman's childbearing experience is more neglected than the postpartum adjustment, especially in the United States. After up to 10 months of being the center of attention, postpartum mothers can feel sidelined as the baby and newborn care take center-stage. Physicians' postpartum medical care has historically been based on only two visits during the puerperium; however, there are many other adjustments that have a daily impact on quality of life, require more attention and span a longer period of time (Johnson 2017). A new mother's love affair with her baby, or one that is seemingly slower to evolve, can affect the baby's and family's development and their relationships for their entire lifetimes. Some new mothers report feeling unprepared for the adjustments, gentleness and ferocity that motherhood ignites. New mothers and their families need reliable, sustained care for many weeks, months and sometimes longer, to maximize postpartum recovery and foster a healthy start to family development. Unfortunately, fragmented, extended families and inadequate social support can leave mothers isolated, with minimal attention to their many postpartum needs. By providing postpartum massage therapy, you can give one-on-one, focused care to new mothers. With your input, you can help ease women through the magical and mundane realities of mothering, truly nurturing her birth and growth as a mother.

In 2018, the American College of Obstetricians and Gynecologists (ACOG) published recommendations for optimizing postpartum care. These included more postpartum contact for new mothers with their physicians within the first three weeks postpartum, followed up with ongoing care as needed, and concluding with a comprehensive postpartum visit no later than 12 weeks after the birth, with a full assessment of physical, social and psychological well-being (ACOG 2018). Consider how physicians might integrate postpartum massage into their patients' office visits, which could improve visit attendance, postpartum care satisfaction and experience.

Integrating Traditional Cultures' Postpartum Wisdom

There is much to learn from traditional cultures worldwide that have remarkable postpartum massage rituals. Their wisdom reflects deference and attunement to the grandeur of pregnancy, birth and mothering. Specific rituals are designed to nourish, nurture and revitalize new mothers. During the "golden month," new parents take the opportunity to rest, recuperate and bond with their new wonders of the world (Johnson 2017). In the Ayurvedic tradition from India, new mothers receive daily *abhyanga*, warm-oil massages that soothe the nerves by calming excess *vata* (wind) after birth (Chopra et al. 2009). In Latin America, mothers enjoy a 40-day *cuarentena*, nestled at home with their belly massaged and wrapped in a *faja*, a cloth sash to stabilize and warm the womb. Household responsibilities are delegated to others to guard against future exhaustion-related conditions and illnesses. In Africa's Ivory Coast, female relatives arrive at new mothers' homes to offer massage in healing shea butter. Malaysians practice *mengurut badan*, massaging new mothers from head to toe with herbal oil and focusing on abdominal care (Johnson 2017). In the Chinese tradition of *zuo yue zi* or "sitting the month," new mothers rest at home for 30 to 42 days after birth, while female relatives take over all daily household tasks. Medicinal broth soups regenerate postpartum bodies and promote

lactation. Other postpartum rituals include: protecting new parents' emotions by limiting visitors; avoiding watching electronic devices so that outside drama does not affect the new family; warming or "roasting" the mother to heal the womb; and avoiding cold air, food and water (Ou et al. 2016).

One of the reasons why these postpartum care traditions are disappearing is that many new mothers return to work as soon as possible, because they have no paid maternity leave (Johnson 2017). Another factor in the loss of these traditions, including massage, was the move of births from home to hospital. In 1900, over 95 percent of U.S. births occurred at home, where the postnatal care rituals of immigrants from around the world were woven into new mothers' lives (Wertz and Wertz 1989). As a massage therapist, consider how you will integrate early postpartum massage therapy into your practice. Share these cultural postpartum massage rituals to provide the much-needed perspective that postpartum massage is a necessity, not a luxury, for new mothers. Talk with your pregnant clients about the benefits of continued massage therapy in the postpartum time and create a new family-friendly environment for her to return to your care.

Caring for all

With thousands of ethnic, cultural and religious groups worldwide, it is essential to understand and honor the critical role that our backgrounds and beliefs play in childbearing (Ricci 2017). People may deem it important to adhere to their culture's traditional practices. Others may bring their traditional practices with them into a different culture or try to conform to another culture's practices – with or without success. Some individuals turn to their religious beliefs to assist them in making healthcare and medical decisions. Faith-based worries regarding modesty can include not receiving care from someone of the opposite sex. Also, some religions have required daily prayers that might affect scheduling sessions (CulturaLink 2016).

Recent research also points to ethnic disparities in maternity care. American women in all minority ethnic groups have poorer experiences of maternity services than white women (Henderson et al. 2013). Black mothers in the United States die at three to four times the rate of white mothers (CDC 2019). In a study of common causes of maternal death and injury, black women were two to three times more likely to die than white women who had the same conditions. The disproportionate toll on black women is the main reason why the U.S. maternal mortality rate is so much higher than that of other affluent countries. Remember to be mindful of where each client is coming from. Expand your cultural competencies, religious acceptance and appreciation for ethnic diversity to effectively care for all.

Being Flexible with Positioning and Equipment

All positions for receiving postpartum massage therapy are safe options – supine, semireclining, sidelying, prone and seated. Some positions will be more comfortable than others, depending on whether your client had a vaginal or Cesarean birth and where she is in her postpartum healing. Most clients need accommodations for breast tenderness and fullness in prone position, with additional breast supports that take pressure off their breasts, and additional upper chest and/or abdominal pillows, rolled towels or a bodyCushion™ with larger breast recesses. After a Cesarean birth, the prone position can be added when she is ready and with her physician's medical consent.

Sidelying positioning, just as in your prenatal sessions, is sometimes the most comfortable for posterior work, especially if your client is breastfeeding her baby or is in the days immediately after epidural or spinal anesthesia during birth (Figures 6.2 and 6.3). The sculptured torso cushion of the Side Lying Positioning System is particularly effective in cradling, not compressing, tender breasts, as outlined in Chapter 3. If the baby is not on the table with her, remember to lift her ceiling-side arm off her breast with a pillow or a bolster at her chest. All the other supports and guidelines for safe and comfortable sidelying positioning explained in Chapter 3 still apply, except that you can eliminate the abdominal support wedge pillow once her uterus has completely involuted and any incision has healed. The supine position is ideal for postpartum abdominal work. Use high knee bolsters to passively reduce her lumbar lordosis. If she is still edematous, also level her feet and calves with her knees.

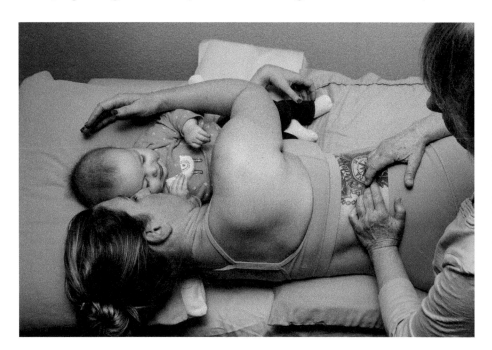

Figure 6.2
Flexibility with client and newborn positioning includes sidelying positioning for posterior work, especially if your client is breastfeeding her baby or in the days immediately after epidural or spinal anesthesia during the birth.

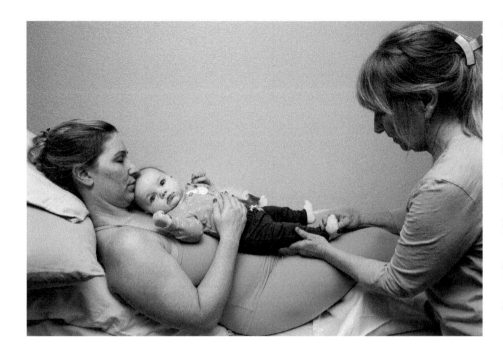

Figure 6.3
The semireclining position offers another position that also naturally supports skin-to-skin contact, breastfeeding and touching.

Immediately after a Cesarean birth, be mindful of position changes to avoid painful movements and to protect the healing, sutured incision. The "log roll" technique can eliminate pain and discomfort when the client moves on and off your massage table or in and out of bed, or changes resting positions. From supine or semireclining, ask the client to rest her head on a pillow and slowly slide one foot at a time toward her hip, bending the knee until both feet are flat on the massage table or bed with knees resting together. Place a small pillow horizontally over the lower abdomen and Cesarean incision, then ask your client to hold it in place with the hand on the same side as the direction she will be turning. Guide her to gently contract the hamstrings and gluteal muscles to bridge her pelvis up slightly off the massage table or bed, then turn to her side as she brings her hips back down. Once she is in sidelying position, leave the pillow at her abdomen to support the uterus and incision. Hospital beds have arm side rails that your client can also hold to use her other hand to assist with turning to sidelying position. When she is ready to get up, guide your client to place the elbow of her table-side arm and her other hand on the massage table or bed and slowly push up toward a seated position. Her head should lift last as she slowly extends her knees and lowers her feet off the massage table or bed. To get her onto the massage table or into bed, reverse the sequence of movements (Creager 2001).

Some mothers may be concerned about breast milk leakage on your linens and table. Even when her baby is not present, the thoughts and sounds of a baby can trigger oxytocin release, which prompts breast milk flow. It is wise to protect your table with a thick towel over its head end, and offer a warm pillowcase for over her chest; she may prefer to keep her bra on during the session. Until lochia flow has ended, a thick towel on your table under her pelvis is ideal, and she will probably keep her undergarment and peripad on. When she requests a complete massage to her back and is wearing a bra for her breast comfort, ask permission to temporarily unfasten and refasten it. Seek the same permission to move her underwear to work with her lower abdomen, sacrum and pelvis, or ask her to move it. As always, clean your linens in accordance with professional sanitary standards to remove these common postpartum bodily fluids, and also sanitize your table and other equipment regularly.

Benefiting from Skin-to-Skin Contact and Touching

In the fourth trimester and beyond, even though the baby is outside the mother's womb, it is essential to continue thinking of them as one – a mother–baby dyad – and to

Chapter 6

foster beneficial skin-to-skin contact, breastfeeding and touching (see Figure 6.3) (Liu 2017). Increased oxytocin levels during birth sensitize both mother's and baby's skin to touch, stroking and warmth. In the fourth trimester, the mother's oxytocin levels increase in response to the baby's skin next to hers, suckling at the breast and their mutual touch. Her breast temperature increases and pulses, thereby raising the baby's skin temperature. Skin-to-skin contact also lowers the baby's cortisol levels and pulse rate, and baby cries less. Mother and baby interact more, and their vocal communication synchronizes. At one year, mothers and babies who have skin-to-skin contact after birth interact more, and in a more intuitive way. Babies who have skin-to-skin contact after birth handle stress better than those who have been close to their mothers, but with clothes on (Uvnäs-Moberg 2014). A groundbreaking 2017 study suggests that early postnatal contact has lasting impacts on newborns' biology by actually changing their DNA. When researchers studied children who received high contact and low contact, they found significant differences at five specific sites in their DNA. The children who experienced less physical contact had cells that were not as developed as they should have been for a child of that age (Moore et al. 2017). We recommend that you offer flexibility in your postpartum sessions for clients to be with their babies, as well as honoring their desire for time and space for just themselves.

What would you do?

Your client appears for her first postpartum massage with her newborn in arms. Her daughter is sleepy after a recent feeding. Your client requests full-body massage with a focus on her back, neck and arms. What sequence of client and baby positions and techniques would allow you to meet her request, given that the baby recently fed? How would you be creative and flexible if her baby cues for interaction and attention? How can you interact with your client, keeping focus on her rather than her adorable baby?

Early Postpartum Adaptations and Adjustments

Endocrine System

As soon as the placenta is birthed, dramatic hormonal changes shift a new mother's body from pregnancy and birth toward mothering and lactation. Birth creates an adrenaline and oxytocin surge, resulting in postpartum euphoria for many. Hormonally driven episodes of involuntary shakiness immediately after the birth are common. Oxytocin and prolactin levels increase, especially if a woman is breastfeeding (Uvnäs-Moberg 2014). With birth of the placenta, circulating estrogen and progesterone drop quickly. Estrogen is at its lowest level a week after birth and, for a breastfeeding mother, remains low until breastfeeding frequency decreases. In a woman who is not breastfeeding, estrogen levels increase by two weeks postpartum. Progesterone levels are undetectable by two days after birth, and production resumes with the first menses (Ricci 2017).

Abdomen and Uterus

Uterine involution is a process of normal, healthy postpartum uterine contractions, also called afterpains. It returns the uterus to a smaller size and reduces postpartum hemorrhage risk at the placenta's prior attachment site. By 10 days postpartum, the fundus is more difficult to palpate, as it has descended back into the pelvis (Figure 6.4) (Ricci 2017). Breastfeeding and uterine fundal massage stimulate involution. Usually, the abdomen is larger than before pregnancy and somewhat pendulous, with stretched, loose skin and connective tissue often etched with stretchmarks. Also, the new mother's core stability may feel weak, uncoordinated and uncomfortable because of the imbalance between hypertonic back and hip muscles, and hypotonic, stretched abdominal muscles, which are often weakened by diastasis recti and where painful trigger points are plentiful (see Figure 6.12). Recovery of abdominal muscular tone and resolution of diastasis recti are related to the mother's activity and self-care, including appropriate exercises (King et al. 2019). A recent study found diastasis recti in 60 percent of primiparous mothers during pregnancy and 12 months postpartum (Sperstad et al. 2016).

Diastasis recti is also more common with multiples and in **multiparous** women (Creager 2001). 🌐

During uncomplicated vaginal birth, average blood loss is approximately 1 cup. Lochia is the tissue discharge from the placenta's healing, prior attachment site that flows out of the vagina for up to six to eight weeks after birth. Client communications during some techniques can be clearer if you know the changing appearance of lochia. For the first few days, lochia looks like heavy menstrual flow with small blood clots (Simkin et al. 2018). Lochia progresses through three stages – lochia rubra for the first four days with deep red tissue discharge, followed by lochia serosa until near 10 days as a pinkish brown tissue, and ending as lochia alba for the remaining weeks with a creamy white, brownish discharge. After Cesarean birth, lochia tends to diminish, as some of this uterine tissue is removed with the placenta. Lochia is heavier when mothers breastfeed, have uterine massage or are overactive too soon after birth (Ricci 2017).

Gastrointestinal System and Pelvic Floor

The new mother may initially experience sluggish gastrointestinal function and constipation. Decreased peristalsis can be a result of insufficient fluid intake, diminished intra-abdominal pressure, and analgesics used in birth. With pelvic floor trauma, she may fear further pain or damage and delay bowel movements (Ricci 2017). The perineum needs her special care after a vaginal birth, as it may be tender, inflamed, edematous and bruised for the first few days. Superficial microtears of the labia or vagina may heal on their own, while a perineal tear or an episiotomy incision has sutures that dissolve in the first month (Simkin et al. 2018). Perineal tissues may take four to six months to completely heal.

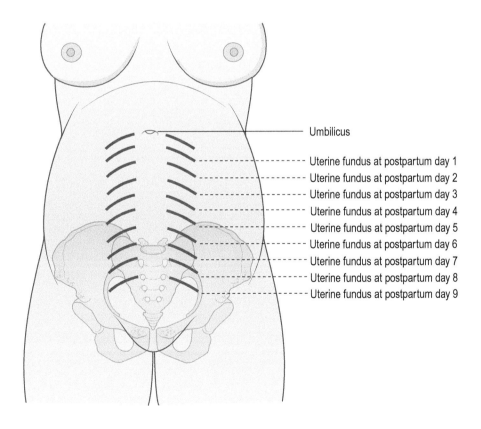

Umbilicus
Uterine fundus at postpartum day 1
Uterine fundus at postpartum day 2
Uterine fundus at postpartum day 3
Uterine fundus at postpartum day 4
Uterine fundus at postpartum day 5
Uterine fundus at postpartum day 6
Uterine fundus at postpartum day 7
Uterine fundus at postpartum day 8
Uterine fundus at postpartum day 9

Figure 6.4
Uterine involution. On postpartum day one, the fundus can be palpated behind the umbilicus and descends about one fingerwidth each day. The fundus may be higher in multiparous women.

Adapted from Ricci S (2017) Essentials of Maternity, Newborn and Women's Health Nursing, 4th edn. New York: Wolters Kluwer.

Pelvic floor muscle tone may or may not return to normal. Your client can experience stress incontinence — both urinary or fecal — and hemorrhoids, which can further affect her daily quality of life. These are more common after perineal trauma, a prolonged second stage of labor and assisted deliveries with vacuum and forceps.

Skin

Striae gravidarum that developed during pregnancy on her breasts, abdomen and hips gradually fade from red or dark lines to silvery ones. The new mother may also experience temporary hair loss (Ricci 2017). Postpartum **diuresis** and **diaphoresis** are also caused by postpartum hormonal changes, retention of excess pregnancy fluids and intravenous fluids administered in birth. Diuresis begins within hours after birth, continues through the first postpartum weeks and returns to normal within a month. Diaphoresis is common in the early weeks, especially at night.

Respiratory System

As the uterus involutes, the ribs, thoracic spine, abdominal organs and diaphragm slowly return home, closer to their pre-pregnancy locations. Respiratory capacity and volume return to normal within one to three weeks; however, pregnancy's facilitated neuromuscular patterns of shallower chest breathing can remain. Cardiac output returns to pre-pregnancy levels by three months postpartum (Ricci 2017).

Circulatory System

Postpartum clotting factors promote coagulation at sheared maternal blood vessels at the placenta's former attachment site. While these protective changes reduce the risk of postpartum hemorrhage, they also predispose the new mother to thromboembolism. Some clotting factors normalize to pre-pregnancy levels by three weeks postpartum; however, the remaining clotting factors may not return to normal levels for eight weeks postpartum or longer (King et al. 2019). Tissue injury after a perineal trauma, Cesarean birth, **tubal ligation** or **hysterectomy**, coupled with the resulting immobility and venous stasis, can further increase thromboembolism risk (Ricci 2017). In these situations, postpartum patients in the hospital may wear pneumatic compression devices on their lower legs to reduce the risk of thromboembolism until fully ambulating (King et al. 2019).

Weight

New mothers can lose as much as 5 pounds (2.3 kg) in the first week, followed by 1 to 2 pounds (0.5 to 1 kg) per week and gradually over several months (Simkin et al. 2018). The rate and amount of postpartum weight loss are determined by the same factors that influence weight loss at any time in a person's life, including existing weight, body mass index, diet, age and activity level (Ricci 2017).

Breasts

Lactation is facilitated by more remarkable hormonal changes. Prolactin levels increase and initiate milk production at the end of pregnancy. At birth, surges of oxytocin promote milk "let down" or movement, and the baby sucking at each feeding provides the continuous stimulus for prolactin and oxytocin release. Skin-to-skin contact immediately after birth allows the baby to use innate reflexes called the **breast crawl**. The darkened skin pigmentation of the abdomen's linea nigra and the breasts' **areolas** are thought to be the baby's roadmap to the mother's breasts. During the first 24 to 72 hours after the birth, the breasts secrete colostrum. Mature breast milk appears between the second and fifth days and is more voluminous (Ricci 2017). Breastfeeding is, on average, a 40-hour-per-week commitment with a single baby, and a new mom can count on overtime with multiples. A newborn's stomach is about the size of a ping pong ball; that means feedings every two to four hours for a total of 8 to 12 feedings a day (KellyMom 2019). The American Academy of Pediatrics (AAP) recommends exclusive breastfeeding for six months, followed by the introduction of appropriate complementary foods and continued breastfeeding for as long as mutually desired by mother and baby (AAP 2012).

If a mother chooses not to breastfeed, or cannot due to prior breast surgery, adoption or fetal demise, she can receive support for suppressing lactation. When a baby dies, suppressing lactation may cause her to experience a "second grieving" for her baby, who cannot have her breast milk. Some mothers choose not to suppress lactation immediately, but express and donate their milk to milk banks and other families in honor of their babies. Others make such donations just because they experience an oversupply (Simkin et al. 2018).

Emotions

As a mother cares for her new, little human being, it is normal for her to feel a full spectrum of emotions. While the stereotype is of the euphoric, smiling mother cuddling a quiet, cute newborn, women may also honestly express some ambivalence, doubts, regrets and sadness as they explore the gaps between the new realities of motherhood, their expectations and the changes to their normal routine. Bonding with a new baby is an evolving process that usually unfolds over weeks and months, not always in a split second immediately after the birth. A new mother's mood fluctuations may also be exacerbated by a disappointing or difficult birth, an unexpected illness or condition in her baby, or a personally stressful situation. Lack of support, feelings of loneliness or isolation, or a personal or family history of mood disorders can further destabilize her emotional world. She is also navigating changes in her relationship and intimacy with her partner, if she has one. Single mothers are often overwhelmed with 24/7 newborn care, and their self-care, especially if they do not have adequate social support. Most mothers experience changes in their self-identity and an emotional transition to their new mother lifestyle (Simkin et al. 2018).

About 80 percent of new mothers, and many new fathers, experience "baby blues," usually in the first week after the birth. Symptoms include crying easily, feeling overwhelmed or out of control, feeling exhausted, anxious or sad, and lacking confidence as a parent. Baby blues are considered normal and appropriate responses to parenthood's profound changes and rarely last longer than two weeks. Symptoms diminish with resting, reducing stress and pain, and providing the new family with plenty of support. About 20 percent of new mothers and some fathers develop perinatal mood and anxiety disorders, which are postpartum complications that require referral for appropriate treatment (see Chapter 7) (Simkin et al. 2018).

Reminder

Postpartum depression is the most common postpartum complication, so stay alert for signs and symptoms in your clients (Chapter 7).

Sleep and Activity

Sleep is another key postpartum adaptation. During the first month, the baby sleeps 60 percent of the day in phases of active, light, rapid eye movement (REM) sleep and deep, quiet sleep. Newborn sleep often consists of short naps, punctuated every few hours by feeding cues − opening mouth, extending tongue and rooting toward the breast. The amount of time the baby spends in awake states − quiet alert, active alert, drowsy and crying − increases during and after the first month of life (King et al. 2019). The resulting maternal fatigue and sleep deprivation can profoundly challenge postpartum recovery. The mothering mantra "sleep when the baby sleeps" reminds us that rest and sleep are top priorities. Integrating more naps and resting, even if not asleep, gives a mother the energy to meet her newborn's round-the-clock needs. Her baby may sleep as much during the day or more than at night − a common, temporary newborn sleep pattern (Simkin et al. 2018). Evidence-based information on "sleepfeeding" can help parents adapt their sleep rhythms and avoid fatigue and sleep deprivation (McKenna 2020). Resting between feedings, eating nourishing foods, honestly talking about their feelings, receiving postpartum massage therapy and connecting with the slower rhythms of Mother Nature help new mothers make a smooth postpartum transition to avoid or reduce these symptoms (Johnson 2017).

Remind your client to listen to inner wisdom respecting her healing postpartum body, as well as follow her physician's or midwife's recommendations about activities, including lifting, driving, stair climbing and exercise. After several weeks to months, she may gradually resume more exercise. Many women push themselves too hard and too fast, contributing to exhaustion, pain, pelvic floor heaviness and increased lochia. Uterine ligaments need time to heal to stabilize the uterus effectively during physical activity. When your client needs more guidance, refer her to a women's health physical therapist or postnatal fitness expert (Simkin et al. 2018).

Musculoskeletal System

The effects of pregnancy, labor and birth on muscles and joints vary widely in women after birth (Ricci 2017). Pregnancy's musculoskeletal adaptions are primarily related to the growing uterus, weight gain, changes in center of gravity, increased postural changes, altered movement and gait patterns and hormonal changes (Chapters 1 and 4). Add the musculoskeletal effort and adaptions during labor and birth (Chapter 5) and consider her **gravidity**, all culminating in the postpartum time. Couple those experiences with the strain of newborn care on stretched, weak or imbalanced joints and muscles – especially in the neck, pectoral girdle, arms, back and pelvis – and the results are apparent and widespread. Approximately half of women have residual back and pregnancy-related pelvic girdle pain after pregnancy and birth, especially in the pubic symphysis, sacroiliac joints and hips (King et al. 2019).

As massage therapists, we would all love to know the exact time that hormones discontinue their relaxing effects on ligaments and joints. The truth is that there is conflicting information, as well as research challenges, that prevent us from understanding these complex, multi-tasking hormones better. Some sources report that pregnancy's joint adaptations "revert back" during the postpartum period. After the birth of the placenta, which makes many pregnancy hormones, the hormones that previously coordinated their efforts to relax the joints – relaxin, estrogen and progesterone – plummet, "resulting in a return of all joints to their prepregnant state" (Ricci 2017). Despite this, some new mothers note a permanent increase in shoe size (Jordan et al. 2014). Some sources report that by six to eight weeks after the birth, joints are completely stabilized and return to normal (Ricci 2017). Other sources report gradually regaining tone and stability, but that can take months to years (King et al. 2019). The physiological roles of relaxin remain poorly understood. Relaxin's ongoing effects may depend upon the amount of circulating hormone and the local endocrinological milieu (Goldsmith and Weiss 2009). We recommend that you palpate and explore your client's body with curiosity to discover her individual postpartum changes. Marry this with your understanding of joints' normal range of motion and communicate with your client about your discoveries across her postpartum time. Look for themes and changes for resolved and unresolved issues in each mother's unique postpartum healing journey.

General Guidelines and Goals for Early Postpartum Massage Therapy

Even one postpartum massage therapy session can be powerful for most clients. After a first session when she experiences deep relaxation, pain relief and a safe space, and also has success synchronizing her massage with her baby's needs, she is often more motivated to schedule another session. These next sections will provide you with general guidelines and goals to choose from for that one postpartum session or, more ideally, for many of them.

Providing Nurturance and Emotional Support

This is a special time to focus on "mothering the mother" in a calming environment, where you actively listen to her feelings with your reflective words, your hands and your heart. In addition to your touch, your caring verbal interaction stimulates oxytocin, also known as the "tend and befriend" hormone. Remember oxytocin's calming effect on mother and baby – stabilizing blood pressure, lowering cortisol levels, increasing trust and facial recognition, and decreasing anxiety and aggressive behaviors (King et al. 2019).

General Guidelines

You can help your client adjust to hormone-driven emotional shifts by focusing on her scalp, face, upper body, abdomen and feet. Promote deep relaxation with quiet, soothing, slow Swedish and Esalen massage styles, energy balancing and connective tissue massage (*Bindegewebsmassage*). Invite time for solitude and recuperative rest.

Your client's birth experience lives on in her mind and emotions as she integrates her prior expectations with all the realities of the birth. She needs to make sense of her birth, reconstructing what happened and how she felt in her own words. Early intervention, with open-minded and open-hearted processing of her birth experience, can enhance its positive aspects and her role in it, and prevent psychological trauma. Delay or avoidance of this sharing misses an opportunity to positively influence a woman's long-term self-esteem and mental health (Simkin 2008). Her satisfaction with her birth experience has lifelong implications for her health and well-being (Karlström et al. 2015).

Your client may share and process her birth story during massage sessions. If so, work slowly at her feet while she recounts her birth. Hold her feet, your palms to her soles, and follow with long, inferiorly directed leg strokes to ground her and move through moments of emotional lability. This may also prompt the unburdening of strong feelings about the birth and her postpartum life. Actively listen, knowing that this processing can emotionally buoy her while she establishes her "new normal."

Be alert for cues about her social support to coordinate that with your between-session recommendations. If she wants suggestions, recommend helpful social supports – posting a helpers' list at home with tasks that visitors can help with; asking a family member or friend to set up a regular meal delivery calendar; and hiring a **postpartum doula**. Perhaps you want to become a postpartum doula so that you can easily integrate massage into your client's home visit care. If she exhibits symptoms of "baby blues" after two weeks, or a possible perinatal mood and affective disorder, remind her that "she is not alone," and discuss referral for professional medical assessment (Chapter 7).

Teach her simple effleurage strokes for her baby's legs, arms and back. Infant massage promotes healthy parent and infant bonding, the infant's growth and development, and supportive family ties (Liu 2017). It can also promote weight gain in premature low-birth-weight babies and also leads to earlier discharge. In one study, babies massaged three times a day, for 15 minutes each time, showed significantly more weight gain starting on the fourth day, and that was followed by earlier hospital discharge (Rad et al. 2016). For infants with colic, a one-week intervention significantly improved symptoms and was more effective than rocking (Sheidaei et al. 2016). Consider taking an infant massage instructor's course to enhance your understanding of and confidence to teach families and caregivers. Encourage your clients to enjoy exchanging back and foot massages with their partners and older children at home.

Keep in mind that while most postpartum people are celebrating a healthy newborn, some are grieving and in pain after a miscarriage, **stillbirth** or fetal/infant death or injury. Remember that women who choose or need to terminate their pregnancies are also in postpartum recovery (Chapter 7). Your compassionate ear, coupled with hands that say, "I am here," are powerful tools in their grief recovery.

Specific Techniques

- Autonomic Sedation Sequence 3–1–1 (see Figures 4.8–4.10).
- Breathing Enhancement (see Figure 4.11).
- Cervical Transverse Rocking (see Figure 4.12).
- Foot Reflexive Zone Therapy (see Figure 4.13).
- Grounding Hold (see Figure 5.11).
- Occiput Traction and Rocking (see Figure 4.14).
- Pectoral Girdle Mobilizations (see Figures 4.24 and 4.25).
- Pelvic Girdle Decompressions (see Figure 4.33).
- Spinal Rocking (see Figure 4.40).

From the treatment room

I entered a postpartum hospital room to offer a first-time mother a 30-minute massage in her hospital bed. She was anxious, reporting a pain level of eight in her back and difficulty connecting with her new baby. Ten minutes into slow spinal rocking and breathing enhancement visualizations with her, we welcomed her crying baby from bedside bassinet to alongside her in sidelying position in the hospital bed. As I began stroking her back again, she began stroking her baby in the *exact* same rhythm. She made eye contact and talked more with her baby between moments of drifting off to sleep. After the massage, she reported her back pain was lower, at a two. She quietly smiled at her baby while stroking his face.

– Michele Kolakowski, therapist

Healing after Labor and Birth

After reading Chapter 5, you understand that labor and birth are like an athletic event for which your postpartum client may now be seeking a post-event sports massage! Muscle exertion and strain, and pelvic ligament and joint strain and pain, coupled with physical and emotional fatigue, make this an opportune time to experience a fabulous postpartum massage.

General Guidelines

Ideally, you can work with your client within her first postpartum days for a short 20- to 30-minute or longer full-body session of Swedish and lymphatic drainage. Massage can soothe the sore areas that worked so hard to give birth and to move about and sustain positions through the hours of her labor and birth. Research suggests that this may happen on a cellular level, decreasing inflammation and increasing the energy-producing organelles of the muscle (Turchaninov 2011). Massage therapy may be an effective way to manage pain, including postoperative discomfort, and reduce opioid use (Simonelli et al. 2018). Connective tissue massage may lower pain perception and increase beta-endorphin production (Bauer et al. 2010).

Massage may help to facilitate diuresis and diaphoresis, as well as a smooth transition to normal postpartum physiology and homeostasis (Andrade and Clifford 2008). Connective tissue massage and reflexive zone therapy also may stimulate the body's return to normal energy and hormonal levels (Enzer 2004). Because the dramatic postpartum physiological changes compound birth's emotional intensity, some people may experience a profound clearing and resetting of their nervous system. They may shiver, shake or sweat profusely during or after a session, especially in the early days. Keep them comfortable and warm, and invite deep, diaphragmatic breaths. To reduce additional gas pain, encourage deep breaths with a forced exhale. When it is not possible to directly massage an area of discomfort or pain, such as that caused by gas, constipation and perineal injury, use reflexive zone therapy. Reassure her of the normalcy and transient nature of these postpartum transitions.

A beautiful closure to a postpartum massage session is a "sealing" (Figure 6.5). Your intention is to create an energetic closing effect, cocooning her within the massage sheets to rest at session's end. Use either the bottom sheet or an additional flat sheet that you placed prior to your session to gradually enclose your client. Beginning at her feet and finishing at her head, bring each side of the sheet over her, twisting it gently yet firmly together at the midline over her body. Hold at each point, particularly where she feels most "open," to energetically seal these places before moving along. Leave an open space at her head so she can breathe easily. After a satisfying rest period, slowly unwrap her from head to foot.

Specific Techniques

- Abdominal Kneading, Vibration, Tapotement and Trigger Points (see Figures 6.9–6.12).

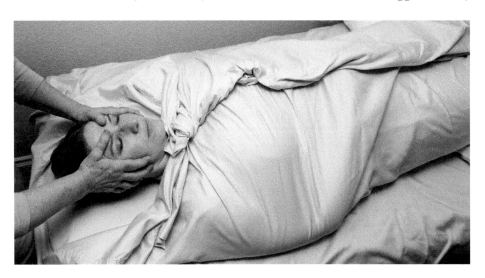

Figure 6.5
Energetic sealing at the end of a postpartum session. Create an energetic closing effect, cocooning the new mother within the massage sheets to rest at the end of a session.

- Breathing Enhancement (see Figure 4.11).

- Deep Tissue Sculpting – Lateral Pelvis, Paravertebrals, Upper Trapezius, Levator Scapulae, Scalenes, Pectoralis Major and Minor, Ribcage (see Figures 4.20, 4.23, 4.26–4.30 and 4.34).

- Foot Reflexive Zone Therapy (see Figure 4.13).

- Hip Infinity Mobilization (see Figures 4.44 and 4.45).

- Hip Joint Decompression (see Figure 4.46).

- Iliopsoas Structural Balancing (see Figure 6.14).

- Laminar Groove Inching (see Figure 4.19).

- Lumbosacral Joint Decompression (see Figure 4.22).

- Sacroiliac Joint Rhythmic Deep Tissue (see Figures 4.38 and 4.39).

- Spinal Seated Fascia Stretching (see Figure 6.15).

- Swedish Massage of Arms and Legs (see Chapter 4).

- Symphysis Pubis Rebalancing (see Figures 4.41 and 4.42).

- Upper Back, Neck and Arm Techniques (see Chapter 4).

- Uterine Fundal Massage (see Figure 6.16).

- Uterine Positioning (see Figure 6.17).

From the treatment room

Rhonda had muscle spasms in her sacral area that "took her breath away" during the last two months of pregnancy and continuing five weeks postpartum. She was afraid to traverse stairs and feared dropping the baby when the pain hit. After a requested infant massage lesson, I sculpted her hip muscles, focusing on tensor fasciae latae and piriformis. She experienced immediate relief for three days, then intermittent spasms returned. Our second session was similar, with additional work in her upper back and pelvis. She then became pain-free with confidence and normal mobility.

– Linda Hickey, therapist

Healing after Cesarean Birth

In the United States, one in three women gives birth by Cesarean section. In some cases, a Cesarean is necessary to protect the mother's and baby's health, but according to the ACOG and the Society for Maternal-Fetal Medicine, Cesarean birth remains too common. Cesareans carry risks of infection or blood clots, and many people experience longer recoveries and difficulty with future pregnancies. Cesareans can also cause problems for newborns, including breathing difficulties that require treatment in a **newborn intensive care unit (NICU)**. Long term, research shows that Cesareans can cause chronic pelvic pain in some people, and babies born by Cesarean are at increased risk of developing chronic childhood diseases like asthma and diabetes (Leapfrog Group 2019).

As such, a person who has given birth by Cesarean has even more need for therapeutic massage, as she is recovering from either planned or unplanned major abdominal surgery. Even a short postpartum massage can have a profound effect on her early postpartum experience. A 2018 study concluded that postpartum women need to remain alert and awake to provide effective care for and feeding of their newborns, develop positive bonds and return to optimal health. Further, researchers found that the use of massage as an integrative postoperative pain intervention reduced first-time mothers' pain, stress and opioid use and increased relaxation after unplanned Cesarean births (Simonelli et al. 2018). In another study, 20 minutes of hand and foot massage for women who birthed by elective Cesarean reduced both pain and anxiety immediately following massage, 60 and 90 minutes later (Irani et al. 2015).

General Guidelines

Research suggests that clients' acute response to massage therapy was equal to a dose of morphine in improving sleep and decreasing anxiety after gynecologic surgery (McRee et al. 2007). In addition to pain, numbness, edema and itching surrounding the incision, they may have severe abdominal and subscapular pain from intestinal gas and air trapped under the diaphragm during and after surgery. As you work, invite deep breaths and focus on stimulating peristalsis. You can also address initial and more painful uterine involution contractions with reflexive techniques until direct Cesarean Scar Massage techniques (see Figure 6.13) are appropriate, as detailed later in Chapter 6.

Let your client know that, when she is ready, early and thorough scar work can reduce pain and numbness, and prevent or reduce fascial shortening and adhesion formation that could lead to visceral dysfunction and other long-term postural imbalance. Scar tissue is inherently different from typical epidermal tissue, having more connective tissue and less epithelium, meaning that it is less flexible and lacks vascularity. As massage therapists, we palpate and massage scar tissue to increase pliability, generate heat, and create movement and sliding of the connective tissue layers (Whitridge 2019; Smith and Ryan 2016).

In Europe, physicians commonly prescribe lymphatic drainage for their postsurgical patients to enhance lymphatic circulation, immunological functioning and parasympathetic stimulation. With a planned Cesarean birth, pre-surgical lymphatic drainage can be beneficial, and post-surgical full-body lymphatic drainage techniques may facilitate postoperative recovery (Chikly and Chikly 1997). After a Cesarean birth, a mother may have pain when moving out of bed to stand and walk and when holding her baby, so use and show her the "log roll" technique discussed earlier in this chapter.

If her labor ended in an unplanned Cesarean, she may have extreme fatigue and, at some point, feel a need to finish the incomplete labor phases. As you address abdominal and pelvic recovery, encourage her to move, grunt and bear down if she expresses that urge. Be prepared for some emotional release and relief as well. Unplanned Cesarean birth is also associated with an increase in pain and stress compared with vaginal birth, so place special focus on these needs.

Surgical incisions and exhaustion after labor and surgery can impair a mother's ability to bond with, breastfeed and nurture her baby (Zanardo et al. 2010), so your extra support toward these goals is key. Emergent or unplanned Cesarean births can have negative effects on breastfeeding, especially during the initial postpartum period (Sakalis et al. 2013), so refer to the additional techniques in this chapter. Offer a referral to a lactation consultant who does home visits for after hospital discharge. With an emergency Cesarean, you may note guarding, protective tension throughout her torso and pelvis, hypervigilance and fear due to her sense of loss of control (see Chapter 7) (Simkin et al. 2018).

Cesarean scar tissue takes many months to fully heal, form and remodel in response to the functional stresses placed upon it. Aim to create a parasympathetic response in a comfortable atmosphere and to develop your client's trust. An essential step in that is to be sure that *she* is ready for scar work to begin. With her consent, you can then offer safe touch to the injured vulnerable area, without being invasive, as you apply the scar techniques detailed in this chapter's Technique Manual. Touch, explore, move and massage the tissues to feel for suppleness, fluidity and flexibility. Prompt and respond to your client's immediate, direct verbal feedback or non-verbal response to your touch. During the session, save time to have her practice the appropriate technique(s) and help her strategize a daily time to do it/them at home. Since changes often occur slowly, her self-care massage can speed the healing process. Also ask your client if she wants to track her scar tissue healing progression by taking a color photograph of the scar at each session. Document her pain level, sensation, adhesion quality and movements, other details of the scar, and any changes. This will create a complete reference to evaluate the effectiveness of your Cesarean scar massage and her self-care massage over time.

Your intention is to give a gentle stimulus to cause a local inflammatory response that will naturally lead to a remodeling cycle. The repeated nature of working with and massaging scar tissue helps condition it to touch and allows the mother to experience less pain and more mobility. People with Cesarean birth scars will likely be cautious, but when it comes to final remodeling, they must create functional pressures into and around the area of vulnerability for proper healing. The earlier we gently and conservatively massage her scar, the better the outcomes tend to be. Positive outcomes depend on expectations, so help her understand this process. Share how massaging the tissue can create a healing inflammatory response that can lead to more and steady remodeling (Whitridge 2019). ⊕

Specific Techniques

- Arms and Legs Swedish Massage Therapy (see Chapter 4).
- Breathing Enhancement (see Figure 4.11).
- Cesarean Scar Massage (see Figure 6.13).
- Foot Reflexive Zone Therapy (see Figure 4.13).

From the treatment room

As my client prepared for a planned Cesarean birth, we integrated lymphatic massage into her session three days before her birth. At our first postpartum session, we began the progression of Cesarean scar tissue massage techniques. Initially, she was nervous, but she experienced dramatic pain reduction and resolution of numbness at each session over three months. Coupled with her self-massage, she was proud of the scar's recovery and appearance. At one year postpartum, she showed her doctor and bragged about how beautiful her baby's "window to the world" was.

– Michele Kolakowski, therapist

What would you do?

Personally, you are a staunch supporter of natural childbirth, but your client arranged to have a scheduled Cesarean birth so that her out-of-state mother could be present and help her postpartum. In the first week postpartum, she calls for you to come to her home to help her with severe headache and back and abdominal pain. What postpartum complications should you be alert for? What further information do you need from her or her doctor? How will you manage your personal "I told you so" feelings regarding her choice of a Cesarean rather than vaginal birth?

Encouraging Abdominal and Pelvic Floor Healing

New mothers may be disappointed when they do not immediately resume their pre-pregnancy state, especially in the abdomen and pelvic floor. Although some may understand the possible pain relief to be gained from a postpartum massage, especially if they enjoyed prenatal massage, their diminished body image may have a profound effect on their openness to consider and willingness to receive massage therapy. With sensitive communication, you may be able to overcome that reluctance so that she reaps the abdominal and pelvic floor benefits of your work. Communicate your intention to "meet her where she is at" with her readiness to receive massage for her abdomen and pelvis. Explain the possible benefits but avoid pressuring her for consent; wait until she is ready (Figure 6.6).

General Guidelines

In the immediate postpartum time, your clients may feel such intense afterpains that they require the focus to be on deep relaxation and diaphragmatic breathing to help manage them. This is especially true during breastfeeding, while a mother is having pitocin administered after birth to manage and prevent **uterine atony**, and with multigravidas (Ricci 2017). The prevalence of diastasis recti is approximately 60 percent both during pregnancy and after childbirth; however, women with and without diastasis recti can report the same amount of lumbopelvic pain at 12 months postpartum (Sperstad et al. 2016). Consider the effect of diastasis recti on her spinal and pelvic alignment, postural dysfunction, and visceral and musculoskeletal pain. As taught in advanced hands-on workshops, help her determine whether she has diastasis recti and measure its extent. Remind her to roll onto one side when rising from a reclining position and to avoid jackknife-like movements, which further strain this vulnerable area. You can also guide her to resources for appropriate abdominal strengthening (Bowman 2016).

With the diastasis recti assessment completed, continue with comprehensive abdominal and pelvic treatment. Focus on reducing pain emanating from trigger points and hypertonicity in each abdominal muscle, iliopsoas,

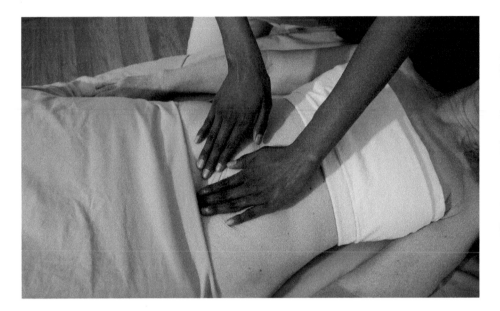

Figure 6.6
Encouraging abdominal healing. A new mother may be disappointed when she does not immediately resume her pre-pregnancy state. Communicate your intention to "meet her where she is at" with her readiness for massage for her abdomen and pelvis.

quadratus lumborum, spinal erectors, and other pelvic and posterior areas. Use connective tissue massage and skin rolling to functionally normalize abdominal skin and connective tissue. Continue to nourish her skin with your massage lubricants, and invite her to do the same at home with her favorite products. If she had a Cesarean birth, integrate Cesarean Scar Massage (see Figure 6.13), detailed in this chapter. Although stretchmarks eventually lose their redness, a reliable method to erase stretchmarks remains unconfirmed, so be wary of choosing products that make this claim.

For her pelvis, integrate reflexive work to facilitate perineal healing. Offer gentle, sustained compression to her pelvic bones to address the openness and instability. "Closing the bones" is a postpartum pelvic healing technique practiced in many traditional cultures. In Central and South America, midwives teach new mothers to wrap a rebozo around their lower abdomen and pelvis (Gonzalez and Vinaver 1997). Take advanced hands-on training that teaches you pelvic work to inguinal ligaments and all lower pelvic attachment sites, including the adductors, which may be sore and strained from labor and birth.

Other local comfort measures that she may take at home include placing ice packs on her perineum, gently spraying water over the pelvic floor with a peribottle, or submerging her pelvic floor in a medicinal sitz bath. Encourage her to strengthen her pelvic floor with appropriate exercise. Women who use pelvic floor muscle exercises fare

much better in their postpartum recovery (Ricci 2017). In 21 research trials involving 1,281 women with postpartum urinary stress incontinence, mothers who used pelvic floor muscle training were 17 times more likely to report cure or improvement and feeling more satisfied with their active treatment. Women also reported better continence-specific quality of life than women who did not use pelvic floor muscle training (Dumoulin et al. 2014).

Specific Techniques

- Abdominal Kneading, Vibration, Tapotement and Trigger Points (see Figures 6.9–6.12).
- Breathing Enhancement (see Figure 4.11).
- Foot Reflexive Zone Therapy (see Figure 4.13).
- Iliopsoas Structural Balancing (see Figure 6.14).
- Lateral Pelvis Deep Tissue Sculpting (see Figure 4.20).
- Lumbosacral Joint Decompression (see Figure 4.22).
- Sacroiliac Joint Rhythmic Deep Tissue (see Figures 4.38 and 4.39).
- Symphysis Pubis Rebalancing (see Figures 4.41 and 4.42).

Supporting Satisfying Feeding of the Newborn

Feeding her baby is often one of a new mother's greatest joys. If a mother is breastfeeding, she has a full-time job with that activity alone, and more with multiples. If she has a rough start with breastfeeding, as evidenced by sore, cracked or blistered nipples, or her breasts become engorged, she may be demoralized and discouraged. A rested, relaxed mother usually has an easier, more satisfying feeding experience.

General Guidelines

Support your client with compassion and be non-judgmental about her choices to breastfeed, bottle-feed or supplement her baby as she chooses. Use all your skills to support her relaxation and increase movement and flexibility in her neck, chest, torso and arms. Swedish massage with passive and active stretching of the pectoral girdle can help, particularly when it addresses the remnants of pregnancy's anterior shoulder rotation with stretching and deep tissue sculpting to pectoralis major and minor. Ribcage myofascial release adjacent to breast tissue with cervical and thoracic spine mobilizations also brings relief. Lymphatic drainage techniques for the upper body can be especially helpful with engorgement and mastitis, as is teaching self-lymphatic massage. Encourage regularly switching arms for feedings and periodically lifting and straightening out the neck.

Whatever feeding positions the new mother adopts throughout her day – reclining, sidelying, seated or standing – assist her in using ideal body mechanics. Show her how pillows to support her neck, arms, back and legs help feeding to be a relaxing experience that minimizes strain on these areas. Show her how looking behind each shoulder periodically while she nurses makes the opposite, balancing and stretching movement. When she is not holding the baby, shoulder rolls, arm stretches, and imagining the area behind her ears lifting skyward help to relax and stretch these muscles (see Figure 4.15). Use reflexive techniques to address both the breast and the lymphatic zones on her feet.

Facilitating a satisfying feeding experience can be greatly enhanced with therapeutic breast massage. Review and comply with your local laws governing the provision of therapeutic breast massage (see "Points of view: Breast massage"). Consider taking a breast massage course to expand your skills and knowledge, and have a handheld breast model to demonstrate breast

massage techniques to your clients. Massage to the breast tissue may improve overall breast health (Simkin et al. 2018). Therapeutic breast massage in lactation is helpful for reducing the acute breast pain associated with milk stasis. Mothers find it helpful both in the immediate term and for managing potential recurring problems (Witt et al. 2015; Bolman 2020). 🌐

During the postpartum time, milk expression or pumping during and after feedings, integrating breast massage and warm compresses may enhance her experience (King et al. 2019). Breast massage, warm showers and heat can ease engorgement, help prevent blockage of milk ducts and help avoid mastitis (Simkin et al. 2018). With mastitis, cool compresses or towels wrapped around each breast can decrease pain and reduce inflammation as the breasts heal. If breastfeeding is problematic, refer your client for advice from a lactation consultant or her local La Leche League. If she is bottle-feeding, breast massage may be a very important self-care practice to

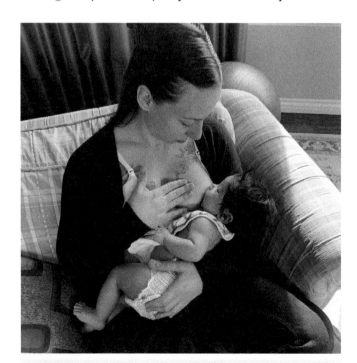

Figure 6.7
Therapeutic self-breast massage. Teach your client to use her fingertips to make slow, rhythmic, circular motions moving over the most peripheral breast tissue and toward, but avoiding, the areola and nipple.

help compensate for the loss of breastfeeding's benefits for long-term mammary health (Curties 2011).

Therapeutic breast self-massage in lactation generally involves teaching the client to use her fingertips to make slow, rhythmic, circular motions beginning around the breast and moving over the breast tissue and underlying structures toward, but avoiding, the areola and nipple (Figure 6.7). Additionally, during feedings, mothers can use pressure and rhythmic compression on each breast to enhance their milk flow. This technique also encourages babies to eat more, especially those who are gaining weight slowly, and entices sleepy ones to continue feeding. It also helps relieve breast fullness and empty plugged ducts during a feeding (Simkin et al. 2018; Bolman 2020).

Points of view: Breast massage

Debra Curties (2011) highlights the many benefits of therapeutic breast massage for general breast health and specific conditions affecting the breast tissue. During breastfeeding and weaning, lactation consultants offer and teach a technique called "therapeutic breast massage in lactation" to quickly resolve breast pain, engorgement, plugged ducts, mastitis and discomfort with weaning (Bolman 2020). Some professionals disagree as to whether massage therapists should perform breast massage. Long-standing debates continue, with the arguments against therapists working in this highly sensitive and sometimes sexualized area of the body including: legal restrictions; heightened possibility of misunderstood intention; crossing of professional boundaries; and injury due to lack of or inadequate training (Polseno-Crawford 1998). Some educators advocate for offering therapeutic breast massage with written consent as a session option due to its many benefits. They also highlight the need for therapists to have improved instruction in breast anatomy and physiology, as well as technical skill. It is essential to learn about clear client communication, informed consent, possible psychological and emotional reactions, and precise draping (Fitch 1998).

From the treatment room

As a self-employed massage therapist, I had planned to return to work when my baby was six weeks old. With my career, the added strain of holding my baby proved too much, and I developed tendonitis. I visited my massage therapist for deep tissue sculpting to my forearms, wrists and hands. Only one session was necessary to comfortably get back to work, and breastfeeding became easier as well.

– **Karen Salas,** therapist

Promoting Sleep and Rest

The postpartum time usually requires new mothers to adapt to new sleep rhythms with their new responsibilities and routines caring for and feeding their babies (Goyal et al. 2009). Of relevance to us as pre- and perinatal specialists, postpartum mothers identify insufficient sleep as a primary stressor during their early postpartum time (Hung 2006). Having adequate sleep and rest is essential because shorter sleep time, more sleep disturbances and great fatigue are associated with depressive symptoms in mothers (Parfitt and Ayers 2014). In one study, new mothers received a single 20-minute back massage session at the same time each evening for five consecutive days. Sessions were administered by a certified massage therapist, and this simple intervention significantly improved the quality of mothers' sleep (Ko and Lee 2016). Research shows that mothers with fragmented sleep – less than four hours at night and less than a one-hour daytime nap – have an increased risk for depression at three months postpartum. Assuring at least a four-hour stretch of sleep was more of a factor than the baby's temperament in decreasing the likelihood of postpartum depression (Goyal et al. 2009).

General Guidelines

Calming any sympathetic arousal may help reduce the mother's anxiety, help her sleep more deeply and, as a result, also help her heal quicker. Observe her recognition of her need for sleep and rest, and how realistic she is about her expectations. If she would like your input, suggestions to promote sleep and rest include napping while the infant is sleeping, and asking a family member or friend, or hiring a postpartum doula or night nanny, to care for the baby some nights. For a breastfeeding mother, the caretaker can "room-service" her baby to her during the night as needed, to maximize sleep durations. Cutting back on visitors, except for those who help with household tasks and care of older children, while also reducing participation in activities outside the home, conserves her energy and allows more rest. For the entire family's well-being, daily routines can be reviewed and clustered to conserve energy and promote rest (Ricci 2017). Review this chapter's suggestions for integrating baby in massage sessions. Consider how a postpartum massage session with baby present to breastfeed, followed by a restful nap for both, or a session with time to herself to sleep deeply on the massage table can accomplish this clustering goal.

Specific Techniques

- Arms and Legs Swedish Massage Therapy (see Chapter 4).

- Autonomic Sedation Sequence 3–1–1 (see Figures 4.8–4.10).

- Breathing Enhancement (see Figure 4.11).

- Cervical Transverse Rocking (see Figure 4.12).

- Foot Reflexive Zone Therapy (see Figure 4.13).

- Grounding Hold (see Figure 5.11).

- Occiput Traction and Rocking (see Figure 4.14).

- Pectoral Girdle Mobilizations (see Figures 4.24 and 4.25).

- Pelvic Girdle Decompressions (see Figure 4.33).

- Spinal Rocking (see Figure 4.40).

Preventing Strain and Pain from Childcare Activities

Infant care is usually love-filled, but can also feel surprisingly strenuous, tedious and mundane, especially to a mother who was previously very active. Diapering, consoling, lifting, carrying and interacting with her baby often involve repeated forward-bending motions and sustained positions throughout each day. A mother spends many hours side-bending and forward-tilting her neck and head, with mostly static use of her upper back muscles, that creates an overuse syndrome that we call "new mother's neck" (Figure 6.8). Further, to securely hold her baby in her arms while seated or standing, a mother sustains her shoulders in lateral and medial rotations, arms in flexion and rotations, with wrists flexed and laterally or medially deviated and with hand and finger muscles flexed, for long hours. A first-time mother who is learning

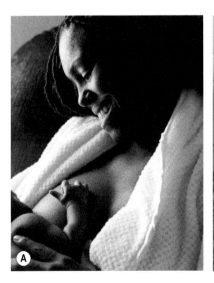
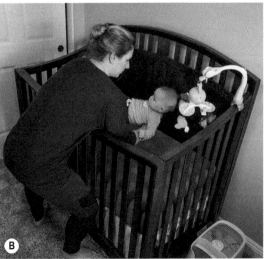

Figure 6.8A–B
Strain and pain from childcare activities. **(A)** "New mother's neck"; **(B)** forward-bending motions.

to breastfeed may initially lean forward and side-bend her torso away from the needed support to bring her breast to her baby. A mother who bottle-feeds may be holding the bottle in a way that stresses her other arm and hand. As a baby develops more head control and motor skills, a mother's body mechanics evolve to include more lifting, putting down, twisting and balancing her active, growing baby on her hip.

The legacy of pregnancy's increased risk of carpal tunnel syndrome can be debilitating, physically and emotionally, for a mother whose gestational carpal tunnel syndrome continues into the postpartum period. Her activity-related and nocturnal hand paresthesia is more likely to be bilateral when compared to the non-pregnant population (King et al. 2019). Her confidence and ability to securely pick up, hold and feed her baby can be severely compromised. And when she does use her hands, it can elicit pain. New research shows that gestational carpal tunnel syndrome can be persistent in women post-pregnancy. Approximately 28 percent of previously asymptomatic women have gestational carpal tunnel syndrome in pregnancy's third trimester. During the first six weeks postpartum, 85 percent of women gradually experience resolution of symptoms. For the remaining 15 percent, it is likely that their symptoms will persist and worsen with time. At 12 months, approximately 5 percent have persistent symptoms that are more severe than their initial ones during their third trimester. Women from minority ethnicities, with higher body mass index, history of smoking and pre-eclampsia, are at increased risk (Mora et al. 2019).

General Guidelines

Postpartum massage therapy can reduce the likelihood of excessive musculoskeletal strain and pain distracting from motherhood's pleasures. Research also shows us that massage therapy is beneficial for many conditions that postpartum people experience, including headaches, back pain, carpal tunnel syndrome and de Quervain's syndrome (Zulak 2018). Your expertise in ideal body mechanics can also assist tremendously in preventing infant care strain and pain. Focus on reducing strain and pain related to the most common infant care tasks as they evolve across the postpartum time. If you are trained in functional assessment, use those tests to make your technique choices more targeted (Zulak 2018).

Most postpartum sessions need to include significant time to reduce upper body strain from childcare activities. The new mother, her partner and other caregivers benefit from lessons in how to lift, hold, carry and bend over. Consider teaching her prenatally, if possible, so she gets off to a good start immediately after birth. Instruct her to lift her baby just as anything should be lifted – protect her spine by bending her knees and engaging her core with a gentle, sustained transversus abdominis contraction; lift from her legs by straightening the knees rather than lifting with the back or pectoral girdle (Figure 6.8B); and when possible, avoid lifting and twisting the spine simultaneously, especially with a car seat's additional weight. Guide her to carry her baby close to her center of gravity and hold under her baby's pelvis whenever possible. This is better for baby's developing motor skills and engages baby's reflexes to be upright, thereby strengthening the torso musculature. By not lifting under her baby's arms, she also avoids wrist and thumb strain that leads to de Quervain's syndrome (Creager 2001).

Give guidance to redirect the common carrying tendency to extend the spine posteriorly, beyond its normal neutral position, as this can painfully compress the lumbar spine and contract back extensors and carrying muscles of the shoulders. If she cannot maintain spinal and pelvic alignment, facing the baby outward at waist level is a good alternative. One of her forearms supports the baby under the pelvis, while the baby leans forward with the tummy on mom's other forearm. The "football hold," with the baby prone and draped over her forearm, is another possibility. Both of these carries have the additional advantage of tummy time – an alternate worldview that is great for baby's development (Creager 2001). Remind her to drop her carrying shoulder to a more relaxed level. Show her alternatives to holding her baby in her arms, such as baby wearing, using ergonomically designed, arms-free baby slings and carriers. The benefits of baby wearing may include a happier and healthy baby, a more confident parent, comfort and convenience, as well as facilitating other potential loving caregivers to give the mother a rest (Blois 2016). Consider taking a baby-wearing workshop to expand your awareness of the options to better serve your clients.

As her baby grows, note any tendency to place the baby on one hip or carry laterally in a baby sling or carrier.

While this provides additional support for the baby, it contributes to excess hypertonicity and trigger points in the mother's quadratus lumborum, erector spinae and oblique abdominals. Remember that, during feedings, mothers need back support, seats with low arms, and sufficient pillows supporting the baby to relax and align her neck, back, shoulders, wrists and hands. If she has lingering edema in her arms and hands from pregnancy or birth, integrate Chapter 4's techniques for her arms, including lymphatic drainage. With carpal tunnel symptoms, blend Swedish, passive wrist movements, cross-fiber friction and sculpting into your session. Consider shorter, more frequent sessions, such as 30-minute massages two times per week. Remember that research suggests that massage therapy works on a cellular level to decrease inflammation and increase the energy-producing organelles of the muscle (Turchaninov 2011) – a viable alternative to carpal tunnel surgery.

As she arrives at and departs from sessions, offer body mechanics tips for getting her baby in and out of the car, using a stroller, and carrying a heavy car seat and diaper bag. Also encourage her to check her home ergonomics by choosing appropriate heights for her baby furniture, stroller and bath, which can all affect musculoskeletal comfort and pain. Focus deep tissue sculpting, passive movement, stretching and trigger point therapy on the sternocleidomastoid, suboccipitals, splenius capitis, levator scapulae, supraspinatus, infraspinatus, subscapularis, teres major and minor, rhomboids and quadratus lumborum. Then work with the trapezius, latissimus dorsi and erector spinae group. Remember to also address the pelvis with attention to the sacroiliac joints, which distribute weight from the upper body down through the legs. Reduce strained and painful areas by stimulating the related reflexive zones of the feet for the back, neck and shoulders.

Specific Techniques

- Arms and Legs Swedish Massage Therapy (see Chapter 4).
- Autonomic Sedation Sequence 3–1–1 (see Figures 4.8–4.10).
- Foot Reflexive Zone Therapy (see Figure 4.13).
- Iliopsoas Structural Balancing (see Figure 6.14).
- Laminar Groove Inching (see Figure 4.19).
- Lateral Pelvis Deep Tissue Sculpting (see Figure 4.20).
- Lumbosacral Joint Decompression (see Figure 4.22).
- Paravertebral Deep Tissue Sculpting (see Figure 4.23).
- Pectoral Girdle Cross-fiber Friction (see Figure 4.31).
- Pectoral Girdle Deep Tissue Sculpting (see Figures 4.26–4.30).
- Pectoral Girdle Mobilizations (see Figures 4.24 and 4.25).
- Ribcage Deep Tissue Sculpting and Trigger Points (see Figures 4.34 and 4.35).
- Sacroiliac Joint Rhythmic Deep Tissue (see Figures 4.38 and 4.39).
- Spinal Seated Fascia Stretching (see Figure 6.15).
- Structural Balancing Education (see Figures 4.15–4.17).
- Symphysis Pubis Rebalancing (see Figures 4.41 and 4.42).

From the treatment room

Hillary had her second baby by Cesarean. Through her third trimester, we addressed her occasional hip pain and problematic left pectoral girdle from carrying her three-year-old. To begin her first postpartum massage, we worked with her standing alignment and alternative ways to carry her baby to protect her recovering left shoulder and back. With her in sidelying position, I integrated rhythmic passive movements, positional releases, deep tissue sculpting and cross-fiber friction to her pectoral girdle and paravertebral muscles. After extinguishing a trigger point, she reported her pain completely resolved. With gentle abdominal and foot work, we finished this session and made a plan to begin Cesarean scar work at our next session.

– Carole Osborne, therapist

Reducing Residual Pain and Promoting Structural Integrity

Pregnancy-related pelvic girdle pain resolves in the majority of women within the three months after birth. By the first year after birth, only 1 to 2 percent of women report persistence of pain, and these are usually women who have had more severe symptoms during their pregnancies (CPWHC 2014). Factors that make a woman more likely to have postpartum back and residual pregnancy-related pelvic girdle pain are a history of back pain, elevated maternal weight, multiples and the length of birth's pushing stage. Onset of symptoms can potentially begin postpartum after awkward, sustained labor positions that can result in mild to severe lumbar, hip, sacral or pelvic pain. A woman's pelvic size and shape and their relationship to her baby's head size and position also affect the degree of pelvic ligament strain during birth (King et al. 2019). With longer-duration labors, women are at greater risk of being symptomatic at 18 months postpartum. For subsequent pregnancies, there is a high risk of recurrence of pregnancy-related pelvic girdle pain; however, this may not be as severe when treated early and well managed (CPWHC 2014). Almost as many postpartum women develop pregnancy-related pelvic girdle pain as develop it during the second trimester (Howard 2000).

In addition to reducing residual pregnancy-related pelvic girdle and back pain, we want to promote structural integrity and reorganization of functional movement patterns. The iliopsoas muscles are pelvic stabilizers, the primary hip flexors affecting the torso and back, and are integrally involved in gait. Ideally, one iliopsoas initiates leg flexion on the pelvis, followed by rectus femoris and other quadriceps muscles' contractions. Simultaneously, the weight-bearing and contralateral iliopsoas stabilizes the pelvis to avoid excess pelvic rotation and tilting. During pregnancy, these two iliopsoas functions adapt as the continuous anterior uterine weight contributes to disuse of the usual iliopsoas functions for walking. Instead, the hip joints begin to externally rotate, and the hip abductors, rather than the iliopsoas, initiate each step. The resulting "duck walk" or "sailor's roll" is characteristic of both third trimester and postpartum, with hypertonic iliopsoas muscles prone to spasm.

General Guidelines

For relieving pelvic and back pain and for promoting structural integrity, work initially on your client's back with broad, sweeping, superficial strokes, progressing to deeper, more specific work. Use craniosacral and connective tissue techniques as well. If she had an epidural or a spinal, you many need to pay specific attention to the administration site, usually at L3 or L4, during the first week postpartum. It is frequently tender, eliciting a psychological protectiveness that immobility and positioning during administration may have caused. Rarely, she may experience spinal headache, but you can position her with feet and hips slightly higher than her head to help alleviate this. If pain at the epidural or spinal site does not resolve, refer her to her physician. Deep tissue sculpting and postural guidance facilitate healing of strained pelvic joints, and release of chronic muscular tension and of shortened posterior fascial planes.

Pay particular attention to the sacroiliac, lumbosacral, symphysis pubis, sacrococcygeal and coccygeal joints. If she had a prior or birth injury, these joints may take some time to heal and require treatment by a women's health physical therapist (Ricci 2017). Studies indicate that strengthening exercise for the smaller pelvic girdle and abdominal muscles, followed by the global muscles, is more effective for reducing pregnancy-related pelvic girdle pain (Bowman 2016; Stuge et al. 2006). Likewise, you should first balance the gluteus medius and other hip movers, quadratus lumborum and iliopsoas. Next, focus on the erector spinae, lumbodorsal fascia, latissimus dorsi, gluteus maximus and minimus, piriformis and tensor fasciae latae. In addition to the iliopsoas, remember that abdominal muscles harbor trigger points that refer to the mid and low back and the sacrum. Extinguish trigger points using neuromuscular therapy, rhythmic and positional movement techniques, and deep tissue methods (see Figure 6.12). If you are trained in functional assessment, use those tests to make your technique choices more targeted (Zulak 2018).

Use imagery and sensitive deep tissue work to guide her in regaining iliopsoas use, resolving hypertonicity or hypotonicity, and increasing her awareness of this important postural muscle. The iliopsoas may also benefit from stretching. Some iliopsoas strengthening occurs when the postpartum woman repeatedly reduces lumbar lordosis by tilting her pelvis posteriorly, using the iliopsoas rather than the gluteal, leg or upper abdominal muscles. As in pregnancy, active and passive pelvic tilts also help relieve lumbar pain. Guide her standing, seated and carrying postpartum postures to re-establish effortless, graceful alignment and to reduce musculoskeletal strain. Correct the typical anterior-tilting pelvis and increased lumbar curvature with your postural guidance. If her uterus is misplaced, consider possible uterine ligament pain referrals into her back and pelvis (see Figure 1.7) while inviting ideal repositioning of the uterus. Address head, spinal and pelvic zone therapy reflexes on her feet. If your client reports symptoms of pregnancy-related pelvic girdle pain syndrome, or difficulty urinating or controlling bowel movements and gas, or pelvic pain during bowel movements or intercourse, or **coccygodynia**, refer her to a women's health physical therapist.

Specific Techniques

- Abdominal Kneading, Vibration, Tapotement and Trigger Points (see Figures 6.9–6.12).

- Breathing Enhancement (see Figure 4.11).

- Foot Reflexive Zone Therapy (see Figure 4.13).

- Hip Infinity Mobilization (see Figures 4.44 and 4.45).

- Hip Joint Decompression (see Figure 4.46).

- Iliopsoas Structural Balancing (see Figure 6.14).

- Laminar Groove Inching (see Figure 4.19).

- Lateral Pelvis Deep Tissue Sculpting (see Figure 4.20).

- Lumbar Lengthening (see Figure 4.21).

- Lumbosacral Joint Decompression (see Figure 4.22).

- Paravertebral Deep Tissue Sculpting (see Figure 4.23).

- Pectoral Girdle Cross-fiber Friction (see Figure 4.31).

- Pectoral Girdle Deep Tissue Sculpting (see Figures 4.26–4.30).

- Pectoral Girdle Mobilizations (see Figures 4.24 and 4.25).

- Pelvic Alignment Education (see Figure 4.32).

- Ribcage Deep Tissue Sculpting and Trigger Points (see Figures 4.34 and 4.35).

- Sacroiliac Joint Rhythmic Deep Tissue (see Figures 4.38 and 4.39).

- Symphysis Pubis Rebalancing (see Figures 4.41 and 4.42).

- Spinal Seated Fascia Stretching (see Figure 6.15).

- Uterine Positioning (see Figure 6.17).

Reminder

The iliopsoas needs considerable postpartum attention to restore and improve its function as a major postural muscle.

From the treatment room

A new client who was 11 days postpartum greeted me at the door bent over and walking like she had been "in the saddle" for months. I immediately taught her a pelvic tilt without clenching the gluteals and abdominals, as she had been doing. Hip, abdominal and low-back deep work were gratefully received, but more than that, the information I had to share was like a lifeline to her. She had been desperately asking every woman she knew "why do I hurt so much, and why can't I stand straight?" She had enough college anatomy training to understand my descriptions, and, when I isolated the psoas muscle, it was like a light going on for her. She got off my table standing 100 percent better, but it wasn't just my work. It was the relief that she now understood what was going on, and she had a tool to deal with it.

– Deborah Donaldson, therapist

The Later Months and Years of Postpartum Massage Therapy

A doctor or a midwife's release from maternity care signals the end of puerperium medical care; however, most women continue their postpartum recovery long after. An appropriate truism is that it takes 40 weeks to make a baby and at least equal time to recover after pregnancy and birth. That is much longer than the traditional short-term view of the postpartum period as lasting for six weeks or approximately "40 days," as some cultures identify postpartum. During these times, your massage therapy sessions can include some of your previous approaches and other modalities. For restoring and improving structural integration and function, this is an excellent time to enjoy a complete series of Rolfing, Structural Integration, Aston Patterning or other structural balancing work. Pelvic ligaments can be slow to recover. Use cross-fiber friction throughout the posterior pelvic ligaments if your client has chronic pelvic pain. Over these months, she can gradually regain muscle strength in her abdominals, iliopsoas and pelvic floor – the core of postural integrity. If she has not already, encourage her to begin a progressive sequence of exercise targeted to these key postural muscles. "Once a mother, always a mother" rings true in some women's bodies. Although their "babies" might be 30 years old or more, women often benefit from sessions of postpartum massage techniques. Ask when symptoms first began, and choose techniques designed to address any long-standing issues.

Precautions for Postpartum Massage Therapy

These are summarized in Box 6.1.

> **Box 6.1**
> Precautions for postpartum massage therapy
>
> - In the early postpartum days, closely observe and communicate with your client to reach her therapeutic relaxation and pleasure-pain level goals. Adapt your pressure and techniques accordingly when she is taking pain medication that may alter her perception of your work, or if she is experiencing a medication side effect such as headache, backache or fever. Keep your eyes open for any possible intravenous puncture, epidural, spinal anesthesia or wound sites and adapt your techniques accordingly.
> - Continue all prenatal precautions with massage therapy for the legs and pelvis for eight to 10 weeks postpartum, including lower abdomen and inguinal areas as thrombi are common in the femoral and iliac veins. The more sedentary the new mother is, the more prudent this more conservative precaution becomes. Those at higher risk are those mothers who had Cesarean births, hysterectomy and tubal ligation.
> - For abdominal techniques, the client will be more comfortable with an empty bladder. With diastasis recti, avoid laterally directed pressure techniques on the area of separation until it is healed. Maintain a trusting connection by making eye contact with her face as she may feel vulnerable, self-conscious and/or emotional.
> - If she experiences an emotional release, slow and stop your technique while you check in with her and actively listen. Normalize her emotional release's expression and validate her feelings.
> - After Cesarean birth, perform abdominal massage techniques after physician's postoperative consent for massage therapy. Thereafter, use impeccable hand hygiene and modify techniques to avoid unintentional hand placement or movement on the incision (see Figure 6.13).

From the treatment room

An active 54-year-old woman suffering from headaches and back pain arrived at my office. Her pain started in her twenties with sporadic headaches after the birth of her two sons, born by Cesarean and now ages 28 and 30. I asked for and received her consent to abdominal massage – her first ever – and to explore this possible connection with her pain, in addition to massaging her back. Her rectus abdominis and iliopsoas were riddled with trigger points that replicated her exact pain. I observed that her Cesarean scar was puckered and deformed with thick adhesions. I pulled up my chair table-side, asked and received her permission to place her hand with mine over her Cesarean scar. Tears welled up in her eyes as she remembered her births. I met her expressed fear, sadness and anger with active listening and diaphragmatic breathing. After her emotional release, she smiled and said, "I never told anyone this." I thanked her for trusting me to share this and finished the massage at her feet, stimulating the reflexive zones for headaches and her entire spine. When I checked in with her by phone two days later, she reported her back pain and headache were gone.

– **Michele Kolakowski,** therapist

This section includes detailed instruction in how to perform selected techniques for postpartum clients. Techniques are alphabetized, rather than organized according to a specified sequence, so that you can be creatively flexible and responsive to your client. Note that the online resources do contain a few specific sequences that may offer you a basic session structure until you gain enough experience to confidently design more individualized sessions. 🌐

Each of the techniques is described as follows:

Hints

Tips for ease, variety or effectiveness. These are pointers for your own body use and ways to adapt the technique, including suggested alternatives for creating the same effect.

Precautions

Safety adaptations and guidelines. Certain techniques require specific guidance – in addition to that in Chapter 2 – so that they are not only effective but also safe.

[Name of Technique]

Intentions

The outcomes or purposes of the procedure. Understanding this underlying rationale will enable you to be more anatomically precise; to create safe and individualized sessions; and to talk with your clients and alleviate any concerns about your work.

Procedure

Precise instructions in how to accomplish the technique (written with a specified client position in mind, if relevant), usually accompanied by a photo of a client and a therapist correctly performing the technique. (Note that, for clarity's sake, the client is usually clothed, rather than professionally draped as shown in Chapter 3.) Most figures have some of the following to convey further details:

- an overlay with the anatomical structures involved
- solid red arrows indicating the vector or direction of your pressure
- dashed red arrows marking the total area to apply the technique
- white arrows showing movement you request of your client
- red dots identifying typical trigger points to locate and extinguish
- an indication of whether to use a professional massage therapy lubricant.

These instructions use the following terms:

- Outside hand = your hand farthest from the table when you are standing beside it. Which hand is "outside" depends on if you are facing the head or the foot end.
- Inside hand = your hand between your torso and the table when you are standing beside it. Which hand is "inside" depends on if you are facing the head or the foot end.
- Ceiling side = the side of your client's body that is highest from the table and usually most available to work with when she is sidelying.
- Table side = the side your client is lying on.

Abdominal Kneading, Vibration, Tapotement and Trigger Points

Intentions

To facilitate relaxation; to lubricate the abdominal skin, reducing dryness and itchiness; to gently mobilize torso joints; to reduce abdominal, pelvic and leg edema; to promote visceral healing through normalization of organ spacing; to reduce abdominal gas and constipation by stimulating peristalsis; to stimulate abdominal muscle tone; to reduce referred pain in the abdomen and back by locating and extinguishing trigger points in all abdominal musculature; to facilitate connection to her postpartum abdomen without the baby and a healthy postpartum body image.

Procedure

All of these abdominal procedures are best performed in supine position with the client's knees bolstered.

Kneading (Figure 6.9)

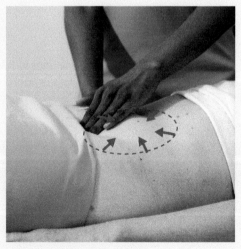

Figure 6.9   Abdominal Kneading.

1. Stand at pelvic level, facing the client's head.
2. Use the heels of your hand and/or fingertips to knead the abdomen in a clockwise direction with peristalsis.
3. Focus on the lateral sides of the abdomen, scooping toward the midline and umbilicus, including the large intestine's splenic and hepatic flexures just inferior to the anterior ribcage.

Vibration (Figure 6.10)

1. Stand facing the client's abdomen, with or without lubrication; place the palm of your non-dominant hand on the abdomen and your dominant hand directly on top.
2. As the client exhales, gradually press into her abdomen and then initiate a vibration movement from your shoulders, creating a deep, high-frequency vibration that penetrates deeply and posteriorly to the spine.
3. Vibrate for 5 to 10 seconds as she completes her exhalation, and then release pressure when she inhales again.
4. Repeat two more times.
5. Relocate your hands and repeat until you have vibrated over her entire abdomen.

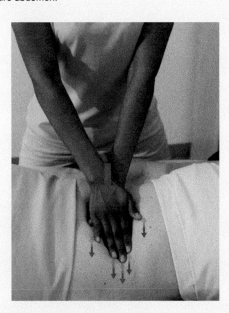

Figure 6.10 Abdominal Vibration.

Tapotement (Figure 6.11)

1. Maintaining loose wrists, tap gently with the fingertips or lateral edge of the fifth metacarpal bones on the rectus abdominis, internal and external obliques and transversus abdominis muscles from the attachments below the ribcage and inferior to just above the pubic bones to activate the proprioceptors and tone muscles.
2. Repeat for 10 to 20 seconds until you feel the abdominal muscles reflexively tightening under your tapotement.

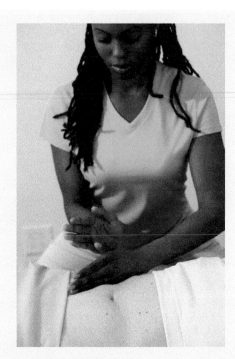

Figure 6.11 Abdominal Tapotement.

Trigger Points (Figure 6.12)

1. Stand at pelvic level, facing the client's head.
2. Ask the client to report any tenderness or painful sensations in the anterior or posterior torso as you friction the abdominal muscle attachments.

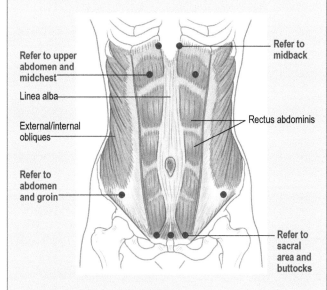

Figure 6.12 Abdominal Trigger Points.

3. Use several fingertips to create a sawing motion to check the locations indicated in Figure 6.12, including:

   - 1 to 2 inches (2.5 to 5 cm) below the xiphoid process
   - Superficial to ribs 8 to 12 and just below the costal border of the ribs
   - Medial to the anterior superior iliac spine
   - Along the anterior pubic bone, avoiding the symphysis.

4. Identify any areas eliciting a jump response from the client.

5. Release your pressure on the point creating that response until the pain is no more intense than pleasure on the borderline of pain.

6. Confirm that any pain in the soft abdomen, off the bony attachments, is actually a trigger point and not organ tenderness. Check by having the client lift her head and/or torso, activating the muscle group. If pain increases with contraction, this is a trigger point, so proceed with extinguishing it. If pain decreases, the pain is likely in an organ and will not respond to trigger point treatment, so release the pressure.

7. Request client feedback on changes in pain intensity. Once pain has dissipated, continue to compress for 7 to 20 seconds.

8. If possible, stretch the trigger point area for 30 to 60 seconds or perform localized fanning strokes over the trigger point.

9. Remember that most abdominal trigger points refer within the abdomen, except those in the rectus abdominis attachments, which refer to the mid-back, sacrum and buttocks.

Precautions

Consult earlier discussions in this chapter to determine when you can safely begin to work on the postpartum abdomen.

Cesarean Scar Massage

Intentions

To create healthy, functional scar tissue by preventing and/or reducing adhesions that may have formed; to reduce edema, support healing, reduce pain and numbness at and around the incision; when performed on older scars, to reduce dysfunctional postural, visceral or other imbalances.

Procedure

Best performed in supine position with the client's knees bolstered to comfort.

1. Review Cesarean birth incisions (see Figure 5.9) to understand the different possible incisions below the skin and through each layer of tissue, to make your work most effective. Offer a series of techniques to the client over a number of sessions, spanning weeks, months or years, at her desired pace.

2. Initially, have the client place her hands on the bandages over "baby's window to the world," directing warmth and healing intention to the area (Figure 6.13A).

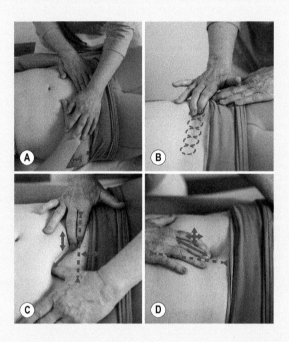

Figure 6.13A–D   Cesarean Scar Massage.

3. For the early weeks after Cesarean birth, teach her to move localized edema above and below the scar toward the inguinal nodes with feather-light fingertip vibration, working from the midline out laterally, one side at a time. Several weeks later, after the skin is healed and closed, place your hands lightly and use warmth, intention and vibration to the level of client tolerance physically and emotionally, creating pleasure and not pain.

4. Once she has post-surgical consent for massage therapy, begin using light fingertip circling with no lubrication to gently move the visible scar on the skin on the underlying superficial fascia. Add pressure to progress to gentle movement of the scar and superficial fascia on the muscle layers beneath.

5. Locate any immobile adhered areas with circling movements (Figure 6.13B). With fingertips and no lubrication, create a tensile stretch on the scar tissue at its maximum comfortable motion, holding each stretch for 30 seconds minimum. Repeat this in multiple directions – horizontal, vertical and diagonal. Note that it is common for one side of the scar to be more painful, numb or adhered than the other. In areas of numbness, move tissue more conservatively until sensation slowly returns over several days and weeks. Dissolvable sutures can sometimes be palpated for several weeks as they dissolve, especially on lateral ends of the incision.

6. Once the superficial layers are mobile, progress to deeper muscular, fascial and visceral levels. Circle from the center of scar, moving up toward the umbilicus, holding a tensile stretch on any immobile area for at least 30 seconds (Figure 6.13C). Remember, most Cesarean births use a horizontal "bikini-line" incision at the skin, as illustrated in Figure 5.9, with the muscles opened vertically at the linea alba as high as the umbilicus and a horizontal incision at the uterus.

7. Return to a superficial level to apply fingertip cross-fiber friction. At each adhesion, compress the scar tissue against the underlying tissue and perform brisk stationary friction for three to five minutes (Figure 6.13D).

8. Moving superiorly from the midline, as in the step above, perform friction to the deeper fascial layers.

9. Using your thumbs and fingertips, lift the scar and gently roll the skin in one long stroke or in sections and in all directions. At adhesions, hold a tensile stretch, lifting the tissue, and gently and slowly move in all directions.

Hints

- Before securing the client's permission, discuss the benefits of these techniques prenatally if she is planning a Cesarean birth or as soon as possible postpartum.

- Demonstrate the next appropriate technique in the progression on your arm or her arm and practice getting her feedback on her comfort.

- Teach the client each technique to continue at home. She may choose to use a scar oil product to help improve the color and appearance of the skin. The darker pigmentation of the incision typically fades by approximately one year postpartum.

Precautions

- Steps 2 and 3 can be performed immediately after birth. Steps 4 to 9 should be performed only after the physician gives postoperative consent for massage therapy.

Foot Reflexive Zone Therapy

Intentions

To create parasympathetic stimulation that promotes systemic relaxation; to promote metabolic functioning and reflexively facilitate postpartum recovery, especially musculoskeletal strain and organic dysfunctions.

Procedure

This procedure may be performed in any position.

1. Use the side of the thumb and/or finger to create a bone-to-bone pressure into the foot. Travel with tiny, overlapping movements, compressing the skin and undifferentiated nerves of the foot against the underlying bones (see Figure 4.13).

2. Rhythmically inch along and across specific reflex areas (zone) or over the entire foot. Press, rather than rub, to achieve the desired effect. Imagine that your finger or thumb moves like a tiny inchworm.

3. Repeat three times in each reflex zone with specific focus on the following postpartum complaint areas: musculoskeletal strain in the neck, upper back, spine, pelvis and sacrum; headache; diaphragm; constipation; hemorrhoids; uterine afterpains; bladder pain; pelvic pain; breast pain. ⊕

Hints

- Choose a seated or standing position as you work to maximize your most efficient, aligned body mechanics.

- Offer warmth to her feet with hydrotherapy, hydrocollator packs or socks after your techniques.

Precautions

- Avoid initiating calf cramps by not plantarflexing the foot.

Iliopsoas Structural Balancing (Figure 6.14)

(Adapted from Maupin 2005.)

Intentions

To reduce iliopsoas spasm; to activate and strengthen iliopsoas awareness and tone; to reduce back pain from improper spinal and pelvic alignment.

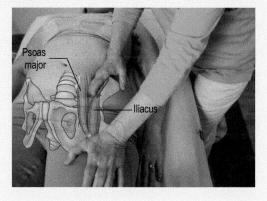

Figure 6.14   Iliopsoas Structural Balancing.

Procedure

This procedure may be performed in the sidelying or supine position (described in supine).

1. Stand at pelvic level, facing the client's feet. Place your outside hand supportively on the anterior upper thigh. Straighten your inside hand; then, leading with your little through middle fingers, use this edge to gradually sink into the pelvic bowl just medial to the anterior superior iliac spine, sliding medially against the ilium as tissue softens and avoiding any unintended, pointed pressure on her abdominal organs.

2. Continue to compress toward and into the iliacus, and eventually the psoas, releasing tenderness and pain. Be patient, work slowly and recognize that your movement into the deeper tissues may occur over several sessions.

3. At each point of entry, maintain a melting compression for at least 30 to 60 seconds.

4. Extinguish iliopsoas trigger points as needed.

Hints

- Teach your client to activate the iliopsoas using imagery that encourages lengthening of her lumbar spine against the table and/or flexion of her thigh on her pelvis. For lengthening, try the imagery in the pelvic alignment education technique (see Figure 4.32) and repeat for as many as 12 times. For hip flexion, have her imagine a string tied to her upper thigh. Place your flat palm over her anteromedial thigh, just inferior of her inguinal ligament. The string continues up toward the ceiling. Ask her to imagine that a giant puppeteer pulls the string, lifting her upper thigh slightly from the table while her lower back lengthens toward the table. After imagining that movement several times, ask her to initiate that movement. Coach her to coordinate her movement with her exhalation if possible.

- After she can do one of the above movements, sink gradually into the iliopsoas and then ask her to imagine and do the movement. During each activation of the iliopsoas, maintain your compression. Coach her movement until you can confirm activation of the iliopsoas under your fingertips. As the tissue softens and lengthens, follow the tissue changes.

- You can similarly release more superior segments of the iliopsoas. Work in mid-psoas, entering at the rectus abdominis's lateral edge at umbilicus level. Sink in just medial of the ribcage's costal edge, avoiding pressure on the xiphoid process, just where the rectus abdominis crosses the ribcage toward its attachments. In these upper areas, pelvic tilting, rather than the hip flexion, is the most productive movement.

- For clients who have experienced a traumatic birth, proceed especially sensitively and carefully, observing the client's protective responses as the iliopsoas is activated in sympathetic "fight or flight."

Precautions

- Do not apply direct pressure in an inferior direction on the inguinal ligament, as it may be weakened, thereby causing a hernia.

Spinal Seated Fascia Stretching (Figure 6.15)

(Adapted from Maupin 2005.)

Intentions

To elongate myofascial tissue and fascial planes; to reduce back pain by re-educating spinal alignment and normalizing spinal curvatures.

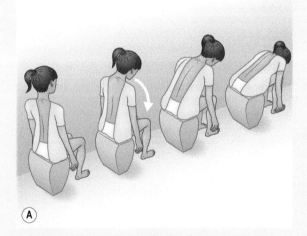

Ⓐ

Figure 6.15A Spinal Seated Fascia Stretching (Client's movement).

Procedure

Performed with the client seated on a sturdy stool or backless chair, adjusted to the right height for her thighs to be parallel with the floor, with her feet flat on the floor.

1. Drape the client to modestly cover her breasts but leave access to her bare back from neck to panty line; use a hospital gown, or a large button-down shirt or robe worn backwards.

2. Instruct your client to perform the following movement – sit upright with the back of her neck elongated, arms at her sides. Begin to move her torso toward her thighs by first dropping her chin to her chest. Gradually roll forward and downward from the top of her spine, one vertebra at a time (Figure 6.15A).

3. When her torso reaches her thighs, or she cannot roll down any further, ask her to reverse, erecting her spine in the opposite order. Instruct her to push her feet into the floor as her sit-bones press into the chair. Let her sacrum and waistline move back first, as a base for erecting her spine, vertebra by vertebra, from the bottom to the top. Finally, guide her to bring her head up and lift through the crown of her head.

4. Observe the fluidity and range of the client's movement. Note where spinal segments are moving as a unit rather than as individually articulating vertebrae.

5. Explain that she will repeat this movement while you use your fists to stroke deeply down both sides of the paravertebral musculature and fascial planes. Stand behind and place your gently fisted knuckles near C7. Direct your pressure caudally and medially. As the client rolls her spine down, let her movement glide you down her back, as shown in Figure 6.15B. Proceed paravertebrally to the coccyx, if possible.

6. Allow the speed of her movement to guide your speed and intensity as you stroke down.

7. When she reverses her movement, as in Step 3 above, help guide more differentiated movement of her vertebral segments by tapping gently on each consecutive vertebra to call her attention to individual movement that stacks her spine from the bottom up.

8. Repeat, using your elbows for a narrower, more medial stroke.

9. Repeat, using a knuckle into the laminar groove.

Precautions

- Do not perform on any client with spine injuries or diseases. Take extra care with scoliosis to make contact with myofascia, not bone.

- Be sure the client is breathing normally throughout this procedure and, if she becomes dizzy or light-headed, discontinue it.

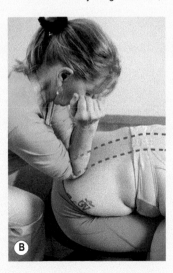

Figure 6.15B Spinal Seated Fascia Stretching (Therapist's movement).

Uterine Fundal Massage (Figure 6.16) 🌐

Intentions

To facilitate relaxation; to reduce the discomfort of uterine afterpains; to facilitate uterine involution and improve uterine tone to prevent postpartum hemorrhage; to facilitate connection to her postpartum abdomen without the baby and a healthy postpartum body image.

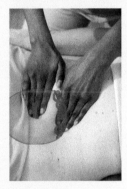

Figure 6.16 Uterine Fundal Massage.

Procedure

Best performed in the supine position with the client's knees bolstered to comfort; with or without lubricant.

1. Stand facing the client's abdomen. Place one hand just superior to the pubic bone with fingertips together and thumb open to stabilize both lateral aspects of the uterus. Maintain a superiorly directed pressure throughout the following steps.

2. Place the fingertips of your other hand at or just above umbilicus level if the technique is performed immediately after birth. For each day postpartum, place them approximately one fingerwidth below the umbilicus toward the pubic bone.

3. Sink to organ level, making contact with the uterine fundus. Perform circular kneading strokes deeply to the fundus until you feel her uterus firm with a contraction and/or she reports uterine contractions (see Figure 6.4 for postpartum changes in fundal level).

4. After two weeks postpartum, change to a bilateral fingertip position over the uterine fundus just above the pubic bone, with the fingertips directed at the pubic bone, and continue circular kneading.

Hints

- With fundal massage, expect some afterpains and some increase in lochia discharge during or right after massage for up to two to three weeks.

- This is a much gentler technique than the fundal massage that physicians and midwives use in the third and fourth stages of labor and birth. Explain your gentler intentions to the client. Teach her this technique to do herself as postpartum self-care as needed, daily and every few hours in the early postpartum weeks.

Uterine Positioning (Figure 6.17)

Intentions

To facilitate uterine involution and improve uterine tone to prevent postpartum hemorrhage; to reposition the uterus and bladder in their ideal positions in their fascial matrix.

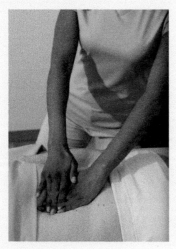

Figure 6.17 Uterine Positioning.

Procedure

Best performed in supine position with the client's knees bolstered to comfort; no lubricant.

1. Stand facing the client's pubic bone and knees. During her exhale, place your flattened distal fingers just superior to the pubic bone at the midpoint and sink to organ level. Without sliding on her skin, shift your body weight toward her head to create a pull on the fascial matrix around the bladder and uterus. Hold for 5 to 10 seconds as she holds her breath, and then slowly release when she inhales again.
2. Repeat two more times.

Precautions

- If any pelvic organ (bladder, uterus or bowel) is prolapsing, this technique is beneficial but also requires a referral to her physician, midwife and a women's health physical therapist.

Chapter Summary

No part of a women's childbearing experience is more neglected in Western cultures than the postpartum period. The early weeks and months can be a thrilling and tiring time as mothers focus on caring for their newborns and simultaneously recover from the remarkable adaptations of pregnancy and the hard work of birth. New mothers and their families need reliable and sustained care for many weeks and months to maximize full postpartum recovery and foster healthy family development. You can be an integral care provider immediately after vaginal and Cesarean births and for the weeks, months and potentially years to come. With caring, knowledgeable hands and your heart, you can help ease clients into and through their transformations as mothers — nurturing themselves and the next generations to come.

Think it through

To deepen your knowledge, go to our online resources, answer the test questions for this chapter and explore further. 🌐

References and Further Reading

AAP (American Academy of Pediatrics) (2012) Breastfeeding and the Use of Human Milk. Available at: https://pediatrics.aappublications.org/content/129/3/e827.full#-content-block [accessed October 31, 2019].

Abbasi S, Hamid M, Ahmed Z et al. (2014) Prevalence of low back pain experienced after delivery with and without epidural analgesia. Indian J Anaesth. 58(2):143–148.

ACOG (2018) Committee Opinion on Optimizing Postpartum Care. Available at: https://www.acog.org/Clinical-Guidance-and-Publications/Committee-Opinions/Committee-on-Obstetric-Practice/Optimizing-Postpartum-Care [accessed October 31, 2019].

Andrade C, Clifford P (2008) Outcome-based Massage: From Evidence to Practice, 2nd edn. Baltimore: Lippincott, Williams & Wilkins.

Bauer B, Cutshall S, Wentworth L et al. (2010) Effect of massage therapy on pain, anxiety, and tension after cardiac surgery: a randomized study. Complement Ther Clin Pract. 16(2):70–75.

Blois M (2016) Babywearing: The Benefits and Beauty of This Ancient Tradition. Amarillo, TX: Praeclareus Press.

Bolman M (2020) The art of therapeutic breast massage in supporting breastfeeding. GOLD Learning Online Continuing Education Webinar. Available at: https://www.goldlearning.com/ce-library/all-lectures/art-of-therapeutic-breast-massage-54r-detail [accessed May 30, 2020].

Bowman K (2016) Diastasis recti. Seattle: Propriometrics Press.

CDC (Centers for Disease Control) (2019) Pregnancy Mortality Surveillance System. Available at: https://www.cdc.gov/reproductivehealth/maternal-mortality/pregnancy-mortality-surveillance-system.htm?CDC_AA_refVal=https%3A%2F%2Fwww.cdc.gov%2Freproductivehealth%2Fmaternalinfanthealth%2Fpregnancy-mortality-surveillance-system.htm [accessed January 30, 2020].

CPWHC (Chartered Physiotherapists in Women's Health and Continence) (2014) Management of pelvic girdle pain in pregnancy and post-partum. Royal Coll Physicians Ireland. Guideline no. 16. Revised August.

Chikly B, Chikly A (1997) Applications of pre- and post-surgical lymphatic drainage therapy. Massage Bodywork. Summer/Fall:64–67.

Chopra D, Simon D, Abrams V (2009) Magical Beginnings, Enchanted Lives: A Holistic Guide to Pregnancy and Childbirth. New York: Three Rivers Press.

Creager C (2001) Bounce Back Into Shape After Baby. Berthoud, CO: Executive Physical Therapy.

CulturaLink (2016) The Impact Religion Can Play in Healthcare. Available at: https://theculturalink.com/2016/10/17/the-impact-religion-can-play-in-healthcare/ [accessed January 30, 2020].

Curties D (2011) Breast Massage. New Brunswick, Canada: Curties-Overzet.

Dumoulin C, Hay-Smith E, Mac Habée-Séguin G (2014) Pelvic floor muscle training versus no treatment or inactive control treatments for urinary incontinence in women. Cochrane Database Syst Rev. 2014(5):CD005654.

Enzer S (2004) Maternity Reflexology. UK: Soul to Sole Reflexology.

Fitch P (1998) The case for breast massage. Massage Ther J. 36(4):64–78.

Goldsmith L, Weiss G (2009) Relaxin in human pregnancy. Ann N Y Acad Sci. 1160:10.1111.

Gonzalez H, Vinaver N (1997) Massage techniques from Mexico. Workshop Presentation at Midwifery Today Conference, San Diego, March.

Goyal D, Gay C, Lee K (2009) Fragmented maternal sleep is more strongly correlated with depressive symptoms than infant temperament at three months postpartum. Arch Womens Ment Health. 12:229–237.

Henderson J, Gao H, Redshaw M (2013) Experiencing maternity care: the care received and perceptions of women from different ethnic groups. BMC Pregnancy Childbirth. 13:196.

Howard F (2000) Pelvic Pain: Diagnosis and Management. Baltimore: Lippincott, Williams & Wilkins.

Hung C (2006) Correlates of first-time mothers' postpartum stress. Kaohsiung K Med Sci. 22:500–507.

Irani M, Kordi M, Tara F et al. (2015) The effect of hand and foot massage on post-cesarean pain and anxiety. J Midwifery Reprod Health. 3(4):465–471.

Jefferies J, Bochner F (1991) Thromboembolism and its management in pregnancy. Med J Aust. 155:253–258.

Johnson K (2017) The Fourth Trimester: A Postpartum Guide to Healing Your Body, Balancing Your Emotions and Restoring Your Vitality. Boulder, CO: Shambhala.

Jordan R, Engstrom J, Marfell J et al. (2014) Prenatal and Postnatal Care: A Women-centered Approach. Ames, IA: John Wiley and Sons.

Karlström A, Nystedt A, Hildingsson I (2015) The meaning of a very positive birth experience: focus groups discussions with women. BMC Pregnancy Childbirth. 15:251.

KellyMom (2019) Breastfeeding. Available at: https://kellymom.com/category/bf// [accessed October 31, 2019].

King T, Brucker M, Osborne K et al. (2019) Varney's Midwifery, 6th edn. Burlington, MA: Jones & Bartlett Learning.

Kitzinger S (1994) The Year After Childbirth. New York: Charles Scribner's Sons.

Ko Y, Lee H (2016) Randomized controlled trial of the effectiveness of using back massage to improve sleep quality postpartum. J Clin Nursing. 25(3–4): 332–339.

Kolakowski M (2018) Massage therapy provides proven benefits to new mothers. Massage Magazine. 267:40–45.

Leapfrog Group (2019) Leapfrog Maternity Care Report. Available at: https://www.leapfroggroup.org/node/1064 [accessed October 31, 2019].

Lett A (2000) Reflex Zone Therapy for Health Professionals. London: Harcourt.

Liu C (2017) The caregiver–infant dyad as a buffer or transducer of resource enhancing or depleting factors that shape psychobiological development. Aust NZ J Fam Ther. 38(4): 561–572.

Maupin E (2005) Dynamic Relationship to Gravity, vols 1 and 2. San Diego: Dawn Eve Press.

McKenna J (2020) Safe Infant Sleep. Washington, DC: Platypus Media.

McRee L, Pasvogel A, Hallum A et al. (2007) Effects of preoperative massage on intra- and postoperative outcomes. J Gynecol Surg. 23(3):97–103.

Moore S, McEwen L, Quirt J et al. (2017) Epigenetic correlates of neonatal contact in humans. Dev Psychopathol. 29(5):1517–1538.

Mora A, Blazar P, Teplitz B et al. (2019) Gestational Carpal Tunnel Syndrome Found to Be Persistent in Women Post Pregnancy. 2019 Annual Meeting of the American Academy of Orthopaedic Surgeons (AAOS), Las Vegas, March 12. Available at: https://aaos-annualmeeting-press-kit.org/2019/research-news/gestational_carpal_tunnel/ [accessed July 1, 2020].

Ou H, Greeven A, Belger M (2016) The First Forty Days: The Essential Art of Nourishing the New Mother. New York: Stewart, Tabori & Chang.

Parfitt Y, Ayers S (2014) Transition to parenthood and mental health in first-time parents. Infant Ment Health J. 35(3):263–273.

Polseno-Crawford D (1998) Why don't we do breast massage? Massage Ther J. 36(4):95–106.

Population Reference Bureau (2014) International Data. Available: https://www.prb.org/international/ [accessed May 29, 2020].

Rad Z, Haghshenas M, Javadian Y et al. (2016) The effect of massage on weight gain in very low birth weight neonates. J Clin Neonatol. 5(2):96–99.

Ricci S (2017) Essentials of Maternity, Newborn and Women's Health Nursing, 4th edn. New York: Wolters Kluwer.

Sakalis V, William T, Hepworth G et al. (2013) A comparison of early sucking dynamics during breastfeeding after cesarean section and vaginal birth. Breastfeeding Med. 8(1):79–85.

Serrallach O (2018) The Postpartum Depletion Cure: A Complete Guide to Rebuilding Your Health and Reclaiming Your Energy for Mothers of Newborns, Toddlers and Young Children. New York: Hachette.

Sheidaei A, Abadi A, Zayeri F et al. (2016) The effectiveness of massage therapy in the treatment of infantile colic symptoms: a randomized controlled trial. Med J Islam Repub Iran. 30:351.

Simkin P (2008) Processing the birth experience with the woman. DONA International birth doula training manual.

Simkin P, Whalley J, Keppler A et al. (2018) Pregnancy, Childbirth and the Newborn: The Complete Guide, 5th edn. New York: Da Capo Lifelong Books.

Simonelli M, Doyle L, Columbia M et al. (2018) Effects of connective tissue massage on pain in primiparous women after cesarean birth. J Obstet Gynecol Neonatal Nurs. 47(5):591–601.

Smith NK, Ryan K (2016) Traumatic Scar Tissue Management: Massage Therapy Principles, Practice and Protocols. Edinburgh: Handspring.

Sperstad J, Tennfjord M, Hilde G et al. (2016) Diastasis recti abdominis during pregnancy and 12 months after childbirth: prevalence, risk factors and report of lumbopelvic pain. Br J Sports Med. 50(17):1092–1096.

Stuge B, Holm I, Vøllestad N (2006) To treat or not to treat postpartum pelvic girdle pain with stabilizing exercises? Man Ther. 11:337–343.

Turchaninov R (2011) How massage therapy heals the body: Part 3 Vasodilation and mechanisms. J Massage Sci. 3(3):4–6.

Uvnäs-Moberg K (2014) Oxytocin: The Biological Guide to Motherhood. Amarillo, TX: Praeclarus Press.

Wertz R, Wertz D (1989) Lying-In: A History of Childbirth in America. New Haven, CT: Yale University Press.

Whitridge P (2019) Scar tissue and massage. American Massage Therapy Association Online Courses. Available at: https://www.amtamassage.org/courses/detail/117/scar-tissue-and-massage [accessed October 18, 2019].

Wisner K, Sit D, McShea M et al. (2013) Onset timing, thoughts of self-harm, and diagnoses in postpartum women with screen-positive depression findings. JAMA Psychiatry. 70(5):490–498.

Witt A, Bolman M, Kredit S et al. (2015) Therapeutic breast massage in lactation for the management of engorgement, plugged ducts, and mastitis. J Hum Lact. 32(1):123–131.

Zanardo V, Sveglido G, Cavallin F et al. (2010) Elective cesarean delivery: does it have a negative effect on breast-feeding? Birth. 37(4):275–279.

Zulak D (2018) Clinical Assessment for Massage Therapy. Edinburgh: Handspring.

Studying this chapter will prepare you to:

1. care more confidently for the growing number of people
   using assisted reproductive technologies

2. recognize warning signs and symptoms of the most
   common high-risk factors and complications of the pre-
   and perinatal period

3. provide safe and effective massage therapy sessions
   modified for clients on bed rest

4. adapt your prenatal and postpartum massage sessions
   and your birth support appropriately for clients with
   special needs, high-risk conditions and complications

5. assist clients with stress management during and in
   recovery from complications and high-risk conditions,
   including cases with traumatic and tragic outcomes.

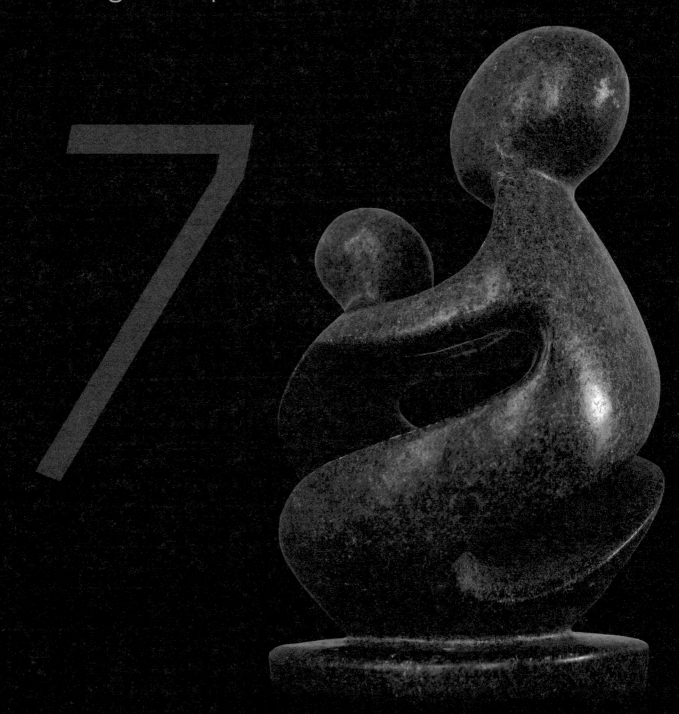

Additional Considerations
Working with Special Needs Clients

7

Chapter Overview

The previous chapters focused on what to expect and how to care for your clients when pregnancy, birth and the postpartum period are normal and healthy. Now we want to begin preparing you for the more complex and unexpected. We will introduce you to a diversity of clients who also need your stress-reducing, safe, pre- and perinatal massage therapy. This includes the special needs of the growing number of people using assisted reproductive technology. Also, approximately one in four pregnant people are diagnosed as having high-risk factors and/or complications (Ricci 2017).

Although these pages are relevant for only a quarter of your potential clients, you must always be aware of and alert for these possibilities for all of your clients. You also want to be conscious of and honor your own feelings. Medical problems in the childbearing years can be scary, and working with such clients may feel daunting – especially if you have had your own difficult health experiences, or someone close to you has. Know that you do not need a medical background to care for these clients, just a willingness to work shoulder to shoulder with them and their medical care professionals to optimize their care and outcomes. In this chapter, we also want to prepare you for possible difficult and tragic outcomes and the grieving so integral to the healing process – for everyone, including you.

Be confident that your skills of observation and communication, along with the specialized pre- and perinatal massage therapy taught in this book, have great potential to support the best possible outcomes for these clients and their babies, despite the difficulties that they face. With your work, you can bring a welcome respite by providing relaxation and reducing the discomforts and side effects of some treatments. If just for the minutes in your care, perhaps you can help your clients feel normal as they undergo their abnormal experiences. These brave, grateful individuals often become some of the most gratifying and appreciative of clients. And we invite you to use this chapter as a constant resource, encouragement and springboard that empowers your confidence, abilities and further study to safely meet these clients' special needs – a most rewarding facet of the pre- and perinatal massage therapy specialization.

Supporting Clients Using Assisted Reproductive Technology

For many people who want to start or grow their families, the dreams of having a child is not easily realized. Since 1981, assisted reproductive technology has been used to help people become pregnant. The most common method is transferring fertilized human eggs into the uterus. For some, deciding whether to undergo and embarking on this expensive, time-consuming and often emotional treatment can be difficult. In recent decades, assisted reproductive technology use has dramatically increased worldwide and has made pregnancy possible for many people. Approximately 2 percent of all infants born in the United States every year are conceived using assisted reproductive technology. Of the approximately 61 million women aged 15 to 44 years between 2011 and 2015, more than 7 million, or 12 percent, received some treatment for infertility. Approximately 7 percent of married women aged 15 to 44 years were unable to become pregnant after at least 12 consecutive months of trying to conceive (ACOG 2016).

In Vitro Fertilization

The most common assisted reproductive technology is **in vitro fertilization (IVF)**. To provide effective, safe and compassionate pre- and perinatal therapy for these clients, the following details about the process are relevant for you to understand. Assisted reproductive technology includes two weeks of several steps and is referred to as a cycle of treatment. The cycle starts when a person begins taking medications to stimulate egg production or starts ovarian monitoring before embryos are transferred. When a pregnancy is conceived through assisted reproductive technology, the date of insemination or embryo transfer is used instead of the typical **last menstrual period dating** (King et al. 2019).

From the treatment room

I have found that it is difficult following an unsuccessful in vitro fertilization for women to return to my massage therapy room with the decorations of baby and pregnancy images. I have given my clients the option to use another treatment room until they felt ready to come back to my room. Even with these sensitive options offered, it is often emotionally difficult for them to return the first time, but they soon find comfort in the familiar setting.

– Linda Hickey, therapist

Some in vitro fertilization practices can increase the risk of multiple gestations, which are considered a high-risk factor (Box 7.1) (CDC 2019a). Also, singletons conceived with assisted reproductive technology may be at higher risk than singletons from naturally occurring pregnancies. The extent to which these associations might be related to the underlying causes of infertility remains unclear. Before initiating assisted reproductive technology, these clients complete a thorough medical assessment with their maternity healthcare providers to ensure that they are in good health and are counseled about the risks. The health concerns of the mother and the expectant couple or egg/sperm donor, including any inherited genetic conditions, are considered, and with the increased risk of higher-order multiples the option of **multifetal reduction** could be discussed. When a client continues a high-order multiples pregnancy, she will need an ongoing obstetric care provider and a hospital specializing in high-order multiples and capable of managing anticipated risks and outcomes (ACOG 2016).

Box 7.1
Pre- and perinatal high-risk factors

Biophysical Factors

- Any history of complications in prior pregnancy (miscarriage, perinatal mood and anxiety disorders, and so on)
- Autoimmune diseases
- Cardiovascular disease, **hemoglobinopathies**, **thrombophilias** and **Rh incompatibility**
- Cervical and uterine abnormalities and diseases **(diethylstilbestrol syndrome)**
- Chromosomal abnormalities
- Chronic hypertension
- Diabetes and gestational diabetes
- Genetic conditions and disorders
- Infections (COVID-19, sexually transmitted, and other viral and bacterial diseases)

- Large-for-gestational-age (LGA) baby or **macrosomia**
- Multiple gestations pregnancy
- Parity – first pregnancies and grand multiparity
- Perinatal mood and anxiety disorders, or a history of depression or mental health disorders
- Placental abnormalities
- Poor nutritional status
- Preterm or post-term labor and birth
- Renal disease
- Respiratory disease, including asthma
- Small-for-gestational-age (SGA) baby
- Thyroid disease
- Underweight (anorexia, bulimia) or overweight maternal status (obesity)

Psychosocial Factors

- Age (younger than 15 or older than 35)
- Alcohol and substance abuse
- Ethnicity – increased risk in non-white people
- History of or current sexual abuse
- Illicit drug use and abuse of medications
- Inadequate support system
- Lack of prenatal, birth and postpartum care
- Marital status – increased risk for unmarried women
- Poverty
- Situational crisis, including falls, accidents, spousal abuse, natural disasters and warfare, and personal stress
- Smoking
- Traumatic birth and/or post-traumatic stress disorder (PTSD)
- Unsafe practices, risky or unhealthy lifestyle, including exposure to **teratogens** (radiation, industrial or household pollutants and chemicals, and second-hand smoke)

Adapted from Ricci S (2017) Essentials of Maternity, Newborn and Women's Health Nursing, 4th edn. New York: Wolters Kluwer.

General Guidelines

- Use all trimester and postpartum appropriate positioning for your client's comfort; remember the benefits of the sidelying position, which easily allows for communication and tracking with a client who may be experiencing more emotional lability (Chapter 3).

- Use massage therapy techniques, environment and your relationship with your client to focus on parasympathetic arousal as a prominent therapeutic intention (Chapters 4 and 6).

- Before insemination or embryo transfer, offer deeper abdominal and pelvic techniques that reduce myofascial restriction and congestion in these areas (Chapter 6).

- After insemination or embryo transfer, follow Chapter 4's trimester recommendations for pregnancy-appropriate abdominal massage. Consider your risk tolerance for any possible perceived association between massage therapy and potentially unsuccessful insemination or embryo transfer, or a miscarriage, when considering abdominal work; if she consents to abdominal techniques, document that consent in your charting notes.

- Use your impeccable active listening to acknowledge and validate the intensities and textures of her feelings about having assistance to become pregnant and any impact on her confidence to maintain her pregnancy, cope with labor and birth, and be a mother.

- Schedule her appointments with sensitivity to the fact that it may be difficult for her to see and hear other mothers with infants or see maternity office decorations.

- With **surrogacy** and a woman who chooses to be a gestational carrier, use relational finesse and emotional awareness to match her balance with her connection with the pregnancy and also, perhaps, her need to maintain some emotional distance. Learn how she is feeling about her pregnancy, taking your cues from her about how much or how little she prefers to connect with the baby. In some cases, you will interact with or perform massages for both the biological mother and the surrogate mother; it is helpful to clearly determine upfront who your client is: surrogate, biological mother or both.

Reminder

Massage therapists do not diagnose high-risk factors and medical complications. Physicians and midwives are responsible for monitoring, screening, diagnosing and treating high-risk factors and complications. Midwives' care focuses on healthy childbearing people with a clearly defined scope of practice that varies from state to state and country to country. In some cases, women's medical care starts with, must be shared with or is completely transferred to physicians who specialize in high-risk factors and complications.

Understanding High-Risk Factors and Complications

High-risk factors include clients' current biophysical and psychosocial issues that suggest a higher likelihood of medical complications developing (see Box 7.1). These people often have more intensive medical assessments and treatments. Most individuals who are identified as having one or more high-risk factors have healthy pregnancies, births and postpartum periods; however, 6 to 8 percent do not and require closely managed medical care (Ricci 2017).

By contrast, complications develop during pregnancy, birth and postpartum, and are an unhealthy condition in an organ or body system and a deviation of physiological or psychological adaptations from normal (Box 7.2) (Nagtalon-Ramos 2014). Many complications can be successfully treated if they are identified early.

Women with high-risk factors or complications have a higher morbidity and mortality compared with mothers in the general population. That status, and that of her baby, can emerge at any moment during the pregnancy, labor, birth and/or postpartum, even in people without any known previous risk (Ricci 2017).

Box 7.2
Common signs and symptoms of pre- and perinatal complications

- Signs and symptoms are grouped together and precede an *italicized* list (with glossary words in **bold**) of the corresponding and most common pre- and perinatal complications.

- Prenatal vaginal bleeding, discharge, gush or slow leakage of amniotic fluid, low back and/or pelvic pain, uterine cramping, contractions, pelvic or thigh pressure: *miscarriage; gestational trophoblastic disease; ectopic pregnancy; cervical insufficiency; preterm labor; premature rupture of membranes; placental abnormalities; stillbirth*

- Severe nausea, weight loss, dehydration: *hyperemesis gravidarum*

- Low or high weight gain, decreased fetal movement: *intrauterine growth restriction (IUGR) or small-for-gestational-age (SGA) baby; large-for-gestational-age (LGA) baby or macrosomia; stillbirth*

- High blood pressure, protein in urine, rapid weight gain, systemic and pitting edema, headaches, vomiting, visual disturbances, blurred vision, upper midback pain especially on right, seizures: *gestational hypertensive disorders*

- Heat, swelling, redness, cyanosis or pain in the arms or legs, particularly unilateral: *thrombi*

- Excessive hunger and thirst, frequent urination, sugar in urine: *gestational diabetes*

- Postpartum bleeding from vagina (more than normal lochia, and soaking through more than one peripad an hour), blood clots the size of an egg or bigger: *hemorrhage*

- Fever of more than 100.4 degrees F (38 degrees C); foul-smelling lochia or an unexpected change in color or amount; breast swelling, redness; swelling, redness or discharge at perineal tear or episiotomy, epidural, spinal or Cesarean incision site; dysuria, or incomplete emptying of the bladder: *infection*

- Shortness of breath or difficulty breathing without exertion; chest pain; disorientation: *cardiovascular disease, acute asthma flare or pulmonary embolism*

- Depression, extreme anxiety, mood swings, difficulty sleeping and eating, weight loss, thoughts of hurting herself or baby: *perinatal mood and anxiety disorders*

- Any abnormal results of blood and other laboratory tests, fetal and maternal monitoring procedures: *any of the complications above*

Adapted from Ricci S (2017) Essentials of Maternity, Newborn and Women's Health Nursing, 4th edn. New York: Wolters Kluwer.

Reminder

Although your client may have a high-risk factor or a complication, in most cases she is still more likely than not to have a normal pregnancy, birth and postpartum time.

How We Can Help

Your role as keen observer of your childbearing clients emerges in multiple beneficial ways. Some clients may have scheduled sessions with you before their maternity healthcare provider even confirms the pregnancy. Some may delay the onset of prenatal and/or postpartum medical care, or skip medical care visits. Further, once pregnancy is underway, you may be the one to notice new signs and symptoms before or between medical care visits. Also, as a pre- and perinatal massage therapist in your sessions or during birth, you have the privilege to observe more of the body and mind, as well as having more time with your client than any other member of her care team. Your thorough written and/or verbal client intake and careful critical thinking (see Chapter 8) round out the many benefits that you offer all your clients, especially those discussed in this chapter.

Reminder

When working with high-risk conditions and complications, consultation with and medical consent from your client's maternity healthcare providers improve your client's care and reduce liability implications for you as the massage therapist.

General Guidelines

Whenever your potential or current client reports, or you notice, worrying signs or symptoms (see Box 7.2), take the following actions and document the results and responses in your charting notes:

- Complete a thorough written and/or verbal client intake, including their maternity healthcare provider's name and contact information (see Chapter 8).

- Assess for other signs of complications by asking further questions during intake or in session, and by palpating and observing her.

- Talk about your concerns calmly, professionally and with a positive intention, thereby avoiding any additional stress caused by an alarmist response. Examples include:

  ○ "I care about your and your baby's well-being. Whenever I have a client with bleeding and back pain, I ask her to connect with her midwife before proceeding with our massage. It's for your well-being having this assessment first."

  ○ "Edema and shortness of breath are common in pregnancy. Thanks for sharing this with me. Have you discussed them both with your doctor, and if so, when? Before our session, would you please discuss them with your doctor, and let me know what they say?"

- Inquire as to whether her physician or midwife knows about what you have observed. If not, have her inform her maternity healthcare provider of those concerns.

- Ask for the date and the results of her most recent visit with her physician or midwife. If medical diagnostic test results are forthcoming, consider rescheduling until after these are available. Or, considering that the results could be positive, negative or inconclusive, proceed with the massage – if safe – and make all necessary adaptations.

- If a diagnosis is already established, consult with the physician or midwife about how to proceed. Adopt his or her level of concern – from none to detailed modifications in the positioning and techniques you will use. If your client is hospitalized, secure the necessary consents and understand the limitations before offering a session.

- Before engaging in phone, email or other communication about a client's care, secure written consent for the release of confidential medical records and your session notes, and for communication between you and the maternity healthcare providers (Chapter 8). If written consent is not possible, ask your client for a verbal report of discussions with physician or midwife about if and how to proceed with you. Document these communications in your charting notes.

Once your preliminary assessments and communications are complete, keep these important general guidelines in mind as you proceed into sessions:

- Ask for thorough updates; perform verbal, visual and palpatory assessments; and complete your charting notes after each session. When necessary, review relevant signs and symptoms in this chapter. Use evidence-based research references to learn more about the condition, causative factors and current treatments available.

- Use critical thinking methods to assist in making good clinical decisions about your clients' care (Chapter 8).

- Consider how to integrate massage therapy during bed rest at home or in the hospital, especially when a baby is in the neonatal intensive care unit (NICU) or your client is separated from her baby.

- Plan your sessions around the likely additional medical appointments these clients have.

- Chronic stress is often a contributing factor to high-risk factors and complications, and frequently a result as well. Focus every interaction with your client, and every technique, on their parasympathetic nervous system activation (Chapters 4 to 6). Teach simple massage techniques to family members so they can offer regular massages too.

- When a client is medically stable – meaning the high-risk condition or complication is being successfully managed and treated – consider any necessary session adaptations. Alternately, when she is not medically stable, further adaptations will be necessary.

- Whenever in doubt about positioning, or without specific instructions, use the left sidelying position.

- If providing massage in a hospital setting, use her hospital bed, just as you would a hydraulic massage table, to properly position her and enable optimal body mechanics for you.

- Teach her how to replicate your massage positioning when at home or in the hospital to extend the benefits of your work.

- Carefully consider every technique's intentions and effects, both positive and negative. If in doubt, err on the side of caution, and you will do no harm.

- Consult evidence-based massage therapy texts about how to adapt your techniques for any medication or treatment and its side effects.

- Since many issues directly involve the baby's well-being and maternal abdominal structures, carefully consider the possible perceptions, implications and liabilities associated with direct abdominal massage and any techniques that indirectly affect the abdomen. You or your employer may decide to forgo such techniques, despite their stress-reducing intention, to reduce legal risk.

- Ask each client about her preference regarding abdominal massage. When your client trusts, is comforted by and consents to abdominal techniques, enjoy and document her consent in your session notes.

- If she prefers to eliminate direct abdominal techniques, use breathing, reflexive techniques and visualizations instead. Visualizing nurturing light, energy or protection around her baby is often beneficial.

- Be mindful of supporting your clients' emotional lability with your kind, calm and non-judgmental active listening.

- High-risk factors and complications can sometimes increase clients' self-care and medical compliance; however, with her postpartum focus on a baby who she worked so hard to bring in, she may ignore her own ongoing care needs. Consider how your work can encourage consistent, meaningful care throughout her childbearing years.

- Think about learning infant massage for medically fragile babies to share the benefits with the family while their baby is in the NICU and if (hopefully, when) the baby comes home.

- When clients experience difficulties outside your scope of practice, ask about their interest in resources and referrals. With her okay, provide robust lists, an office resource notebook, a follow-up phone call or email, or your website's resources page.

- Secure your own professional, confidential support, especially with difficult outcomes.

What would you do?

You volunteer to provide massage at a local organization that serves teenage mothers. What risk factors and complications might you encounter in this situation? What types of technique and positioning modifications might you make? If a client there is considering whether to keep her baby as a single mother or relinquish her baby for adoption, how would you support her contemplations while staying within scope of practice?

Bed Rest

Before exploring common high-risk factors and complications in more detail, let's discuss bed rest – a common treatment for many of these and relevant to our pre- and perinatal massage therapy adaptations. To manage a high-risk condition or complication, 1 in 5 women is prescribed bed rest by their maternity healthcare providers for some period after the 20th week of pregnancy. Depending on the seriousness of the condition and the week of pregnancy, some people may be confined to their homes or a hospital bed for days, weeks or months. Some women are hospitalized on bed rest after birth as well. Bed rest is intended to increase the probability that the pregnancy will continue, and to stabilize her condition until and after the birth (Gilbert 2011). Bed rest has been traditionally prescribed in the hopes of reducing uterine activity, based on the logic that physical activity could prompt preterm birth; however, bed rest has adverse effects that we need to be aware of (Box 7.3). Two recent studies found no evidence to support or refute the use of bed rest at home or in the hospital to prevent preterm birth (Sosa et al. 2015).

Box 7.3
Bed rest and its effects

Conditions for which Bed Rest is Commonly Prescribed

- Cervical changes prior to full-term pregnancy
- Gestational diabetes
- History of pregnancy loss, stillbirth or preterm birth
- Hypertensive disorder
- Multiples (twins, triplets and high-order multiples)
- Placental insufficiency, placenta abruptia, placenta previa, and placenta accreta, increta and percreta
- Poor fetal growth
- Preterm labor
- Vaginal bleeding

Some Negative Side Effects of Bed Rest

- Muscle weakness and stiffness
- Muscle atrophy within six hours, with the greatest atrophy occurring in three to seven days
- Muscle volume loss of more than 25 to 30 percent in five weeks
- Prolonged physical postpartum recovery with muscular and cardiovascular deconditioning
- Increased blood coagulation
- Heartburn, reflux and constipation
- Glucose intolerance and insulin resistance
- Weight loss despite controlled caloric intake and reduced activity
- Blood volume and plasma decrease by about 7 percent of body weight
- Decreased cardiac output and stroke volume
- Increased feelings of isolation, guilt, resentment, loneliness, boredom, anxiety, depression, inadequacy and dependence on others
- Increased concerns about health, body image, family status and disruption of routine
- Increased family/marital stress and possible loss of mother's income

Adapted from Gilbert E (2011) Manual of High-risk Pregnancy and Delivery, 5th edn. St. Louis: Mosby.

General Guidelines

- Ask the client about the diagnosis for which bed rest is prescribed; use the pre- and perinatal massage guidelines detailed in this chapter's relevant sections for how to best work with her, given that diagnosis.

- Depending on your client's level of restriction, perform the massage in her home or her hospital room.

- If in the hospital, use her hospital bed just as you would a hydraulic massage table, with the same client positioning and your ideal body mechanics. If at home, check to see if she can transfer to your treatment table or not.

- When in the hospital, be mindful of any medical equipment, ports, tubes and intravenous puncture sites.

- Discern if the left sidelying position is required to maximize fetal circulation. Ask her maternity healthcare provider's consent to use other positions, including semireclining or right sidelying, to relieve compression and pain from the prescribed extended periods on her left side.

- Focus on relaxation, centering and nurturing. Address bed rest effects (see Box 7.3). Integrate craniosacral therapy, and focus on Swedish and lymphatic drainage work on the torso and arms. Guide her to deeper breathing. Perform gentle foot, head and neck massages for relaxation, but avoid zone therapy on the feet if there is a high risk of thrombi (Enzer 2004).

- Use only superficial strokes on her legs as you respect the increased risk of thrombi. You may want to consult with her medical care team about the level of thrombi risk for both her legs and her arms, and adapt accordingly.

- Further reduce her musculoskeletal pain with appropriate myofascial, passive movement, stretching and trigger point techniques, especially her spine and pectoral and pelvic girdles.

- Allow generous session time to listen or address her needs for caring interaction that you can meet within professional boundaries. Encourage her to use this "time out" to tune in to her baby, and to have her physical and emotional needs fully met. In addition to pre- and perinatal massage, self-care for clients on bed rest can include journaling, relaxing, meditating and/or praying (Figure 7.1).

- Coordinate your care with any home- or hospital-based physical therapy that focuses on stretching and exercise in bed, and reduce myofascial restrictions that make these activities more difficult or painful.

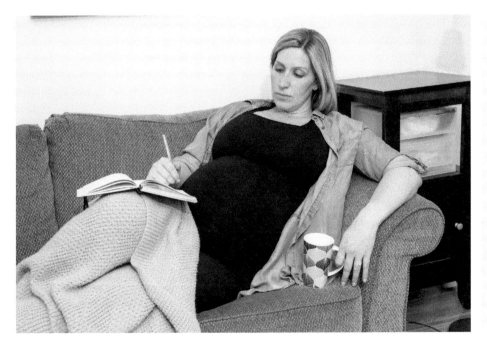

Figure 7.1
Client self-care during bed rest. Women with high-risk factors or complications who are on bed rest often find journaling, online community and other forms of self-care beneficial.

High-Risk Factors and Complications

For the duration of the chapter, we will explore the most common high-risk factors and complications that may emerge during pregnancy, birth and the postpartum period for some clients. For your ease of reference, these are listed in alphabetical order. Each section includes a brief highlight of the condition, its signs, symptoms and prevalence, and its impacts on mother and baby. Each section ends with massage guidelines. Some conditions have enormous and obvious impacts that require substantial adaptations in our pre- and perinatal massage, while we might not even notice other conditions during a session, but they still require some adaptation. But for all of these conditions, there are ways, whether big or small, of adapting your sessions to play a critical role in the care of these clients.

Abnormal Fetal Growth and/or Movement

Successful fetal growth is dependent on genetic, placental and maternal factors. About 10 percent of infants are large for gestational age and another 10 percent are born small for gestational age. These deviations may be the result of genetic predisposition, or the newborns may have grown above or below the norms due to maternal illness or other gestational conditions. Babies who experience intrauterine growth restriction have reduced oxygen, nutrients and other building blocks for growth, resulting in smaller-than-expected sizes. This stunting of growth can be due to placental insufficiencies, hypertension, poorly controlled insulin-dependent diabetes and other disease processes, or lifestyle choices such as tobacco and alcohol use. A smaller-than-normal fetus can suggest that growth is not proceeding well and there is a higher risk for preterm birth, unstable temperature and oxygen balance, and future challenges. In multiple-gestation pregnancies, it is common for one or all of the babies to be smaller than average. A bigger-than-normal or large-for-gestational-age baby (macrosomia) can put the baby at higher risk for hypoglycemia and a potentially challenging birth, as well as future health challenges (Ricci 2017).

Fetal movement is also considered an indicator of the baby's well-being. Smaller babies often move less to conserve energy. Other babies, though growing normally, indicate distress by reduced intrauterine movement. This distress could be the result of maternal use of medications, kidney and other fetal malfunctions, or just their own sleep cycles. A woman may note that intrauterine movement typically stops during her baby's 20- to 40-minute sleep cycle and gradually increases at night. The quality and quantity of fetal movement is a general indicator of fetal well-being, so a woman learns to closely attend to her baby's movements (Ricci 2017).

General Guidelines

- Use the left sidelying position only to maximize fetal circulation.

- Secure the maternity healthcare provider's consent to use other positioning for your client's comfort.

- Guide her in visualizing nurturing light, energy or protection around her baby; invite connection to the baby.

Amniotic Fluid Imbalances and Infections

Amniotic fluid is sterile, fetal urea that the baby swallows, passes through its digestive system and urinates into the amniotic sac cushioning the baby and the umbilical cord during pregnancy. **Polyhydramnios**, also called hydramnios, is a condition in which there is too much amniotic fluid surrounding the baby between 32 and 36 weeks. Approximately 18 percent of all diabetic pregnant women develop polyhydramnios. Overall, it is associated with an increased incidence of preterm births, **umbilical cord prolapse**, breech presentation and Cesarean births. Conversely, **oligohydramnios** is a decreased amount of amniotic fluid between 32 and 36 weeks. One in eight women whose pregnancies continue past 40 weeks develop oligohydramnios as amniotic fluid levels naturally decline at term (Ricci 2017). Reduction in amniotic fluid can reduce the baby's ability to move freely without risk of cord compression and resulting hypoxia (Queenan et al. 2015). Amniotic fluid should be clear. During labor and birth, when the amniotic sac spontaneously or artificially ruptures, cloudy or foul-smelling amniotic fluid indicates infection. Green or brown amniotic fluid indicates that the baby has passed **meconium** in utero. While this is considered normal for a baby in a breech presentation, for other babies it can be a stress response to hypoxia, post-term pregnancy, cord compression, intrauterine growth restriction, maternal hypertension, diabetes or **chorioamnionitis** (Ricci 2017).

General Guidelines

- Use the left sidelying position only to maximize fetal circulation; if mother and baby are stable, continue to use the left sidelying position to maximize fetal circulation, and secure the maternity healthcare provider's consent to use other trimester- or postpartum-appropriate positioning for your client's comfort.

- Guide her in visualizing nurturing light, energy or protection around her baby.

- With infection, follow the guidelines for infections later in this chapter.

Asthma

Asthma is an allergic inflammatory respiratory response to a variety of stimuli that constrict the lungs' bronchioles. Symptoms include breathlessness, wheezing, coughing, chest tightness and mucus production that further limit air movement and make breathing more difficult. Approximately 13 percent of pregnant women worldwide are affected by asthma, and that number is rising; however, the effect on each unique pregnancy is unpredictable. For one-third of pregnant women, their asthma severity worsens; in the next third, it improves; while in the last third, there is no change (Ricci 2017). Severe persistent asthma is associated with maternal complications, including hypertension, pre-eclampsia, oligohydramnios and uterine hemorrhage, as well as fetal complications (Vanders and Murphy 2015).

Asthma attacks can happen anytime, but are most likely to occur during weeks 24 to 36. Interestingly, flare-ups are rarer during the last four weeks of pregnancy and during labor (AAAAI 2015). In pregnant and laboring people, asthma is usually treated aggressively to ensure continuous oxygenation for the baby's health and to prevent fetal hypoxic episodes. Inhaled corticosteroids are the preferred medical treatment for most. The benefits of averting an asthma attack outweigh medication risks (NAEPP 2015). During labor and birth, asthma medication is usually continued, and the woman's oxygenation saturations are closely monitored alongside more frequent or continuous electronic fetal monitoring. Also, pain management with an epidural can further reduce potential stress that might trigger an acute asthma attack (Ricci 2017). Asthma usually returns to the pre-pregnancy level of severity within three months postpartum (Bolz et al. 2017).

As detailed in Chapter 1, all pregnant people experience profound physiological and anatomical changes that affect their respiratory systems, which often are made more severe when complicated by asthma. Hyperventilation tends to increase at full-term pregnancy by as much as 48 percent due to high progesterone levels. Estrogen creates more nasal mucus. Further, as the baby grows, the mother's diaphragm has limited space for its normal motion, resulting in a conversion from abdominal breathing to more thoracic breathing.

General Guidelines

- Remove any asthma triggers in and near your work environment and her birthing room, including strong odors, air pollutants and smoke. If animals come into your work space, be sure to ask clients about any allergies.

- If mother and baby are stable, secure the maternity healthcare provider's consent to use trimester- or birth-appropriate positioning for her comfort. Often, semireclining may make breathing easier.

- When in doubt or if mother and baby are not stable, use the left sidelying position only to maximize fetal oxygenation.

- Focus on autonomic sedation and facilitating more ease and less strain in the breathing musculature, including the scalenes, sternocleidomastoid, pectoralis major and minor, intercostals and ribcage attachments (Chapter 4).

- Guide her to a more upright posture and relax hypertonic muscles that might restrict a lifted, vertical alignment, including the erector spinae, suboccipitals, and pectoralis major and minor (Chapter 4).

- Offer space and time for her to use her prescribed asthma medications before, during and after sessions.

Reminder

With many high-risk factors and medical complications, the left sidelying position provides the additional assurance of maximum circulation to the fetus.

Cardiovascular Disease and Hypertensive Disorders

In the United States, cardiovascular disease is now the leading cause of death in pregnancy, birth and the postpartum period. It constitutes nearly 27 percent of pregnancy-related deaths, with higher rates of mortality among women of color and women with lower incomes. In addition to pre-existing cardiac conditions, there are also acquired heart conditions, which are by far the most common and can develop silently and acutely during or after pregnancy. Currently, **peripartum cardiomyopathy** is the leading cause of maternal mortality, accounting for 23 percent of deaths in the postpartum period (ACOG 2019). Signs and symptoms include chest pain and shortness of breath or difficulty breathing without exertion.

Another related group of complications, collectively named gestational hypertensive disorders, remain the most common pre- and perinatal complications, impacting up to 15 percent of childbearing women. Detailed below, all these hypertensive disorders are on the rise and are associated with higher rates of maternal, fetal and infant mortality and with severe morbidity, especially in cases of severe pre-eclampsia, **eclampsia** and **HELLP syndrome** (Ricci 2017). Severity can range from a mild elevation of blood pressure to severe pre-eclampsia and eclampsia (Ricci 2017). Gestational hypertensive disorders include:

- Chronic hypertension: hypertension that exists prior to pregnancy or that develops before 20 weeks' gestation.

- Gestational hypertension: blood pressure elevation (140/90 mm Hg) identified after 20 weeks' gestation without **proteinuria**.

- Pre-eclampsia: the most common hypertensive disorder of pregnancy, which develops with proteinuria after 20 weeks' gestation. Signs and symptoms include rapid weight gain, systemic and pitting edema (Figure 7.2), headaches, vomiting, visual disturbances, blurred vision, and upper right abdominal or mid or low back pain. It is a multisystem disease process, which is classified as mild or severe, depending on the severity of the organ dysfunction. Pre-eclampsia complicates about 3 to 5 percent of pregnancies. Worldwide, 76,000 women and 500,000 babies die from pre-eclampsia and hypertension each year (FIGO 2019).

- Eclampsia: onset of seizure activity in a woman with pre-eclampsia.

- Chronic hypertension with superimposed pre-eclampsia: this occurs in approximately 20 percent of pregnant women, with increased maternal and fetal morbidity rates (King et al. 2019).

- HELLP syndrome: an acronym for Hemolysis, Elevated Liver enzymes and Low Platelet count, a life-threatening variant of the pre-eclampsia/eclampsia syndrome that occurs in 10 to 20 percent of severe cases (King et al. 2019).

General Guidelines

- Use the left sidelying position to maximize fetal circulation.

- For pitting edema, consult "Points of view: Edema."

- With pre-eclampsia, eclampsia and HELLP syndrome, consider possible liver and kidney referred pain patterns versus musculoskeletal pain. Note that a change in activity or position does not give significant relief to the persistent organ pain often associated with these conditions. Liver problems typically refer as right upper quadrant abdominal pain, or mid back to shoulder pain, especially on the right side. Kidney pain typically refers to the mid and lower back.

Points of view: Edema

Edema (also known as lymphostatic edema or non-pitting edema), particularly in the arms, hands, lower legs and feet, is a normal result of prenatal hormonal and circulatory system changes, the pressure of the growing uterus on pelvic vessels, and a person's activity levels. Pre- and perinatal massage therapy instructors generally agree that this type of edema, which is secondary to a healthy pregnancy, responds well to what we generically refer to as lymph drainage techniques. These are superficial rhythmic strokes, primarily directed toward the terminus of the lymphatic system at the left subclavian vein, and performed on

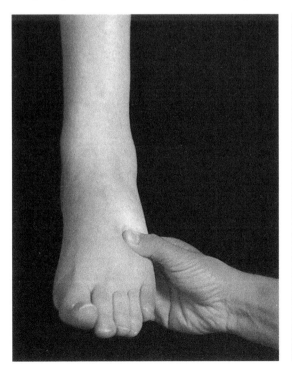

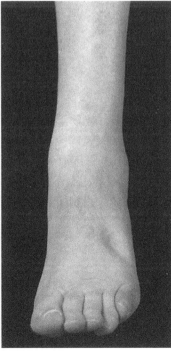

Figure 7.2
Pitting edema. With pitting edema, the area where you press will blanch and take longer than 10 to 30 seconds to refill.

proximal areas before moving further distally. Some emphasize a critical first step of stimulating the lymph nodes throughout the body, whereas others think that the axillary and inguinal nodes must be stimulated for mobilizing edema and lymph from the arms and legs, respectively.

There are considerable differences of opinion about whether to begin or end with this lighter work. Both those advocating beginning superficially and those preferring to finish in this way make the argument that other deeper techniques will compress lymphatic channels, thus obstructing fluid flow. Applying this reasoning, deeper work followed by more superficial techniques would seem to make the lighter strokes ineffective; lighter work followed by deeper is believed to cause the lymphatic channels to compress again, contributing to a rapid return of excess fluid. As a result, some educators warn against deep pressure on any part of an edematous limb at any time during pre- and perinatal massage.

Pitting edema can be evidence of dysfunction in the kidneys, heart or liver due to an underlying medical condition, or, more commonly, due to pre-eclampsia or eclampsia. Here, there is agreement that the maternity healthcare provider should evaluate and make individual recommendations. When edema results from tissue damage or organ malfunction, and when hypertension is untreated and/or uncontrolled, superficial pressure is essential. A well-trained and certified manual lymph drainage specialist may be best for working with these cases.

Of course, attempting to force lymph through edematous limbs is counterproductive. On the other hand, some clients with little or normal pre- and perinatal edema have a greater need for relief of muscular tension, fascial restriction in the extremities, and joint restrictions in the extremities. Automatically eliminating all but the most superficial techniques might deprive these clients of the possible relief created by deeper Swedish and deep tissue techniques and selected myofascial work. These modalities are otherwise safe on healthy clients' legs, except on the medial aspect, and including the other limitations described in Chapter 2. When there are other contraindications to deep leg work, such as severe varicose veins, bed rest or elevated thrombi risks, then deep pressure should be avoided for those reasons. Remember, optimal pelvic alignment helps to open the anterior torso so that lymph can more easily flow past the inguinal ligament. Less stress and pain and, in most cases, more activity also help relieve and prevent edema. Your work should focus on those intentions throughout your client's body. As with many debates in pre- and perinatal massage, each educator is applying her best knowledge and reasoning to a situation in which few actual massage therapy data are available (Stager 2010; Stillerman 2008; Yates 2010).

Gestational Diabetes

Gestational diabetes is glucose intolerance that begins or is first detected during pregnancy, usually around the 24th week. In the United States, the incidence of gestational diabetes is increasing and the condition affects up to 10 percent of pregnancies. Signs and symptoms include excessive hunger and thirst, frequent urination, and sugar in the urine. Gestational diabetes is associated with neonatal complications such as macrosomia, hypoglycemia and birth trauma, or maternal complications such as pre-eclampsia and Cesarean birth. The current understanding of the pathophysiology of gestational diabetes is that it is an unmasking of pre-existing pancreatic dysfunction prior to pregnancy that is revealed during pregnancy's normal adaptation of insulin resistance. Pregnancy can be viewed as a glucose homeostasis mechanism stress test – the woman's body ensures that her baby has an ample nutrient supply by increasing peripheral resistance to insulin. This adaptation is orchestrated by placental hormones that create compensatory increases in insulin secretion to maintain normal blood glucose levels. A favorable pregnancy outcome requires commitment on the woman's part to more frequent prenatal visits, dietary changes, self-monitoring of blood glucose levels, frequent laboratory tests and more intensive fetal monitoring (Ricci 2017).

General Guidelines

- If gestational diabetes is not being successfully treated, lying on the left side is your best option; when well managed with stable blood glucose levels, use all recommended pregnancy and postpartum positioning options.

- Focus on pain complaints associated with a potential sedentary lifestyle or a newly prescribed exercise regime; reduce musculoskeletal and swelling pain with postural guidance, myofascial and deep tissue techniques at pain sites, trigger point therapy and other joint techniques.

- When blood glucose levels are unstable, adapt your pressure to make it lighter on her extremities until levels are stable.

- Support healthy functioning of affected organs – pancreas, liver, gastrointestinal tract, brain and kidneys – by stimulating the corresponding reflexive zones on her feet (see Figure 4.13).

- Offer space and time for your client to check blood glucose levels before and after sessions; encourage healthy fluids and snacks at her sessions.

From the treatment room

I was initially alarmed when I developed gestational diabetes, but my therapist helped calm me. She taught me to breathe more deeply, and I was better able to tune in to my body signals. That helped me to better notice blood sugar fluctuations and to eat according to my nutritionist's guidelines.

– Rosalea, client

Hyperemesis Gravidarum

At least three out of four of women experience nausea and vomiting during their pregnancies (Castillo and Phillippi 2015). Studies show that nausea and vomiting during pregnancy are actually associated with improved fetal outcomes, such as lower rates of miscarriage (Ayyavoo et al. 2014). Such morning sickness symptoms usually disappear after the first trimester; however, hyperemesis gravidarum is a pregnancy complication with persistent, uncontrollable nausea and vomiting that begins in the first trimester and causes dehydration, ketosis and loss of more than 5 percent of pre-pregnancy body weight. The resulting dehydration, weight loss and electrolyte imbalance often requires hospitalization (Taylor 2014). Hyperemesis gravidarum occurs in approximately 2 percent of pregnancies with increased prevalence in **molar pregnancy** and multiple gestations. The peak incidence is at 8 to 12 weeks of pregnancy, and symptoms usually resolve by 20 weeks of pregnancy (Maltepe et al. 2015).

Although the exact cause is unknown, the effects of hyperemesis include decreased placental blood flow, decreased maternal blood flow, and acidosis that can threaten both mother's and baby's health. Dehydration can also lead to preterm labor (Smith et al. 2016). Theories as to the etiology of hyperemesis include high levels of human chorionic gonadotropin and estrogen, vitamin B6 deficiency, genetic factors and psychological stress; however, few studies have produced evidence to identify one cause. It is likely that multiple factors contribute (Ricci 2017).

The most conservative care at home focuses on dietary and lifestyle changes, but if these fail to stop the nausea and vomiting, hospitalization is required, with bed rest, "gut rest," intravenous fluids, antiemetic medication and nutritional feeding tubes. Recent research has reported positive results from using acupressure on the Pericardium 6 (PC-6) acupuncture point to reduce nausea and vomiting (Figure 7.3) (Ozgoli and Naz 2018). Few people experience complete relief of symptoms from any one therapy (Ricci 2017).

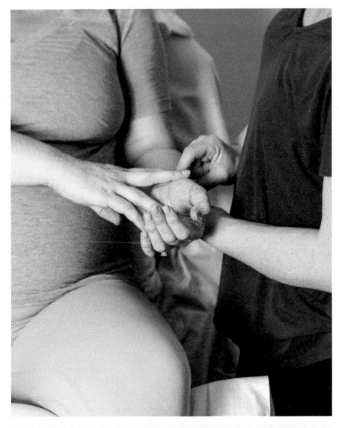

Figure 7.3
Acupressure relief for hyperemesis gravidarum. Locate the Pericardium 6 (PC-6) acupuncture point and apply deep, rhythmic thumb or fingertip acupressure to this point on each forearm, four times daily for 10 minutes each application, as needed.

General Guidelines

- Use the left sidelying position only to maximize fetal circulation; if mother and baby are stable, continue to use the left sidelying position to maximize fetal circulation. Secure the maternity healthcare provider's consent to use other trimester-appropriate positioning for your client's comfort. Some clients may be less nauseous in more upright positions that reduce upward pressure on the esophageal sphincter and stomach.

- Remember that pregnancy's common response to strong odors is nausea; avoid strong odors, scents and smoke on you or in your work environment.

- Locate the Pericardium 6 (PC-6) acupuncture point between the flexor carpi radialis and the palmaris

longus muscle tendons on the anterior surface of the forearm, two client fingerwidths proximal to the wrist crease. Teach her to apply deep, rhythmic thumb or fingertip acupressure to this point on each forearm, four times daily for 10 minutes each application. Teach this technique to her and her family members (see Figure 7.3).

- Eliminate any rocking or motion techniques that might inadvertently increase her nausea.

- Keep an empty trash can and a wipe-up towel accessible, should vomiting occur.

Infections

The most common infections during pregnancy, birth and postpartum include urinary tract infections, infections in healing wounds or surgical sites, mastitis and **endometritis**. Common signs and symptoms of infections include fever (temperature higher than 100.4 degrees F), local swelling, redness, or discharge that is foul-smelling or in which there is an unexpected change in color or amount. Antibiotic therapy continues to be the mainstay of treatment for these types of infection.

Urinary tract infections are caused by bacteria that are often found in bowel flora, and is accompanied by dysuria. Inadequate voiding, urinary catheterization after epidural or spinal anesthesia, frequent vaginal examinations and perineal trauma increase the likelihood of a urinary tract infection, and this is the most common cause of a fever in postpartum mothers.

Any break in the skin or mucous membranes during childbirth is susceptible to possible infection, including site wounds and surgical incisions – Cesarean birth surgical incisions, episiotomy and perineal tears. Wound infections are usually not identified until a person has been discharged from the hospital because symptoms may not appear until 24 to 48 hours after birth (Ricci 2017).

Mastitis is inflammation of breast tissue; it is most common in the first three weeks postpartum but can occur at any stage of lactation. The incidence of mastitis in Western women is 20 percent; however, mastitis is not as common in countries where frequent breastfeeding is the norm. Mastitis may come on quickly, and usually affects only one breast (KellyMom 2018). Flu-like symptoms are often the first clues in the mother, along with a breast that is red, tender and warm to the touch. As well as causing significant discomfort, mastitis is a common reason for mothers to discontinue breastfeeding. Mastitis results from milk stasis as a result of insufficient drainage of the breast, oversupply of milk, pressure on the breast from a poorly fitting bra, a blocked milk duct, missed feedings, breakdown of the nipple via fissures, cracks or blisters, and rapid weaning. A breast abscess may develop if mastitis is not treated adequately with effective milk removal, pain medication and antibiotic treatment (Ricci 2017).

Endometritis is an infection of the endometrium, decidua and adjacent myometrium of the uterus. The amniotic sac is a sterile environment; however, during labor and once rupture of the amniotic sac occurs, the uterus becomes more susceptible to bacterial colonization and infection, especially in prolonged labors (Ricci 2017). The risk of endometritis increases dramatically after Cesarean birth and it complicates 10 to 20 percent of Cesarean births. It occurs within the first two days postpartum or as late as two to six weeks postpartum (King et al. 2019).

Other infections, such as **cytomegalovirus**, **rubella**, **genital herpes**, hepatitis B, varicella zoster virus, parvovirus B19, group B streptococcus, **toxoplasmosis**, HIV/AIDS and sexually transmitted infections, can also negatively affect pregnancy, birth and the postpartum period. As of this book's writing, implications during pregnancy, labor, birth and postpartum, and for the newborn, of the newly emerged coronavirus, COVID-19, are still unclear. Consult evidence-based resources to learn more about these infections.

From the treatment room

During the COVID-19 pandemic, I kept in virtual contact with my pregnant and postpartum clients at the same intervals that we would have had our hands-on sessions. I worked together with them to stay current with emerging facts and best practices while helping them manage the additional stress of this new, unknown infection.

– Carole Osborne, therapist

General Guidelines

- Use trimester- or postpartum-appropriate positioning for your client's comfort and to avoid pressure on infected areas.
- Avoid direct contact with areas of infection; address those areas using reflexive techniques until infection is resolved.
- With Cesarean incision infections, follow the guidelines in Chapter 6 on Cesarean Scar Massage (see Figure 6.13).
- With mastitis, follow the guidelines in Chapter 6 on Self-Breast Massage (see Figure 6.7).
- Follow all current equipment requirements, sanitation and hygiene recommendations applicable to the individual infections that your client experiences, including delaying massage.

Labor Dystocia and Precipitous Labor

Labor dystocia is a complex and unpredictable complication of labor. Also called dysfunctional labor, failure to progress, arrest of labor and arrested descent, it refers to a labor that does not progress normally, and stalls and stops. The timing of the dystocia is a key consideration when determining the cause and selecting possible medical interventions. If labor progress stops or stalls, labor augmentation may be chosen to stimulate her uterus, typically with pitocin. Continuous electronic fetal monitoring is required during labor augmentation (Ricci 2017).

Labor dystocia is the most common reason for **primary Cesarean birth**. Labor dystocia also contributes indirectly to repeat Cesareans, especially in countries where vaginal births after previous Cesarean (VBAC) rates are low. The American College of Obstetricians and Gynecologists (ACOG) estimates that 60 percent of all Cesareans in the United States – primary and repeat – are attributable to labor dystocia. Preventing primary Cesarean births for labor dystocia can significantly lower the number of repeat Cesarean births, and reduce other costly or risky obstetric measures. Preventing labor dystocia also spares women the physical challenges and the emotional disappointment and discouragement that may accompany a prolonged and/or complicated birth (Simkin et al. 2018).

While a woman might fantasize about having a short labor, **precipitous labor**, lasting three hours or less, can come with its own complications. Perineal tissues may not have the requisite time to soften and stretch, so the baby is at greater risk for head or nerve trauma and lack of oxygen due to rapid contractions with little rest in between (Ricci 2017). The surprise, intensity and pain of precipitous labor can result in a panicked, discouraged or angry laboring woman who is overwhelmed and caught off guard. She may well have previously been preparing for the average 12 to 18 hours of active labor, as described in childbirth books and education classes for first-time mothers.

The causes of labor dystocia are listed in Box 7.4.

Box 7.4
Causes of labor dystocia

Labor may delay, slow or stop for any of a number of reasons at any time in labor – in early or active labor, or during the second or third stage of labor. Sometimes several causal factors occur at one time.

Intrinsic causes (also known as the "5Ps," coined by Penny Simkin)

- Powers (uterine contractions)
- Passage (pelvic size, shape and joint mobility, and birth canal stretch and resilience)
- Passenger (fetal head size and shape, fetal presentation and position)
- Pain (and the person's ability to cope with it)
- Psyche (the laboring person's emotional state)

Extrinsic causes

- Environment (feelings of physical and emotional safety created by the people around the laboring woman)
- Ethno-cultural factors (degree of sensitivity and respect for her culture-based needs and preferences)
- Hospital or caregiver policies (degree of flexibility, family or woman centered and evidence-based care)
- Psycho-emotional care (priority given to non medical aspects of the childbirth experience)

Adapted from Simkin P, Ancheta R (2018) The Labor Progress Handbook, 5th edn. Oxford: Blackwell Science.

General Guidelines

- If mother and baby are stable, time and patience are the best interventions and allies.
- When your client is considering other labor augmentation to stimulate progress, ask if she and her medical provider want to try non-medical augmentation methods (see Chapter 5, "Points of view: Induction and augmentation of labor"). Experimenting with these methods has several advantages – treating her as the "key to the solution, not the key to the problem," and creating or strengthening the cooperation between the mother, her support people and her healthcare providers. These actions also carry less risk of harm or undesirable maternal and fetal side effects; reduce riskier, costlier and more complex interventions; and may increase her emotional satisfaction with her experience of birth. The choice of solutions depends on the causal factors, if known, but trial and error is sometimes necessary when the cause is unclear. The greatest drawbacks are that the woman may not want to try these interventions; they sometimes take time; and they may not augment labor.
- When labor stalls or stops, focus on minimizing emotional distress. Promote physiological measures that maintain progress, and encourage rest as well as movement and position changes (Tully 2020). Massage therapy can help reduce the maternal distress that is often at the root of the problem, and that almost certainly will come with labor dystocia. Remember that massage therapy offers a viable complement or alternative to medical interventions, and it may help mothers to cope with the intensity and stress these interventions may create (Simkin et al. 2018).
- Choose client positions and comfort measures with respect for all the medical equipment used to treat labor dystocia (Chapter 5).
- Work closely and cooperatively with her and her partner and her maternity healthcare providers to help her feel safe and achieve the best outcome possible.
- When your client loses confidence and focus, offer your direct, leading guidance to help her regain a rhythmic coping response until she is able to regroup. Stay close, and speak and act firmly, calmly, confidently, kindly and optimistically. Gently insist that she open her eyes to make eye contact with you,

and use rhythmic talk and touch to help her pace her breathing and vocalization (Simkin et al. 2018).

- With precipitous labor, focus on helping her cope with its intensity and speed. Use bilateral compression on her feet, legs or shoulders. Note where she may be tensing against the pain, and hold bilateral pressure there. Be mindful of your own body mechanics to improve your quality of touch and safeguard your body during this intense work.

- While not in your scope of practice, be prepared, as a Good Samaritan, for the slim but real possibility that you must assist a precipitous birth. If her partner and medical care professionals are not available, call 911 (or equivalent in other countries), and encourage her to lie on her left side and pant or blow with her chin up when she feels the pushing urge. As you await the maternity healthcare provider's arrival, reassure her, remain calm and turn up any heat source. Wash your hands, if possible, preparing to assist the baby up to her mother's chest. Encourage her to hold and briskly rub her baby with warm clothing to dry amniotic fluid off the skin. Patiently wait for the placenta's birth, and save it for later medical evaluation. Ask her permission to begin Uterine Fundal Massage (see Figure 6.16) and, if baby is not yet at the breast, have her or her partner stimulate her nipples to release oxytocin to prevent hemorrhage (Simkin et al. 2018).

From the treatment room

Grief is a very real part of mothering. Every mother will experience grief in different ways and to different degrees. Grief can be felt in the loss of her identity, who she was before she had a baby, or realizing that the idea of the mother she thought she would be does not match the reality of the mother she is. Grief can come with the surprise that her baby is an unexpected gender. And grief is inevitable when her baby dies. We cannot force a mother through her grief, and we certainly have no right to judge her journey. I do my best to allow my massage room to be a space where she can be in her grief, and I meet her where she is at.

– Andrea Engi, therapist

Miscarriage and Stillbirth

Childbearing loss may affect mother and family for a lifetime. The need to grieve, share, and regain strength is universal for all families dealing with loss (Ricci 2017). Miscarriage, also known as spontaneous abortion, is the most common complication of early pregnancy (Tulandi and Al-Fozan 2015), and refers to the loss of a fetus prior to the 20th week and resulting from natural causes – that is, not elective or therapeutically induced by a procedure. Miscarriage often happens so early in pregnancy that a woman may not yet realize that she is pregnant. Heavy bleeding is the most common sign, often accompanied by uterine cramping. Of recognized pregnancies, 15 to 20 percent result in miscarriage, and about 80 percent occur within the first trimester. Women may express a wide spectrum of feelings from relief to sadness and despair (Ricci 2017).

A stillbirth is the loss of a fetus after the 20th week of gestation and up to and during labor and birth. Stillbirths are much less common than miscarriages, occurring in one out of every 160 pregnancies (March of Dimes 2015b). Signs and symptoms include reduced fetal movement, preterm uterine contractions, loss of amniotic fluid and vaginal bleeding. Sometimes, there is little or no warning and no preparation for the impending grief. Approximately 90 percent of mothers will go into spontaneous labor within two weeks of fetal death. Once intrauterine fetal death is confirmed, most mothers choose to immediately undergo induction of labor (Green 2016).

With the death, a mother's dreams and hopes for her expected baby suddenly dissolve. Deep emotions of sadness, sorrow, emptiness, anger, anxiety, loneliness, helplessness, disbelief, unreality and powerlessness are common. The grieving process spans a long and varying period of time, and for some it is never complete. For many mothers, emotional healing takes much longer than physical postpartum healing. Grieving generally moves through phases of:

- accepting the reality of the loss

- feeling the pain but moving through suffering from the loss

- adapting to her new environment without the baby

- emotionally relocating the baby as a part of her history and moving forward with her life (Grunebaum and Chervenak 2014).

Stillbirth is associated with post-traumatic stress disorder (PTSD) in subsequent pregnancies (Robinson 2014).

General Guidelines

- With any threatened loss, use the left sidelying position to maximize fetal circulation; if loss is confirmed, continue to use trimester- and postpartum-appropriate positioning for your client's comfort.

- Focus on her postpartum recovery goals. Full-body sessions of Swedish or passive movement methods can convey a sense of wholeness, as can craniosacral and other energetic work.

- Be mindful that massaging an area where she feels the loss of her baby – abdomen, chest and arms – can elicit a flood of emotions. Integrate the sealing technique (see Figure 6.5) into your session.

- Eliminate all abdominal techniques except in cases of postpartum uterine atony, in which case Uterine Fundal Massage is indicated (see Figure 6.16).

- Acknowledge and validate the varying intensities and textures of her grief with impeccable active listening, including attentive silence, a heartfelt "I'm so sorry" or "What can I do to help you?," and a comforting touch as she talks or cries.

- Use somato-emotional integration techniques at her neck and throat when full expression of her emotions is her goal, but honor the fact that some people may completely inhibit their grief, and others delay feeling grief to "take care of business" – usually another infant or older child.

- Schedule her appointments with sensitivity to the fact that it may be difficult for her to see and hear other mothers with infants or see baby-related office decorations.

- Be flexible in your scheduling, if possible, to accommodate her need to tell her story; as she talks, work on her hands and feet to help her feel more grounded.

- Provide referrals to mental health professionals and support groups that specialize in perinatal loss and partner/relationship support after loss. Know that with skillful intervention, the bereaved family is better prepared to experience their grief and move forward. ⊕

- If you have the privilege to support a stillbirth, use your touch as appropriate, such as holding a hand or touching a shoulder to comfort the mother through labor and birth (Figure 7.4). Be prepared for her maternity healthcare providers to offer the family the opportunity to see, touch and hold the stillborn infant, to validate the death and provide time for the family to be together and grieve.

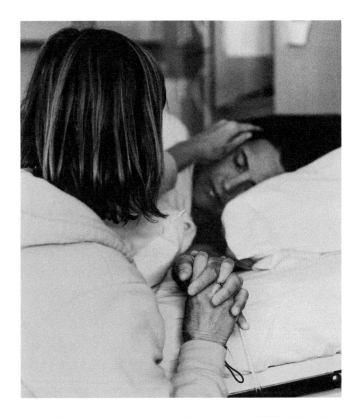

Figure 7.4
Supporting stillbirth. If you have the privilege to support a stillbirth, maintain calm physical contact with your client to comfort her through labor.

- Learn more about perinatal grief and deal honestly with your own feelings about loss and death to be better able to help your clients.

From the treatment room

I had two miscarriages prior to receiving bodywork. Through the course of my sessions, I discovered a lot of stored-up feelings regarding a child I'd carried and delivered many years prior to these losses. I was able to process my feelings regarding that baby and the feelings around the miscarriages. My next pregnancy produced my precious Brittany.

– **Courtney**, client

Multiple Gestations

Multiple gestation is defined as a pregnancy with two or more fetuses. This includes twins, and higher-order multiples such as triplets and quadruplets. In the United States, the number of multiple gestations has increased dramatically in the past two decades due to assisted reproductive technology and people choosing pregnancy at older ages. About one-third of live births from assisted reproductive technology result in more than one infant, and twins represent 85 percent of all multiples (De Sutter 2015). The overall prevalence of twins is approximately 12 per 1,000, and two-thirds are identical twins (March of Dimes 2015c). The two common types of twin are **monozygotic** (identical) and **dizygotic** (fraternal). Triplets can be monozygotic, dizygotic or **trizygotic**.

Mothers of multiples are at higher risk for preterm labor, polyhydramnios, hyperemesis gravidarum, anemia, pre-eclampsia, perinatal depression, and antepartum and postpartum hemorrhage. Risks and complications for the babies include prematurity, respiratory distress syndrome, birth asphyxia, congenital anomalies, **twin-to-twin transfusion syndrome**, intrauterine growth restriction and becoming conjoined (Martin et al. 2014).

General Guidelines

- Consider moving into second- and third-trimester-recommended positioning earlier in a multiples pregnancy to maximize the benefits of sidelying and semireclining, and to avoid supine hypotensive syndrome.

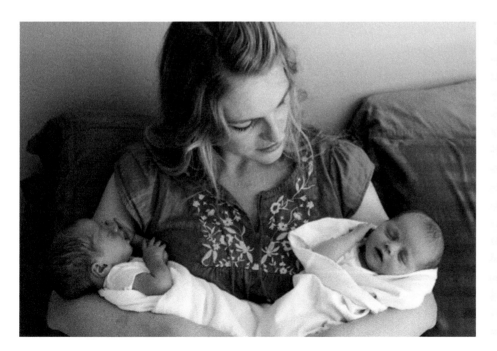

Figure 7.5
Multiple gestation with twins. Twice the joy and twice the strain of newborn care mean these mothers need your healing postpartum massage.

Chapter 7

- Consider the many hormonal, physical and emotional adaptations that may happen earlier with multiple gestations.

- Focus on postural changes, giving special attention to your client's pelvis and all weight-bearing myofascial structures and joints, including her feet.

- Offer extra abdominal care as her soft tissue may be more stretched and hypotoned, especially if she comes close to term pregnancy.

- In the postpartum time, provide focused work to her neck, shoulders, arms and back because of the increased infant care with multiples, and support her as she tries to regain core strength and integrity (Chapters 4 and 6).

From the treatment room

Because I was carrying triplets, I was on total bed rest from week 22 until their birth at 35 weeks. I got so stir-crazy. I was either in pain or generally achy all the time. The last weeks of pregnancy, I got massages each week, and they were the highlight of each week. I never would have carried my babies as long without it. Massage helped me maintain the pregnancies and my sanity.

— **Kristen**, client

Perinatal Mood and Anxiety Disorders (PMADs)

Perinatal mood and anxiety disorders are the most common complication of the childbearing years and are a leading cause of maternal morbidity and mortality. They can begin any time during or after pregnancy, after a pregnancy loss or after an adoption. As discussed in Chapters 1 and 6, emotional lability is a normal prenatal experience; the "baby blues" are considered normal, appropriate responses to parenthood's profound changes and rarely last longer than two weeks. Symptoms diminish with resting, reducing stress and pain, and providing the family with plenty of support (Simkin et al. 2018). At least 1 in 7 mothers experience serious depression or

anxiety during pregnancy or postpartum, and 1 to 2 out of 1,000 have postpartum psychosis. And let's not forget that 1 in 10 fathers and partners also experience postpartum depression or anxiety.

Signs and symptoms often appear well before the postpartum period (Box 7.5). Thirty percent of people who showed signs of depression after birth had previously experienced an episode before their pregnancies. Forty percent had an episode of depression during pregnancy, and more than two-thirds also had signs of an anxiety disorder. Of those with postpartum depression, 1 in 5 of the women had thoughts of harming themselves. Suicide is the second leading cause of death in postpartum

---

Box 7.5
Signs and symptoms of perinatal mood and anxiety disorders (PMADs)

- Anxiety, depression and mood swings
- Loss of confidence and feelings of guilt and failure as a mother
- Loss of appetite, weight loss, constipation
- Low mood, especially in the morning, sadness, tearfulness
- Low energy, exhaustion that is not relieved by sleep, and sleep difficulties (insomnia)
- Irritability, indecisiveness, diminished concentration
- Compulsive and obsessive thoughts
- Loss of joy, pleasure or libido
- Poor personal hygiene
- Despair and low interest in life
- Bleak and pessimistic view of the future
- Lack of response to the infant's cues or cries for care
- Social isolation (does not answer the door or the phone)
- Thoughts of hurting herself or the baby

Adapted from Ricci S (2017) Essentials of Maternity, Newborn and Women's Health Nursing, 4th edn. New York: Wolters Kluwer.

people. All of these sobering statistics point to the need for early universal screening for perinatal mood and anxiety disorders.

Mandatory screening of pregnant and postpartum women for perinatal mood and anxiety disorders is now recommended by the ACOG, the American Academy of Pediatrics and the American Medical Association, following recommendations of the 2019 United States Preventive Services Task Force. Another group, Postpartum Support International, recommends universal screening using an evidence-based tool such as the Edinburgh Postnatal Depression Screen (EPDS) or Patient Health Questionnaire (PHQ-9). These are free, self-administered, easy to complete, translated into many languages, and a reliable and valid measure of mood in mothers, fathers and partners.

Of course, screening by itself does not improve outcomes for mothers and their families. It is necessary to have appropriate follow-up and treatment with professional behavioral health providers specializing in perinatal mood and anxiety disorders (Postpartum Support International 2019).

Reminder

Each person with a perinatal mood and anxiety disorder deserves a customized, multidisciplinary care plan specific to her needs – individual and group behavioral health therapy, nutritional adjustments, supplements, medication, and a mixture of integrative modalities including massage therapy (King et al. 2019; Ricci 2017).

Numerous research studies point to massage therapy having great potential for depressed and anxious mothers and their babies. One study suggests that pregnant women diagnosed with major depression who received weekly prenatal massage had reduced depression prenatally and postpartum. Their newborns were also less likely to be born preterm and with low birth weight, and had better neonatal adjustment (Field et al. 2010). Another small study of depressed second-trimester women documented

reduced back and leg pain, lower levels of stress-related neurotransmitters and less reported anxiety. Their babies were less likely to be premature and scored better on newborn assessment scales than control babies whose mothers were also depressed but received only relaxation guidance (Field et al. 2004).

Recent research also points to the link between inflammation and maternal mental health (Achtyes et al. 2020). Inflammation is associated with the onset of major depressive disorders independent of the pre- and perinatal period. Various sources – from stress to refined sugar to chemical exposure – can cause inflammation in the brain and gut, impacting the production of mood-boosting neurotransmitters such as serotonin (Deans 2017).

General Guidelines

- Use trimester- or postpartum-appropriate positioning for your client's comfort.

- Integrate postural guidance and integrity techniques (see Figures 4.15–4.17) to address the typical "closed body" posture that is often an expression of suppressed mood.

- Remind her that "she is not alone and deserves to and can feel better." Tell her that you care about her and her family. Make lists of professional behavioral health providers specializing in perinatal mood and anxiety disorders available to all your clients, and offer a referral and assistance to connect with them when clients seek this help. With the client's prior permission, notify her maternity healthcare provider as well.

- Encourage her seeking social support for herself and her family from her family and friends.

Placental Abnormalities

Placenta previa means "afterbirth first" and refers to when the placenta implants and develops over or near the cervical opening, or os. Placenta previa is classified as total, partial, marginal or low-lying, depending on coverage of or proximity to the cervix (Ricci 2017). The risk of placenta previa in a first pregnancy is 1 in 400, but it rises to 1 in 160 after one Cesarean birth; 1 in 60 after two; 1 in 30 after three; and 1 in 10 after four Cesarean births. Placenta previa is associated with hemorrhage, placenta abruptia or emergency Cesarean birth (Joy and Temming 2015). With the increase in Cesarean births, coupled with higher maternal age and more infertility treatments, the incidence of placenta previa has risen dramatically.

Prenatal care and timely diagnosis of placenta previa on ultrasound can improve outcomes. Bleeding in the last two trimesters of pregnancy is a very worrying symptom requiring immediate medical care. Choice of medical treatments depends in part on the extent of bleeding and the degree to which the placenta covers the cervix, if the baby is developed enough to survive outside the womb, and if the woman is or is not in labor (Yeomans 2017). If the mother and baby are both stable, medical care may include "expectant management" – a "watchful wait-and-see," either at home with no bleeding or in a hospital antepartum unit for continuous care and monitoring.

Also, placental vascularization can be defective, with the placenta attaching deeper and directly into the uterine muscle layers. The mildest cases are diagnosed as placenta accreta; those deeply attached to the uterine muscle layers are called placenta increta; and the most severe, infiltrating the uterine muscle layers, are referred to as placenta percreta.

Placenta abruptia is the premature separation of a normally implanted placenta, after the 20th week of gestation and prior to birth, followed by concealed or apparent, mild, moderate or severe hemorrhage (Ricci 2017). The baby's blood supply is compromised, and **fetal distress** develops proportionally with the degree of placental separation. Placenta abruptia is a significant cause of third-trimester bleeding and occurs in about 1 percent of all pregnancies worldwide. It is potentially lethal, with 50 percent fetal mortality, and 6 percent maternal mortality related to Cesarean birth, hemorrhage and coagulopathy (Jaju et al. 2014). Risks to the mother include hemorrhage, blood transfusions, emergency hysterectomy, **disseminated intravascular coagulopathy** and renal failure (Mukherjee et al. 2014).

General Guidelines

- If the mother is currently bleeding, refer her to her maternity healthcare provider before massaging.

- Use the left sidelying position only to maximize fetal circulation.

- If mother and baby are stable, continue to use the left sidelying position to maximize fetal circulation, and secure the maternity healthcare provider's consent to use other trimester- or postpartum-appropriate positioning for her comfort.

Preterm Labor and Birth

A developing baby grows throughout pregnancy, including in the final weeks, when the brain, lungs and liver fully develop. Labor is considered preterm when the baby is born before 37 weeks of gestation. The same signs and symptoms of full-term pregnancy labor occur – change in vaginal discharge indicating possible premature rupture of membranes or bloody show; rhythmic, dull low backache; regular or frequent uterine contractions; increased pelvic pressure; diarrhea; and a shortening cervix with changes in effacement and/or dilation – but they come too early. A woman is at greater risk of preterm labor if she had a prior preterm birth, is pregnant with multiples, has cervical insufficiency, is a smoker and has not had prenatal care (King et al. 2019). In 2018, preterm birth affected 1 of every 10 infants born in the United States. Persistent racial and ethnic differences in preterm birth rates are illustrated by a 14 percent preterm birth rate among African–American women versus 9 percent among white women.

Babies born preterm and before 32 weeks have higher rates of death and disability. In 2017, preterm birth and low birth weight accounted for about 17 percent of infant deaths. Infants who are born prematurely have higher rates of **cerebral palsy**, sensory deficits, learning disabilities and respiratory illnesses compared with children born at term, and can have lifelong or life-threatening health problems. Preterm births can also take an emotional toll on and create a financial burden for families (CDC 2019c). Treatment is typically directed at keeping the baby growing in utero if possible, with bed rest, tocolytic medications that slow or stop uterine contractions, and corticosteroids to help mature the baby's lungs (King et al. 2019).

General Guidelines

- Use the left sidelying position only to maximize fetal circulation. If mother and baby are stable, continue to use the left sidelying position to maximize fetal circulation, and secure the maternity healthcare provider's consent to use other trimester-appropriate positioning for your client's comfort.

- When she is on bed rest, follow our recommended guidelines.

- Use additional towels or a waterproof covering on your table, in case further leakage occurs during your session.

Traumatic Birth and Post-Traumatic Stress Disorder (PTSD)

Sometimes giving birth is traumatic. Much depends on how the woman perceives events, rather than on how others perceive them (Beck et al. 2013). A woman is more likely to experience her baby's birth as traumatic if labor pain exceeds her ability to cope with it, if the birth is complicated (such as preterm labor, hemorrhage, unexpected hysterectomy, life-threatening pre-eclampsia or eclampsia, perineal trauma, emergency Cesarean birth), if she or her baby goes to the NICU, or if the baby has unexpected birth defects or dies. A mother may anguish over her fragile child fighting for life. She may feel shocked, guilty, and torn between bonding and distancing herself, hoping to minimize her pain if the baby dies. Hopes for survival and worries about whether her baby will be normal can upend joyous expectations with anxiety and grief over the loss of the ideal infant that she dreamed of while also suffering separation from her baby.

Traumatic childbirth occurs in as many as 25 to 34 percent of births (PATTCH 2019). Research from a variety of countries shows that a person is also more likely to experience giving birth as traumatic if she perceives the medical professionals as uncaring, if she feels disrespected or that her dignity has been stripped away, or if

it seems that she has no control over what is done to her or her baby.

Approximately one-third of these people may develop post-traumatic stress disorder (PATTCH 2019). Often, they experience an extreme sense of helplessness, isolation, lack of care, fear and anxiety (Simkin et al. 2018). Signs and symptoms include persistent increased arousal (irritability, difficulty sleeping, hypervigilance, exaggerated startle response); avoidance of stimuli associated with the birth, including thoughts, feelings, people, places and details of the event; intrusive re-experiencing of a past traumatic event with anxiety and panic attacks, flashbacks or nightmares; and feeling a sense of unreality and detachment (PATTCH 2019).

In 2014, the World Health Organization (WHO) issued a statement called "Prevention and Elimination of Disrespect and Abuse During Childbirth." It reports that "Many women experience disrespectful and abusive treatment during childbirth in facilities worldwide. Such treatment not only violates their rights to respectful care, but can also threaten their rights to life, health, bodily integrity, and freedom from discrimination. In addition to physical and psychological harm, this treatment can lead to poor labor progress and fetal distress. Although young, unmarried, poor, or ethnically excluded people are particularly likely to receive cruel treatment, middle-class well-educated women are also treated this way." WHO lists the following as elements of respectful, competent maternity healthcare: "social support through a companion of choice, mobility, access to food and fluids, **confidentiality,** privacy, informed choice, information for women on their rights, and high professional standards of clinical care" (WHO 2014).

Also, survivors of previous sexual trauma are more susceptible to perceiving childbirth events as dangerous, and being retraumatized as a result (Poote et al. 2015). The sexual nature of pregnancy, birth and breastfeeding, coupled with bodily exposure, pelvic penetration, pain, and possible damage to sexual parts of the body, can be very real during both sexual abuse and childbearing. Some experience trauma-related flashbacks, anxiety and intrusive thoughts, which add greatly to their fear and anxiety before, during and after labor (Seng and Taylor 2015; James 2015). Meta-analyses of studies from many countries show that 1 in every 5 childbearing women has experienced sexual trauma between early childhood and age 18. Physical and emotional abuse is also common. Trauma in adulthood – rape or intimate partner abuse – also takes a heavy toll on the childbearing person. Even years afterward, some individuals may have post-traumatic stress disorder (Simkin and Klaus 2011).

Reminder

Some of your clients are probably trauma survivors, whether they tell you or not. Your work can help them to navigate those effects and their childbearing with helpful body awareness and less stress and pain.

Our life experiences strongly influence our perceptions of unfamiliar places, people and events as safe or threatening, reasonable or unreasonable, helpful or not. Survivors of sexual trauma may involuntarily experience intense fear or tension during medical care. This may be triggered by stimuli that other women consider ordinary, such as being asked to remove their clothing, lie on their backs, have cervical examinations and being attached to monitors with belts. They may find the normal sensations of labor overwhelming. Even with pain relief, a sexual abuse survivor may feel violated with her legs in stirrups, private areas being exposed and people staring at her (Beck et al. 2004). Whether a woman has experienced prior trauma or not, a traumatic birth experience adds distress and can diminish confidence at a time when she needs all her resources for postpartum recovery and infant care (Simkin and Klaus 2011).

Because so many childbearing people have experienced trauma as children or adults, trauma-informed care is an essential strategic approach to reducing fear and increasing trust. Many professionals now suggest that trauma-informed care become a "universal precaution" in perinatal care (Box 7.6). Not only is trauma-informed care well received by most people, but it can begin to heal the effects of traumatic experiences (Simkin et al. 2018). If a person feels respected, supported and informed, included in decisions, and adequately in control of what

---

Box 7.6
Basics of trauma-informed pre- and perinatal care

- Screen new clients for possible trauma history. Normalize the client's experience of being asked by sharing "About one in four women has been sexually abused in childhood, and sadly it also happens to adults too. Because these experiences can affect your pregnancy, birth and postpartum time, I ask all my clients about unwanted sexual experiences." Allow the client control over what she says, and when she says it, in order to keep her emotional defenses intact. Refer clients who disclose trauma to mental health professionals who specialize in pre- and perinatal post-traumatic stress disorder.

- Identify the many opportunities to adapt your client's care. Allow her to maintain control with careful attention to your respectful language, obtaining permission and sharing decision making.

- Make reducing her fear and stress a primary goal of your sessions.

- During labor and birth, provide more intensive support and communication that helps to increase her sense of control and safety.

- In the early postpartum time, allow time and space for her to make sense of the birth, reconstructing what happened and how she felt in her own words; remember that her perception is her reality. Use reflective listening skills and express empathy. Remember that early intervention, with "unhurried, open-minded and openhearted processing of her birth experience, can enhance the positive aspects of the birth and her role in it, and prevent trauma. Delay or avoidance of this sharing misses an opportunity to positively influence a woman's long-term self-esteem and mental health" (Simkin et al. 2018).

- Support postpartum wellness and healthy touch and attachment in her family.

Adapted from King T, Brucker M, Osborne K, Jevitt C (2019) Varney's Midwifery, 6th edn. Burlington, MA: Jones & Bartlett Learning and Simkin P, Klaus P (2011) When Survivors Give Birth, 2nd edn. Seattle: Classic Day.

is happening to herself and her baby, she may experience frightening or challenging clinical events without being traumatized. In fact, she may feel that her clinical professionals were especially supportive and skilled. Trauma-informed care supports this type of outcome, and helps prevent trauma responses and post-traumatic stress disorder (Poote and McKenzie-McHarg 2015).

Simkin and Klaus (2011) summarize this eloquently in their work. A satisfying birth experience, as the woman defines it, can be healing and empowering when the care given is respectful, kind and individualized to the woman's needs. If a woman was abused in childhood, trauma-informed care also helps reduce the risk that her own children will be abused. Appropriate massage and bodywork can help pregnant survivors to reduce anxiety and pain; reach deeper relaxation states, improve body awareness and embody positive touch experiences; resolve and discharge traumatic memories and feelings; and physically and emotionally prepare for childbirth and mothering.

General Guidelines

- Use all trimester- and postpartum-appropriate positioning for your client's comfort. Remember that the sidelying position easily allows for communication and tracking with a client with a trauma history.

- Consider better positioning options than prone, especially when working near and with her pelvis, to facilitate her sense of control and create a positive touch experience.

- Review and integrate the basics of trauma-informed pre- and perinatal care (see Box 7.6) in your sessions. Pursue additional training in trauma-informed care and prenatal, perinatal and birth post-traumatic stress disorder.

- Refer her to and consult with mental health professionals who specialize in prenatal, perinatal and birth post-traumatic stress disorder.

Vaginal Bleeding

There are many possible causes of vaginal bleeding, and one usual maternal response – fear. Vaginal bleeding, from light blood staining to hemorrhage, can occur any time before birth. During labor and birth,

vaginal bleeding beyond the normal bloody show or third-stage bleeding is worrying. In the postpartum period, vaginal bleeding in excess of normal lochia discharge warrants your client's prompt call to her maternity healthcare provider.

Up to 20 percent of expectant women have vaginal bleeding during the first trimester, but only about half of these women actually have a pregnancy loss (Gilbert 2011). Causes of first-trimester bleeding include implantation bleeding, miscarriage, ectopic pregnancy, molar pregnancy, subchorionic hemorrhage, cervical examination, pap smear or sex (Grindell 2019). Conditions associated with vaginal bleeding after 20 weeks of pregnancy include placenta previa, placenta abruptia, and placenta accreta, increta and percreta (Ricci 2017).

General Guidelines

- Whenever a client has bleeding – with or without pelvic, back or abdominal pain – attempt to determine if any pain is musculoskeletal in origin. If not, pain may be referred from uterine contractions that suggest a threatened miscarriage or preterm labor.

- Use the left sidelying position only to maximize fetal circulation until bleeding has resolved.

- Eliminate all abdominal techniques except in cases of postpartum uterine atony, in which case Uterine Fundal Massage is indicated (see Figure 6.16).

- If your client shows signs of hemorrhage, call 911 (or equivalent) immediately and with her consent to call; continue Uterine Fundal Massage until medical care arrives (see Figure 6.16) (Simkin et al. 2018).

Chapter Summary

Working with clients with special needs, high-risk factors and complications can challenge and expand your abilities as a pre- and perinatal massage therapist. We understand that it may feel daunting and scary; however, we encourage you to consider the incredible reward – for both you and your clients – when facing your fears and opening to life's challenges as empowering opportunities for growth. Further your understanding of the medical aspects of childbearing so that your massage therapy can skillfully complement your clients' medical care. Continue your pre- and perinatal massage therapy education with ready access to a medical glossary and additional resources on high-risk factors and complications. Revisit this chapter when these opportunities present to safely care for these clients, who are so deserving and in need of your thoughtful, attentive and healing pre- and perinatal massage therapy.

Think it through

To deepen your knowledge, go to our online resources, answer the test questions for this chapter and explore further.

References and Further Reading

AAAAI (American Academy of Allergy, Asthma & Immunology) (2015) Asthma and Pregnancy. Available at: http://www.aaaai.org/conditions-and-treatments/library/asthma-library/asthma-and-pregnancy.aspx [accessed February 2, 2020].

Achtyes E, Keaton SA, Smart L et al. (2020) Inflammation and kynurenine pathway dysregulation in post-partum women with severe and suicidal depression. Brain Beh Immun. 83:239–247.

ACOG (American College of Obstetricians and Gynecologists) (2014) ACOG Task Force on Hypertension in Pregnancy – A Step Forward in Management. Contemporary OB/GYN. Available at: https://www.contemporaryobgyn.net/view/acog-task-force-hypertension-pregnancy-step-forward-management [accessed July 27, 2019].

ACOG (American College of Obstetricians and Gynecologists) (2016) Perinatal risks associated with assisted reproductive technology, Committee Opinion, no. 671, September. Available at: https://www.acog.org/Clinical-Guidance-and-Publications/Committee-Opinions/Committee-on-Obstetric-Practice/Perinatal-Risks-Associated-With-Assisted-Reproductive-Technology, [accessed November 15, 2019].

ACOG (American College of Obstetricians and Gynecologists) (2018) ACOG Practice Bulletin No. 196: Thromboembolism in pregnancy. Obstet Gynecol. 132(1):e1–e17.

ACOG (American College of Obstetricians and Gynecologists) (2019) ACOG Practice Bulletin No. 212: Pregnancy and heart disease. Obstet Gynecol. 133(5):e320–e356.

American Pregnancy Association (2019a) Bed Rest During Pregnancy. Available at: https://americanpregnancy.org/pregnancy-complications/bed-rest/ [accessed October 30, 2019].

American Pregnancy Association (2019b) Pregnancy Concerns. Available at: http://www.americanpregnancy.org/main/statistics.html [accessed July 31, 2020].

Ayyavoo A, Derraik JB, Hofman PL et al. (2014) Hyperemesis gravidarum and long-term health of the offspring. Am J Obstet Gynecol. 210(6):521–525.

Beck C, Driscoll J, Watson S (2013) Traumatic Childbirth. New York: Routledge.

Bolz M, Körber S, Reimer T et al. (2017) Treatment of illnesses arising in pregnancy. Dtsch Arztebl Int. 114:616–626.

Castillo MJ, Phillippi JC (2015) Hyperemesis gravidarum: a holistic overview and approach to clinical assessment and management. J Perinat Neonatal Nurs. 29(1):12–22.

CDC (Centers for Disease Control) (2019a) Infertility services. Available at: https://www.cdc.gov/nchs/nsfg/key_statistics/i.htm#infertilityservices [accessed November 15, 2019].

CDC (Centers for Disease Control) (2019b) Pregnancy Complications. Available at: https://www.cdc.gov/reproductive-health/maternalinfanthealth/pregnancy-complications.html [accessed October 15, 2019].

CDC (Centers for Disease Control) (2019c) Preterm birth. Available at: https://www.cdc.gov/reproductivehealth/MaternalInfantHealth/PretermBirth.htm [accessed November 15, 2019].

Cornell S (2015) Continual evolution of type 2 diabetes: an update on pathophysiology and emerging treatment options. Ther Clin Risk Man. 11:621–632.

De Sutter P (2015) The Challenge of Multiple Pregnancies in Reducing Risk in Fertility Treatment. London: Springer, pp. 1–17.

Deans E (2017) Microbiome and mental health in the modern environment. J Physiol Anthropol. 36:1.

Enzer S (2004) Reflexology: A Tool for Midwives. Pymble, Australia: Susanne Enzer.

Field T, Grizzle N, Scafidi F et al. (1996) Massage and relaxation therapies' effects on depressed adolescent mothers. Adolescence. 31:903–911.

Field T, Diego MA, Hernandez-Reif M (2004) Massage therapy effects on depressed pregnant women. J Psychos Obstet Gynecol. 25:115–122.

Field T, Diego M, Hernandez-Reif M et al. (2009) Pregnancy massage reduces prematurity, low birthweight and postpartum depression. Infant Behav Dev. 32(4):454–60.

Field T, Diego M, Hernandez-Reif M (2010) Prenatal depression effects and interventions: a review. Infant Behav Dev. 33(4):409–418.

Field T, Diego M, Hernandez-Reif M (2012) Yoga and massage therapy reduce prenatal depression and prematurity. J Bodyw Mov Ther. 16(2):204-9.

FIGO (International Federation of Gynecology and Obstetrics) (2019) Predicting and Preventing Pre-eclampsia: The Challenge. Available at: https://www.figo.org/figo-releases-new-guidelines-combat-pre-eclampsia [accessed May 20, 2020].

Genetic and Rare Diseases Information Center (2018) Diethylstilbestrol syndrome. Available at: https://rarediseases.info.nih.gov/diseases/1859/diethylstilbestrol-syndrome [accessed July 25, 2020].

Gilbert E (2011) Manual of High-risk Pregnancy and Delivery, 5th edn. St. Louis: Mosby/Elsevier.

Green CJ (2016) Maternal Newborn Nursing Care Plans, 3rd edn. Burlington, MA: Jones & Bartlett Learning.

Grindell S (2019) What Causes First Trimester Bleeding? An OB-GYN Weighs In. Available at: https://www.romper.com/p/what-causes-first-trimester-bleeding-ob-gyn-weighs-in-18662834 [accessed November 12, 2019].

Grunebaum A, Chervenak FA (2014) Counseling Parents After Fetal Demise and Stillbirth. Available at: https://www.uptodate.com/contents/stillbirth-maternal-care?-search=counseling%20parents-after-fetal-demise-and-stillbirth&source=search_result&selectedTitle=1~150&usage_type=default&display_rank=1 [accessed November 12, 2019].

Hung T, Lo L, Chiu T et al. (2010) A longitudinal study of oxidative stress and antioxidant status in women with uncomplicated pregnancies throughout gestation. Reprod Sci. 17(4):401–409.

Ingram J, Domagala C, Yates S (2005) The effects of shiatsu on post-term pregnancies. Complement Ther Med. 13:11–15.

Jaju KG, Kulkarni AP, Mundada SK (2014) Study of perinatal outcome in relation to abruptio placentae. Int J Recent Trends Sci Tech. 11(3):355–358.

James S (2015) Women's experiences of symptoms of post-traumatic stress disorder after traumatic childbirth: a review and critical appraisal. Arch Womens Ment Health. 18(6):761–771.

Joy S, Temming L (2015) Placenta Previa. Available at: http://emedicine.medscape.com/article/262063-overview [accessed November 4, 2019].

KellyMom (2018) Mastitis. Available at: https://kellymom.com/bf/concerns/mother/mastitis [accessed November 7, 2019].

King T, Brucker M, Osborne K et al. (2019) Varney's Midwifery, 6th edn. Burlington, MA: Jones & Bartlett Learning.

Kleiber B, Dimidjian S (2014) Postpartum depression among adolescent mothers: a comprehensive review of prevalence, course, correlates, consequences, and interventions. Clin Psychology: Sci Pract. 21(1):48–66.

Maltepe C, Popa M, Bertucci C et al. (2015) The effects of counseling and predictors of pregnancy outcomes in women with hyperemesis gravidarum. Obstet Gynecol. 316(125):101S.

March of Dimes (2015a) Asthma During Pregnancy. Available at: https://www.marchofdimes.org/complications/asthma-during-pregnancy.aspx [accessed February 2, 2020].

March of Dimes (2015b) Pregnancy Loss. Available at: https://www.marchofdimes.org/complications/stillbirth.aspx [accessed October 30, 2019].

March of Dimes (2015c) Multiples: Twins, Triplets and Beyond. Available at: https://www.marchofdimes.org/complications/being-pregnant-with-twins-triplets-and-other-multiples.aspx [accessed November 8, 2019].

March of Dimes (2017) Signs and Symptoms of Preterm Labor. Available at: https://www.marchofdimes.org/complications/signs-and-symptoms-of-preterm-labor.aspx [accessed November 10, 2019].

Martin R, Fanaroff A, Walsh M (2014) Fanaroff & Martin's Neonatal Perinatal Medicine, 10th edn. Philadelphia: Elsevier Health Sciences.

Mukherjee S, Bawa A, Sharma S et al. (2014) Retrospective study of risk factors and maternal and fetal outcome in patients with abruptio placentae. J Nat Sci Biol Med. 5(2):425–428.

NAEPP (National Asthma Education and Prevention Program) (2015) Available at: https://www.nhlbi.nih.gov/science/national-asthma-education-and-prevention-program-naepp [accessed May 28, 2019].

Nagtalon-Ramos J (2014) Maternal-Newborn Nursing Care: Best Evidence-based Practices. Philadelphia: F. A. Davis.

Osborne C (2009) Pre- and Perinatal Massage Therapy: Survey of Massage Therapists. Available at www.bodytherapyeducation.com [accessed June 10, 2010].

Osborne C (2015a) Postpartum Depression and Massage Therapy: Selected Research. Available at: https://www.massagemag.com/postpartum-depression-massage-therapy-selected-research-33226/ [accessed October 10, 2019].

Osborne C (2015b) Postpartum depression: physical and emotional benefits of massage. Massage Magazine. November.

Ozgoli G, Naz MS (2018) Effects of complementary medicine on nausea and vomiting in pregnancy: a systematic review. Int J Prev Med. 9:75.

PATTCH (Prevention and Treatment of Traumatic Childbirth) (2019) Resource Guide. Available at: http://pattch.org/resource-guide [accessed November 10, 2019].

Poote A, McKenzie-McHarg K (2015) The experience of post-traumatic stress disorder following childbirth. J Health Visiting. 3(2):92–98.

Postpartum Support International (2019). Available at: https://www.postpartum.net/learn-more/pregnancy-postpartum-mental-health/ [accessed May 16, 2019].

Preeclampsia (2019) Women and Families. Available at: https://www.preeclampsia.org/women-and-families [accessed October 30, 2019].

Queenan J, Spong C, Lockwood C (2015) Protocols for High-risk Pregnancies: An Evidence-based Approach. West Sussex: John Wiley & Sons, pp. 315–328.

Ricci S (2017) Essentials of Maternity, Newborn and Women's Health Nursing, 4th edn. New York: Wolters Kluwer.

Robinson G (2014) Pregnancy loss. Best Pract Res Clin Obstet and Gynaecol. 28(1):169–178.

Seng J, Taylor J (2015) Trauma Informed Care in the Perinatal Period: Protecting Children and Young People. Edinburgh: Dunedin Academic Press.

Serrallach O (2018) The Postpartum Depletion Cure: A Complete Guide to Rebuilding Your Health and Reclaiming Your Energy for Mothers of Newborns, Toddlers and Young Children. New York: Hachette.

Simkin P, Ancheta R (2018) The Labor Progress Handbook, 5th edn. Oxford: Blackwell Science.

Simkin P, Klaus P (2011) When Survivors Give Birth, 2nd edn. Seattle: Classic Day.

Simkin P, Whalley J, Keppler A et al. (2018) Pregnancy, Childbirth and the Newborn: The Complete Guide, 5th edn. New York: Da Capo Lifelong Books.

Smith J, Refuerzo J, Ramin S (2016) Nausea and Vomiting of Pregnancy: Beyond the Basics. Available at: http://www.uptodate.com/contents/nauseaand-vomiting-of-pregnancy-beyond-the-basics [accessed October 15, 2019].

Sosa C, Althabe F, Belizan J et al. (2015) Bed rest in singleton pregnancies for preventing preterm birth. Cochrane Database Syst Rev. 3:CD003581.

Sperlich M, Seng J, Li Y et al. (2017) Integrating trauma-informed care into maternity care practice: conceptual and practical issues. J Midwifery Women's Health. 62(6):661–672.

Stager L (2010) Nurturing Massage for Pregnancy. Baltimore: Lippincott, Williams & Wilkins.

Stillerman E (2008) Prenatal Massage. St. Louis: Mosby/Elsevier.

Taylor T (2014) Treatment of nausea and vomiting in pregnancy. Aust Prescr. 37(2):42–45.

Tulandi T, Al-Fozan H (2015) Spontaneous Abortion: Management. Available at: http://www.uptodate.com/contents/spontaneous-abortion-risk-factors-etiology-clinical-manifestations-and-diagnostic-evaluation [accessed November 1, 2019].

Tully G (2020) Changing Birth on Earth. Bloomington: Maternity House Publishing.

US Preventive Services Task Force, Curry SJ, Krist AH, et al. (2019) Interventions to Prevent Perinatal Depression: US Preventive Services Recommendation Statement. JAMA. 321(6):580–587.

Vanders RL, Murphy VE (2015) Maternal complications and the management of asthma in pregnancy. Womens Health. 11(2):183–191.

Wisner K, Sit D, McShea M et al. (2013) Onset timing, thoughts of self-harm, and diagnoses in postpartum women with screen-positive depression findings. JAMA Psych. 70(5):490–498.

WHO (World Health Organization) (2014) Prevention and Elimination of Disrespect and Abuse During Childbirth. Available at: https://www.who.int/reproductivehealth/topics/maternal_perinatal/statement-childbirth/en/ [accessed November 10, 2019].

WHO (World Health Organization) (2010) The Worldwide Incidence of Preterm Birth: A Systematic Review of Maternal Mortality and Morbidity. Available at: https://www.who.int/bulletin/volumes/88/1/08-062554/en/ [accessed November 13, 2019].

Yates S (2010) Pregnancy and Childbirth: A Holistic Approach to Massage and Bodywork. Edinburgh: Elsevier.

Yeomans E (2017) Cunningham and Gilstrap's Operative Obstetrics, 3rd edn. New York: McGraw-Hill.

Studying this chapter will prepare you to:

1. plan the foundations and growth of your pre- and perinatal business

2. choose from the many possible marketing activities to promote your business

3. collect relevant client health information by performing effective client interviews and managing an effective charting system

4. think logically and critically to create useful, safe sessions

5. communicate with other maternity healthcare providers

6. sustain your business and overcome common obstacles to success

7. contemplate different work environments and models for your practice, based on successful therapists' stories.

Practice Considerations
Growing a Satisfying Career

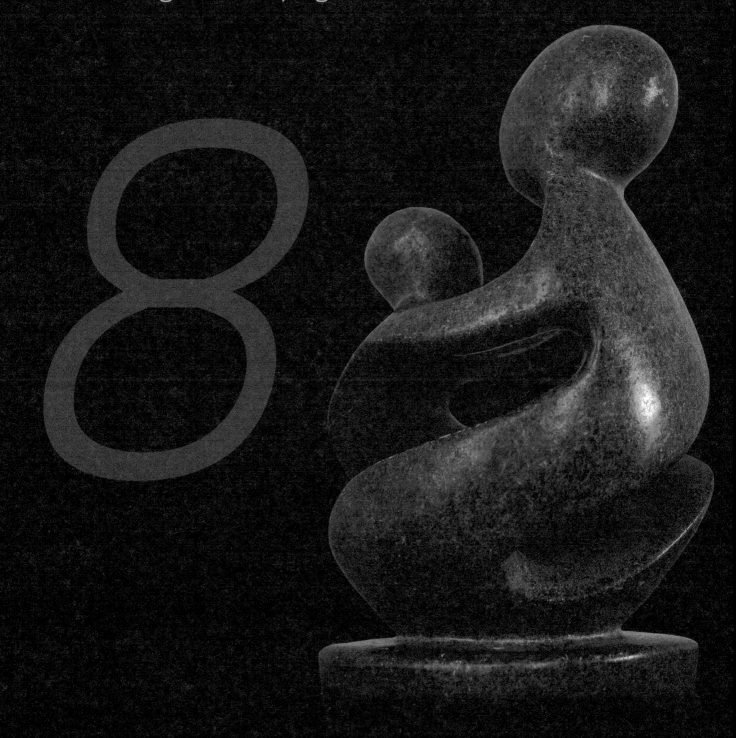

Chapter Overview

The previous chapters have presented general knowledge and specific techniques for childbearing-related needs. Now we will zero in on the practicalities of growing and running a pre- and perinatal massage therapy business. Our decades of working with this special population have given us concrete wisdom that we want to share – a variety of promotional ideas, how to acquire and record important health intake information, strategies to organize your thinking, and ways to create safe, effective sessions. You will learn how to enhance clients' experiences through educational activities, how to expand and diversify for a long-lasting perinatal practice, and how to overcome internal and external obstacles to success.

Because over one-third of massages are received in a therapist's office (AMTA 2018), this chapter focuses on that practice setting; however, most of the ideas and insights here are applicable in other work environments too. Opportunities abound in maternity massage and integrative healthcare centers, in hospital-based programs, in obstetrical, midwifery and other healthcare providers' offices, in spas and resorts, onsite and in franchise massage locations too. At this chapter's end, read the wisdom and insights of therapists who have worked in these various settings.

Getting Started

Prenatal, labor and postpartum massage therapy flourishes in so many settings that the possibilities ahead of you are numerous. But growing a satisfying practice requires persistent self-reflection (see Chapters 1 to 3 in Bower's *The Accidental Business Owner*, 2018) and a promotional foundation that establishes identity, credibility and trust. These questions need thoughtful, complete answers:

- **What will you call yourself?** If you intend to specialize with a prenatal and perinatal clientele, you may want to emphasize this in your title – consider "maternity massage therapist" or "pre- and perinatal massage therapist."

- **What gives you credibility as that specialist?** Many employers and clients seek therapists with more than basic prenatal massage therapy training. They want therapists with a comprehensive, hands-on pre- and perinatal education that has been verified by respected instructors and/or entities. Complete the training you need and plan to use that education and experience, and your professional affiliations – as well as your appearance, demeanor, communications, public image and the testimonials of others – to add to your credibility.

- **What modalities will you offer and during what parts of the childbearing cycle?** Discover what modalities you excel at and lean into promoting the benefits of those skills. Some therapists offer labor massage therapy, and many relish delivering the much-needed benefits of postpartum therapy for a continuum of care through the childbearing years.

- **How will you introduce yourself?** Aim to explain your work briefly and without excessive jargon. Here are two examples:

  o "I offer my pregnant and postpartum clients opportunities to relax, feel better and nurture healthier babies. I use soothing, appropriately deep techniques on painful muscles, and soothing strokes for tense spots, and I adapt my pressure to make it a safe, effective experience for all."

  o "I massage mothers during their labors and births. I also love teaching their labor support people to give relaxing, pain-relieving touch."

Reminder

Writing down your answers to the questions included in this section takes you another step closer to a successful maternity massage therapy practice.

Promoting Your Business

Marketing your work is as simple as "letting the world know you exist so the people who need you can find you" (Bowers 2018). It should be less about selling a product and more about showing who you are and your passion for your work. Our online resources and the sections below offer you specific ways to do just that.

Referrals

Word-of-mouth referrals work exceptionally well because pregnant people tend to talk about and share tips and resources with others – on blogs and social media, at pre- and postnatal exercise, yoga and childbirth education classes, and at baby fairs, as just a few examples. Be sure your current non-pregnant clients also know of your specialized skills. Above all else, make spreading the good word about your services easy: at the least, have a basic but informative website and current business cards ready. Offer complimentary phone or email consultations to potential clients. Make gift certificates available for your current clients and others to give to expectant family members, friends and co-workers.

Reminder

Notify your current clients that you are prepared to work with expectant clients. Consider also including an incentivizing discount on any gift certificates that they purchase for pregnant or postpartum mothers.

Networking

Develop a relationship with a variety of maternity professionals: prenatal exercise and yoga teachers, childbirth educators, birth and postpartum doulas, midwives, birthing centers, obstetricians, family practice physicians, hospitals, lactation consultants, home healthcare nurses, chiropractors, physical therapists, acupuncturists, and psychologists specializing in childbearing issues. Explore ways to mutually benefit each other. Keep them stocked with your promotional materials. Write articles for their blogs. Make educational presentations, a complimentary introductory session and discounts for additional sessions available for their staff or clientele. Build

your reputation in your community as a go-to expert with this client population.

From the treatment room

I joined a local online network group. For a small fee, they list me on their site. They also have local meetings and monthly "Meet the Doula" nights. At these events, I handed out information and talked to expecting parents about the benefits of prenatal massage therapy. I have given discount coupons with my business card and have found people very responsive.

I have built my professional reputation by being good at what I do. The word spreads quickly if you are good (or if you are not!). As I have also worked with the local birthing centers' midwives and nurses in their labor room over the years, they have gotten to know me. They can see that I am knowledgeable, professional and ethical.

– Nanci Newton, therapist

Internet Marketing

Most pregnant people today Google everything, and ask Alexa, and generally find their self-care and health-care via the Internet. At the very least, you need an informative website and a social media presence that highlights your pre- and perinatal services. Online appointment scheduling may help too. You can convey your expertise and demeanor in a blog. (See online resources for some of our favorite sites and blogs.) You may want to develop a niche within the childbearing realm – surrogates, those conceiving through assisted reproductive technology, LGBTQIA clients, military families, later-in-life moms, survivors of childhood or physical abuse, people on bed rest, mothers of multiples – just to name a few. If so, submit blog articles or become a regular contributor to that niche's relevant sites and social media outlets.

Your own client database is the beginning of an email marketing campaign. You also can purchase lists if you need a larger pool of contacts. Consider subscribing to one of several Internet businesses that specialize in circulating your **e-mail blasts** of announcements and e-newsletters. This will help you market responsibly and avoid your emails being filtered as spam. Find help with **search engine optimization**, **banner ads** and other aspects of **electronic advertising**. The Internet can feel complex – do whatever you need to remain focused and undaunted in navigating it.

Reminder

Maintain a lively Internet presence with a website and appropriate social media. Send meaningful information and offers via e-mail blasts. Subscribe to newsletters and follow reputable professionals and organizations.

Print Marketing

Despite our reliance on the Internet, most therapists still use a business card. A print brochure also is helpful to explain your services and their benefits. Feature most prominently, yet succinctly, the benefits clients seem to seek most: lower back pain relief, relaxation and help with sleeping, and upper back, neck and sacral pain reduction (Osborne 2009). You might consider developing and distributing information packets of articles, testimonials and relevant research. Tailor one for prospective clients and their partners, another for physicians and midwives, and yet another for other perinatal professionals. Have electronic files and print copies of all the above.

Explore options for writing for local newspapers, newsletters or other print publications too. **Bulk mailing** of postcards, using a mailing service and the tightest targeted geographic addresses near your workplace, can make using the postal service more economical and effective.

From the treatment room

Before I worked in a hospital setting, I visited OB-GYN offices in the vicinity and placed materials there, introducing myself to the receptionist. Now that I work in a hospital with patients on bed rest, I have a flyer listing the benefits of receiving a massage even if a patient is high risk. I give copies of these and the magazine *Sidelines* (a publication for women on bed rest) to each of the moms on bed rest and simply speak with them as I give those who would like it a hand massage. Most moms on bed rest are feeling restless and alone so that kind of contact is enormously powerful for them. This approach and word of mouth have been enough for generating the number of clients that I need to keep busy.

– **Mia Harper**, therapist

Reminder

Purchase or develop a brochure to convey the benefits of your pre- and perinatal services and a complementing business card.

Presentations

Nothing conveys the feel of what you do and who you are better than an in-person talk, demonstration or class. Touch as many of your audience as are receptive. Feeling the warmth, connection and confidence of your professional touch is worth the proverbial thousand words and accompanying websites. Some of your best venues are birth and postpartum doula meetings, a segment in a childbirth education class, a lunchtime presentation at an obstetrical or midwifery office, or after a prenatal exercise class.

Speeches and demonstrations give you anywhere from 3 to 20 minutes to educate and sell your audience. A class for one to several hours highlights your knowledge breadth and depth, and your interaction style, both key factors clients consider when choosing a therapist (Fogarty et al. 2020). Inform your students rather than sell your sessions, and you will likely net clients from every class that you teach. Some appropriate maternity-related class ideas are: one to three hours of simple techniques for relaxation to mothers and their partners; an hour of self-massage for women's health at a community center; or a short course on "family massage" in an adult education program.

Teach lay people only those techniques that an untrained hand and mind can do. That means omitting any techniques that require advanced anatomical knowledge or refined palpatory skills. Inform and reassure so that, as you give safety precautions, you are not spreading alarm. Be sure to coordinate to complement the other instructors' course material rather than usurping or contradicting it. (See online resources for class plans and tips.) ⊕

Client Education

Self-care instruction is a powerful means to improve your clients' outcomes that also serves in making them ardent promoters of your work. Teaching everyday ways to ease discomfort conveys your knowledge and your caring, which are part of developing a trusted reputation. You can incorporate this informative sharing before, during and after sessions, on your website, in social media and videos, and at special educational events. You can make books, other media and resources readily available too.

Here are a few of many topics to consider offering to your clients or in your communities:

- alignment and supports for maximum sleep comfort
- stretching, self-massage and other daily habits to ease stress and muscle tension
- coping with swollen feet, legs and hands
- massage for comfort and relaxation during labor and birth
- connecting with and massaging baby, older children and/or partners
- pillows, posture, self-massage and stretching for easier feeding and other childcare activities.

Notice that all these topics fall within the usual scope of practice guidelines for massage therapists (Sefton et al. 2011). (See online resources for examples of client education on therapists' websites.) ⊕

Create a practice environment rich in educational value for your clients. Post notices of local events such as lectures, screenings and support groups. Create a resource list of preferred providers of maternity care specialties and referral websites and numbers for services clients may feel reluctant to ask about, such as domestic abuse hotlines and WIC (the Special Supplemental Nutrition Program for Women, Infants, and Children). Provide this resource list to every maternity client as part of her care.

In addition to a lending library of books, periodicals and media, you can obtain informative pamphlets to give away from La Leche League or other breastfeeding support groups, the U.S. Department of Health and Human Services, and other agencies. You may want to sell products that can soothe and relax your clients – massage oils, belly pillows or lumbar support belts.

Reminder

Develop client education activities and materials for better outcomes and as a marketing activity to attract and keep more pre- and perinatal clients.

From the treatment room

I built my professional reputation by writing articles and speaking whenever I could. I have written for a local natural birth association that I am a member of, and I spoke at a few of their conferences. I also presented at a childbirth educators' conference, labor nurses' professional development day, teachers' professional development day, early childhood intervention staff development day, special needs parents' organizations, etc. Whenever an opportunity came up, I said enthusiastically "YES!"

– Linda Hickey, therapist

Advertising

Print advertising can be costly. But a niche publication – from a relevant club, community organization or healthcare provider – might be inexpensive and targeted enough to be worthwhile. Online advertising can be less expensive but confusing for some therapists. As with all Internet endeavors, seek out help from friends and professionals alike.

Adapting Your Business

You and any administrative staff at your workplace will be more effective if you adapt your business to fit the needs of your maternity clientele. Ways of doing this include how you gather and chart client information, communicating with healthcare providers, and insurance and liability issues. Whole books and Web resources such as those in this chapter's references are devoted to each of these activities. Here we will outline a few key adaptions specific to maternity clients. ⊕

First Contact

Information intake ideally begins when a pre- or perinatal client first inquires or schedules an appointment. The basic questions to ask for effective, safe sessions are:

- I want to provide you with the best possible care. May I ask you a few questions?
- What do you hope to get from this massage therapy?
- How far along are you in your pregnancy or postpartum time?
- Have you had any medical complications or any low- or high-risk factors? If so, what are those concerns? Have they resolved?
- And for postpartum clients: When and how did you give birth? Were there any complications?

Seek the information you must have without making her feel interrogated. Listen in a professional manner that conveys receptivity, genuine concern and knowledge.

With these fundamental facts, you can determine whether you need further information or documentation from her or her maternity healthcare provider before seeing her. Plan to obtain that necessary paperwork or authorization (Box 8.1), hopefully prior to her

---

Box 8.1
Healthcare provider communication example

To: Maternity Healthcare Providers

Re: Therapeutic Massage During Pregnancy/Postpartum

Your patient, _____, has requested prenatal/postpartum therapeutic massage. Therapeutic massage is provided prenatally and perinatally as adjunctive healthcare by a massage therapist who has met written and practical examination criteria. It is our policy to work with her only if her maternity healthcare provider has reviewed this request with her. In addition, if her pregnancy is high risk, or if she has experienced any prenatal or postpartum complications or contraindicated conditions, we require a written communication from her healthcare provider stating any specific limitations or precautions that you feel to be appropriate.

Please verify your clearance of massage therapy with your signature below. This verification can be modified or withdrawn at any time, should her health status change. I welcome this opportunity to work with you in providing our respective forms of prenatal care to your patient. Thank you for your time and assistance.

Patient's pregnancy is:___ normal progression___high risk

Specific limitations or precautions: _____

You may contact me directly for clarification or concerns regarding this patient. _____Yes _____No

Signature: _____ MD DO Midwife _____
Date: _____

Please print your name: _____

Name of preferred point of contact: _____

Office phone: _____ fax: _____ email:_____

first appointment. Later, we will discuss using this information to clarify your therapeutic approach and make optimal decisions about positioning, techniques and precautions.

Once she is at your business, remember how important it is for her to feel cared for. Yes, her swelling belly or her new baby will draw your attention but attend to her. She is your primary client to interact and communicate with. "Hello, how are you?" rather than "Wow, look at this belly!" is usually a more client-centered greeting. Ask "How are things going for you?" instead of "How's the baby doing?" Resist your urge to touch her belly; shake hands instead. Give her ready access to the restroom. During your intake, offer water, a stool to prop her legs and a breastfeeding pillow (for your postpartum clients).

Intake and Assessment

With each client, your aim should be to recognize her strength and abilities, assess any potential problems, and then alter your own work to best honor her needs. Prior chapters have detailed the many considerations integral to this aim. When they feel comfortable, most clients readily provide all the information you need about their maternity and general health history. Whenever possible, we recommend that you elicit these details through oral interviews, taking your own notes as your conversation progresses. Listen to what lies between the lines: you will obtain the necessary information along with a more subtle awareness of how she is feeling and thinking.

Alternately, a written intake form, completed prior to your first session, has the advantage of ensuring a written record that is not subject to your own interpretations, misunderstandings or memory. Decide which works best for your practice – maybe you will do both.

Here is the information you need from prenatal clients to ensure critical thinking and effective treatment planning:

1. What discomforts, pain or other needs are you hoping to have addressed?

2. What activities or positions worsen or lessen your discomforts?

3. In what week of your pregnancy are you?

4. Are you regularly seeing a physician, nurse-midwife or midwife? Name? Contact information?

5. When was your most recent visit with your provider? When is your next?

6. Have you previously discussed your pain or concerns with your provider? What have they said about this?

7. Has your provider identified any medical complications at any point in your pregnancy?

8. Does your provider consider your pregnancy to be at low or high risk of developing medical complications? If so, why? (See Box 7.1.)

9. Have you had any of the following: bleeding, cramping, amniotic fluid leakage, swelling, high blood pressure, rapid weight gain, protein in urine or other abnormal laboratory test results, vision disturbances, severe nausea/vomiting or headaches, abnormal fetal growth, heartbeat or movements, high blood sugar, depression or anxiety? (See Box 7.2.)

10. Do you have any underlying medical conditions? (See Box 7.1.)

11. Are you experiencing any injury, disease or disorder of any type, but particularly a cold or other virus, bladder, kidney, breast or other infection, skin irritation, or varicose or spider veins?

12. What changes, actions, limitations or treatments has your provider recommended/prescribed for any of the conditions in the questions above?

13. How does your current level of activity compare with your normal activity level?

14. What limitations on your daily life are you experiencing from your discomforts?

15. Do you have a birth plan that you would like me to consider as I create appropriate sessions for you?

16. What pronouns do you prefer me to use in referring to you? She/her? They/their? He/his? Other?

17. Are there any other aspects of your health or life situation of concern to you?

For postpartum clients:

1. What discomforts, pain or other needs are you hoping to have addressed?

2. What activities or positions worsen or lessen your discomforts?

3. Did you give birth vaginally or by Cesarean? How long ago?

4. Were there any complications during your labor and birthing?

5. Have you seen your perinatal care provider since giving birth? Have you been released from postpartum care?

6. Do you have any of the following: fever, excessive bleeding, headaches, pitting edema, hypertension, or signs of depression, anxiety or mental illness? (See Box 7.2.)

7. Are you breastfeeding? Any difficulties with feeding?

8. Do you have any underlying medical conditions? (See Box 7.1.)

9. Are you experiencing any injury, disease, disorder or infection of any type, but particularly a cold or other virus, bladder, breast (mastitis), scar or other infection, skin irritation, or varicose or spider veins?

10. What changes, actions, limitations or treatments has your provider recommended/prescribed for any of the conditions in the questions above?

11. What limitations on your daily life are you experiencing from your discomforts?

12. How does your current level of activity compare with your normal activity level?

13. What pronouns do you prefer me to use in referring to you? She/her? They/their? He/his? Other?

14. Are there any other aspects of your health or your life situation of concern to you?

Allot 10 to 20 minutes to acquiring at least the information listed above. (See online resources for form examples.) Although some of these questions repeat what was initially asked when scheduling, she will often share more as she begins to feel your professional attentiveness. Furthermore, ask all the basic questions that you usually ask of any client. Be sure to invite any questions that she has and ask what might make her session more enjoyable and effective. Occasionally, additional critical information might not emerge until you are into your massage. If this happens, you may need to tactfully alter your session for a health issue or creatively address a previously unreported need.

There is so much to observe from her movement, posture, breathing, facial expressions and general energy level. Make these informal observations as she moves through your intake process and into the session. Many clients signal you about where they hurt with their comforting hand over an aching sacroiliac joint or under their belly.

We have focused so far on verbal and visual information gathering, but tactile examination is equally revelatory. As she points out a painful spot, ask whether you may touch it to get a palpatory first impression. Verify what you have heard and seen with contact to more precisely confirm her complaints; your hands can identify if the "hip" pain she is referring to actually is at her hip joint or, more likely, at her sacroiliac joint!

Palpatory expertise is crucial for your success. Dive into the research, theory and intriguing exercises in Leon Chaitow's remarkable book, *Palpation and Assessment in Manual Therapy*, to enhance your tactile perception (Chaitow 2017). This same book also will improve your ability to perform functional assessments of your clients with systematic resisted, passive, active and other range-of-motion tests and physical examinations. David Zulak's *Clinical Assessment for Massage Therapy* offers a foundation for informed consent, treatment planning, goal setting, treatment, reassessment, medical/legal reports and charting (Zulak 2018).

In addition to seeking information, you need to give her some. She needs orientation to your office, approach, expectations and policies. Tell her or give her materials to read, whichever seems appropriate for you. Giving her written materials allows her to refer to the information later and to educate and reassure others with it. It also creates a record that you both can refer to if any miscommunication develops. Remember that a client may be stressed and/or sleepy, and might unintentionally omit relevant details.

Of course, a shortened update of the above information must take place each time that you work together.

Reminder

Design and use an intake form and/or methodology that keeps you current and complete in your knowledge about your maternity clients.

What would you do?

You are accustomed to taking a thorough health and pre- and perinatal history on your private practice clients. At your part-time spa job, scheduling and company policies do not easily allow for this type of client intake before your massage session begins. How can you secure the information that you need to design safe and effective sessions for these clients? What strategies might you try to make changes at your spa toward more information gathering? ⊕

Critical Thinking

Once you have thorough intake information and performed necessary assessments, you are ready to reason your way to the safest, most effective treatment plan. Sound clinical decision making considers these crucial categories of information:

- The client's goals, needs, preferences and health conditions, the input of her maternity healthcare provider and the results of any assessments that you performed – what you have acquired in your intake process.

- Your knowledge of current research, the applicable anatomical, physiological and functional realities of pregnancy, labor, birth and postpartum, and potentially effective techniques – what prior chapters have explained and ideally you have learned with an expert's hands-on instruction.

- Your experiences with similar clients and your awareness of relevant patterns – the wisdom achieved from doing, repeating, adapting and learning.

Synthesizing that volume of detailed information in the limited time available can be challenging. Some therapists consider the safety and efficacy recommendations that they know, along with whatever intake information they have, and get started. Here are a few more structured ways to organize your thoughts to create treatment plans that are evidence-based, safe, effective and individualized.

The Alphabet Soups

An informal, yet useful format that we have created to organize your thoughts follows the mnemonic HERS. This memory-friendly structure works especially well when you have little time for a more nuanced, complex treatment design. A bonus – it centers you on your client. The work you are creating must be for **HER**!

- H = Highlights of intake: the top three most relevant details from the client, your assessments, and their goals for the work.

- E = Essential safety: positioning, pressure, area precautions, trimester and postpartum week considerations, risks and complications to ensure client's and baby's safety.

- R = Relevant research and evidence: what data, anatomy, physiology and functional parameters are specifically applicable to this client today.

- S = Session options/ideas: positioning, modalities, techniques and/or educational activities likely to create desired outcomes.

See Box 8.2 for an example of the HERS method of clinical decision making.

Box 8.2
HERS clinical decision-making example

H = Highlights of intake: 30 weeks primigravida. No high risks, medical comp or history illness. Childhood history hip "clicking" (can't remember which hip) and repeated sprains R ankle. Seeking relief – persistent superficial numbness and pain R lateral thigh, sacral achiness – and relaxation.

E = Essential safety: prevent supine hypotension. Avoid iliac pressure when treating for possible lateral femoral cutaneous nerve (LFCN) entrapment. Maintain alignment during hip range of motion (ROM) and other mobilizations, and check for excess ligamental laxity hip and ankle, fibrosis in ankle. Autonomic sedation with pacing, moderating pain level.

R = Relevant research/evidence: neuropathy pattern of LFCN. Effects of relaxin/progesterone. Increased likelihood thrombi. Normal ROM hip and ankle joints. Field studies re: reduced leg and back pain. Meta-analysis pain studies.

S = Session options/ideas: semireclining for maximum access to inguinal ligament and femoral fascial sheets and for hip circumduction and other mobilizations to reduce pressure on LFCN. Sidelying: spinal rocking, lumbosacral stretch, sacroiliac joint releases, inching spinal intrinsics, Swedish to back, infinity hip joint with positional releases and stretches. Approach to R ankle dependent on stability and fibrosis found. Teach passive pelvic tilt and posterior breathing emphasis. End with lumbar lengthening.

Box 8.3
Session records examples

Client No. 1 5/7/19

S = Client's second visit in 7 days. Pregnancy going well. Complains of low back pain and tailbone pain when sits. Also, c/o leg pains, joint pains and anxiety. Hx of hypoglycemia, cysts on vocal cords, gastric bypass in 2003; doc is here at the hospital. Due date next week; primigravida.

O = Excess lumbar lordosis with extensor tension. Overall client seems overwhelmed by the physical aches, pains of pregnancy. 30/30 minutes R and L sidelying. Full-body massage with focus on pelvic/SI, QL and hip joint work. Client had great relief from SI joint decompressions and subtle rocking. Plans to try acupuncture for anxiety.

A = Less pain when seated and during workday, particularly with prolonged standing; better sleep so rested for labor.

P = Continue treatments to sacrum, SI and hip jts and lumbar spine. Reinforce instruction in standing structural balance and breathing patterns. Homework: attention and improving alignment and breathing periodically every day. Showed her how her husband can sit against her knees for at home SI decompression and how to perform L-S decompression. She'll return on her due date if she hasn't given birth by then.

Same Client 5/27/19

S = Vaginal birth 5/15 with long labor after water broke, resulting in baby having a fever/infection. Baby remains hospitalized. Client suffering headaches, leg swelling and nerve pain down R leg. Brought doctor's authorization for massage.

O = Lumbar lordosis less pronounced but persisting. Swelling non-pitting and localized to lower legs bilaterally. Supine/bolstered knees and lower legs. Neck/upper back Swedish, deep tissue. Client asleep almost immediately.

Many therapists use the Subjective, Objective, Assessment, Plan (SOAP) method of charting their massage therapy sessions (Thompson 2018). This methodology also encourages thoughtful treatment and session planning. If this is your preferred documentation system, follow this outline and see Box 8.3 for an example:

Abdominal kneading and effleurage then inguinal myofascial and superficial drainage for legs. L sidelying for R gluteal and piriformis deep tissue; hip joint infinity mobilization. Reported headache gone and less R leg pain after session.

A = Fewer headaches. Normalization of fluid.

P = Reminded re: propping legs when seated until edema resolved. Suggested daily 5–10-min walks to maintain mobility. Suggested breath awareness and deepening for daily stress reduction. Loaned infant massage DVD to help with bonding. Return as needed; discussed options for having baby on table with her.

Client No. 2 Wellness Charting

History and needs: Client 35+ years but no other notable health history or complications. Physician gave her the verbal OK for massage but promises to bring me the signed authorization next time she comes. 21 weeks, no problems with pregnancy, second baby. C/o low back fatigue and occasional headache. Loves deep work.

Treatment: 30 minutes semireclining, 25/25 minutes L and R sidelying. Broad, deep sculpting work at traps, LS, supraspinatus with traction, scalp and occiput work in semireclining. Brief leg work, but thorough foot zone therapy. Sidelying emphasis: Swedish to back and hips with spinal rocking and LS decompression repeated several times as requested. Client able to relax immediately and slept some. Upper back and paravertebrals tense but responsive.

After reported less back pain; no headache at start so no changes. Reminded her of value of walking or swimming for maintaining mobility. Return as necessary/desired.

- S = This refers to the subjective information provided by your client during intake.

- O = What you observe, palpate and test for provides a portion of the objective category; add to that the results of your critical thinking, your session work and your client's immediate responses to the session.

- A = Assess the effectiveness of the work thus far, based on your and your client's desired goals and outcomes.

- P = Finally, record how you and she plan to go forward in subsequent sessions and her at-home care.

Decision Trees

Another way to manage an elaborate amount of information is to break it down into smaller units and arrange those units visually. Respected educator and author Tracy Walton has created such a method, tailored for massage therapy – a decision tree design that guides therapists in how a client's medical condition intersects with massage therapy guidelines (Walton 2011).

As we know, pregnancy and postpartum are not medical conditions; however, the numerous and vast changes require us to consider each development and how our work changes accordingly. When high-risk factors exist and complications develop, a decision tree to help us reason through what to do and what not to do would be useful. Pre- and perinatal massage decision trees have yet to sprout, but perhaps you might want to start creating some.

Other texts offer additional templates and flow charts for creating treatment plans (Thompson and Brooks 2016; Zulak 2018). Regardless of your method, be sure to consider all relevant safety and efficacy recommendations along with whatever intake information you have gathered.

Creating Sessions

Thorough information and thoughtful consideration of it are the foundation ensuring the client's safety and benefit. If you have coupled this with a full repertoire of the previous chapters' specific techniques, you are ready to formulate your massage session. Why do we not just give you a preferred routine or a "signature" massage session in this book? Because maternity massage therapy sessions are best when specifically developed for each unique client. We want you to explore the endless possibilities for adapting each session to the evolving needs at each stage of pregnancy and motherhood. Let your clients' unique and varied needs elicit your creativity!

That said, here are our suggestions and guidelines:

- Develop a method to analyze and summarize the findings from your intake and assessments.

- Decide if regional treatments or a full-body sequence will best meet the client's needs and expectations, and the session's time, equipment and other constraints.

- Determine limitations, preferences and the positioning most likely to facilitate the desired outcomes. Confirm that you have adequate equipment, according to Chapter 3's guidelines.

- Choose appropriate techniques. Each technique described in the prior chapters begins with its intentions; with a deep understanding of each technique's expected effect, you can choose those most likely to address your client's needs.

- Augment your session with other techniques not taught here, but only after thoughtfully considering all the questions in Box 2.4 regarding prenatal adaptations.

- Sequence your work coherently, considering the multiple trajectories of a massage session: assessment–treatment–post-assessment; superficial to deep; general–specific–general; lubricant-free prior to lubricant application; proximal then distal techniques (when edema relief is a desired outcome).

- Include techniques unique to specific structures, as well as others that you will repeat to transition and connect your session and create general autonomic sedation.

- Remain aware, in your mind and your hands, of necessary adaptations to pressure, speed, rhythm, areas of application and other parameters discussed in prior chapters. Remember to follow each technique's precautions to ensure safety.

- Working slowly and mindfully. Fewer techniques performed well will be more effective and appreciated than an abundance of poorly executed techniques. Remember the physiological realities that make each technique effective (myofascial change, for example, usually requires a minimum of 30 to 60 seconds).

- Attend to specific structures as much as the client needs, but also create some balance – between left/right, upper/lower, anterior/posterior – when one part requires more time and attention.

- Consider how your technique sequence will complement any other treatment modalities the client will receive, from heat/cold applications to herbal wraps to chiropractic or physical therapy treatments.

Sometimes we are unable to collect or contemplate client information and create an individualized session. In those undesirable circumstances, having a few fallback "routines" can be helpful (see online resources for examples); however, without thorough client input, we highly recommend that you avoid complex or deep pressure techniques or those with many precautions. Instead, simply prioritize relaxation through autonomic sedation. ⊕

Maintaining Client Records

Pre- and perinatal session recordkeeping requires the same documentation, communication and reflection as for your other clients. Use whatever form of session notes you are accustomed to or are required to use by your employer. Some good choices are the SOAP and wellness charting methods (see Box 8.3), or you might prefer an unstructured narrative style for recording how each session progressed.

Whatever your format, be sure to at least write the week of pregnancy or postpartum, your client's concerns and your session response to them. Also include her summary of any tests or diagnosis her midwife or physician has made.

You also may want to ask to see her birth plan (see Chapter 5) or find out if she has labor preferences. Whether you will be massaging her during labor or not, understanding her vision helps to tailor sessions towards her current needs and her goals for labor and birth, and maybe offers hints of what her postpartum concerns may be.

For the unique parameters of labor massage, typical session note formats are inadequate. Try a pocket notebook to jot down important details and progress reports as soon as possible after they are given. Every few hours, make quick notes of difficulties, progress, interventions and techniques used. Within a few hours of leaving the new family, fill in the gaps and compose a more organized "story" of the labor and birth. These will help complete your records and prompt you to sift back over the difficulties and triumphs, noting any unresolved feelings or issues you might have. Also make note of the labor events that your client might need you to attend to in postpartum sessions. Some therapists like to offer their version of the baby's birth story for inclusion in the family's baby book to come.

Communicating with Other Providers

There are both treatment benefits and business benefits to connecting with your clients' maternity healthcare providers and other professional care providers (Box 8.4). These professionals may include midwives, physicians, nurse-practitioners, nurses, physical therapists, mental health clinicians and chiropractors – and maybe even her

---

Box 8.4
Communications with other providers

Effectiveness Benefits

- Provides further information
- Secures guidance on medical issues
- Produces more individualized application of precautions and guidelines
- Increases efficacy of care and client satisfaction

Business Benefits

- Demonstrates medical necessity, functional outcomes and cost efficiency
- Acts, in part, as marketing and networking for your practice
- Informs providers about pre- and perinatal massage therapy
- Provides some evidence of due diligence if liability questions develop

---

childbirth educator, lactation consultant, birth and postpartum doula, athletic trainer or yoga teacher as well. Consider your client's needs and if the possible treatment or business benefits of these communications are desirable. You may decide to request a full consultation, a simple verbal affirmation or something in between.

Particularly when complications develop or when there are high-risk conditions, we recommend that you seek the knowledgeable, individualized insight of the client's physician or midwife (see Box 8.1). If you are unsure whether you should begin or continue massage with a client, seek your client's written permission to communicate with their provider. Then request a consultation to discuss how massage should fit into prenatal or postpartum care for their patient who is your client. Periodically update a client's provider on the progress of those therapy sessions. Build a collegial relationship through your respectful demeanor, and by maintaining your scope of practice and professional code of ethics in all you do.

Observe professional client/patient confidentiality standards as you consult with and build cooperation with any and all practitioners. Be sure to determine if you are subject to Health Insurance Portability and Accountability Act (HIPAA) regulations. (See Thompson 2018 for guidance.) ⊕

Liability

Minimize your legal risks, particularly those relevant to a maternity pre- and perinatal practice. Many of your clients may have trouble seeing their feet when they walk, can be more prone to imbalances that cause missteps and falls, and are far heavier than they are used to. Alter your treatment room and any waiting area or lobby to minimize the possibility of hazards, equipment failures and other fall risk issues to reduce your chance of physical, medical and/or loss liability. Remember that a standard homeowner's policy does not cover liability if someone visiting your home for business purposes is injured (Sohnen-Moe 2016).

As discussed in Box 2.3, contemplate your and your employer's level of risk tolerance about practice liability and think about how to minimize your chances of being implicated in allegations of wrongdoing.

With our combined 90 years of perinatal massage therapy practice and the experiences of the 5,000-plus therapists we have trained, we think that you and your clients will steer clear of legal troubles by:

- operating in an ethical, professional manner always

- continuously expanding your knowledge with pre- and perinatal massage therapy education that is comprehensive, hands-on and evidence-based

- staying current with emerging data on the childbearing implications of diseases, and with general advancements in obstetrics, midwifery and early parenting, especially following current recommendations made by the American College of Obstetricians and Gynecologists

- adhering to the safety guidelines and precautions described throughout this book

- practicing conservatively, thoughtfully, and with utmost attention to the individual realities of each client in your care

- maintaining written practice records of policies, procedures, consent, intake and session notes.

Of course, maintaining adequate malpractice liability insurance is necessary as well. That insurance is the type that you may purchase for your own protection. In addition, you must also consider if you want, and are able, to accept insurance reimbursement for your maternity massage services – a complex matter beyond the scope of this book but well covered in several books in this chapter's references.

Expanding Your Business

As you grow your business, there are many obstacles that can get in the way. Some of those obstacles emerge from potential clients and their perceptions of you. Some emerge from you. In either case, we have insights to manage those relevant to you.

Financial Obstacles

Obviously, financial stresses increase when a new family member is on the way. Ways to make your sessions more affordable include the following:

- flexible pricing and package discounts (Box 8.5)

- gift certificates or a special for couples planning a "babymoon," a get-away together before the birth

- an add-on complimentary mini-massage or a package series that includes a partner massage

- multiple payment method options (Bowers 2018).

Box 8.5
Pricing and packaging

We believe that pregnant clients should not be charged additional fees for prenatal sessions, which suggests that working with this client population is somehow a burden. However, specialists catering to childbearing clients sometimes charge higher rates than non-specialists for their additional expertise and the maternity-conducive environment they maintain. Weigh these factors to set prices: your overall experience and maternity expertise, your education, **target market**, geographic variables, the current economic milieu and your market's average fees.

Many find packaging their services is economically sound and effective for quality client care. With a package, the client typically pays in full at the start for a bundle of sessions, and then receives a discount as a result. Here are a few package ideas:

- three sessions distributed over each of the three trimesters for 5 percent off

- three sessions – the first scheduled in the last trimester, an hour of labor massage or labor massage instruction, and a final postpartum session – for 5 percent off

- five sessions – one in each trimester; an hour massage during labor, labor massage instruction or a partner session; and a postpartum session – for 10 percent off

- five sessions – three scheduled whenever needed prenatally, a postpartum session, and a lesson in infant massage – for 10 percent off

- 10 sessions, scheduled as needed within a year of purchase, either for the price of eight with the last two "complimentary," or for 20 percent off

- five sessions, paid at regular price at session time, and then a sixth session for free

For labor massage, most therapists charge their hourly rate up to a maximum of 8 to 10 hours of labor. Your client can arrange ahead of time for you to be there for a set number of hours or for the entire labor. With such an arrangement, any additional hours of your care (remember you will be with her until she no longer needs you after the birth) incur no additional charges. Some therapists prefer to base their fee upon the local norm for maternity care. Determine your fee by first surveying the obstetricians and midwives serving your target market. Considering that their flat fee usually covers all necessary prenatal and postpartum visits, charge one-fourth or one-third the average of these healthcare providers, based on their level of education. This will be your total fee, regardless of the length of time you stay with the laboring mother. Alternately, others charge in the range of what birth doulas in their area do.

From the treatment room

Here is how I prevent losing clients once they have given birth. I offer a package: buy four massages, get one complimentary postpartum massage. If you get a client early enough in the process, she may accumulate several postpartum sessions. I stress the importance of self-care after the baby is born. I also offer a postpartum home visit, with breastfeeding support (I took a basic breastfeeding support class). Once clients stop associating you only with pregnancy massage, they are more likely to schedule postpartum.

– Rebecca Leary, therapist

Reminder

Maximize your flexibility to reduce financial and convenience obstacles for potential clients.

Scheduling Difficulties

Setting appointments with clients early in their pregnancies, when they are feeling uncomfortable, or after giving birth can be challenging. Try these ideas:

- Offer times when she is less nauseated or tired, has childcare or can take time off work.

- Make home calls to clients with challenges (those on bed rest and early postpartum when resting).

- Schedule the client's first postpartum session as a home visit without a travel fee.

- Find a trusted person with income limitations to provide infant care at your office; compensate them via session discounts.

- Accommodate the mother–infant dyad on your table, in your treatment room and throughout your business (see Figures 6.2 and 6.3).

Ignorance about Massage Therapy

Consumer surveys point to continued medical acceptance of and recommendations for massage therapy, particularly as a form of non-pharmacological pain relief and for other medical reasons (AMTA 2019). Despite that growing awareness, concern for the safety of both the mother and the baby can cause women, their partners and healthcare providers to hesitate about pre- and perinatal massage therapy. In addition, some people consider it a frivolous indulgence.

A recently published qualitative study investigated what makes pregnant people receiving massage feel safe. Five main themes emerged:

1. Autonomy – able to voice my needs and be heard.

2. Pregnancy massage is more than just a massage.

3. When my therapist is experienced and qualified, I feel safer.

4. The continuity of the massage industry's message about the safety of massage.

5. Decision-making around massage safety (Fogarty et al. 2020).

Given those findings, and our decades of experience, here are suggestions for overcoming ignorance and ensuring a feeling of safety:

- Complete comprehensive, hands-on training in pre- and perinatal massage therapy. Have your knowledge and skills verified through testing and display those credentials.

- Convey your knowledge and expertise in varied sources: your printed materials, blogs and websites (Fogarty et al. 2020).

- Hone your ability to talk and write about the benefits of maternity massage therapy, citing appropriate research studies to document your claims and acknowledging where more data are needed.

- Share maternal, medical and midwifery testimonials with your clients.

- Introduce yourself and send an informative packet of materials to local perinatal specialists.

- Practice conservatively for safety – and boldly for effectiveness. Communicate those standards as you promote your work.

- Assess your clients thoroughly and involve them in decisions about their sessions, especially by soliciting and utilizing their feedback on their experiences with you (Fulton 2015).

- Consult with clients' doctors and midwives for their expertise and knowledge of the client and send your brochure, along with any necessary forms.

- Tell pregnant clients about the value of postpartum work. At your last prenatal session, schedule her first postpartum session.

- Call or send a card to a client after her due date to remind her of how postpartum massage therapy helps her to take care of herself and her family.

Reminder

Educate doctors, midwives and clients about the potential benefits of pre- and perinatal massage, and your ability and qualifications to safely provide those benefits.

Internal Attitudes

The final and most complex obstacle to success is *you*. We all have our beliefs and biases about life in general, and those specifically related to mothering. We have all had a mother, no matter whether we are mothers or not. Examine yourself by answering the following questions:

- If you cannot or do not want to have children, do you feel inadequate? Angry? Sad? Glad? Neutral?

- Have your own pregnancies and parenting created emotional and mental "baggage" you carry into your therapy room?

- Have you witnessed traumatic births that left you with fear, anger and/or grief?

- Do you distrust doctors? Do you think midwives are underqualified?

- Do you fear or like hospitals? Think homebirth is dangerous or the best? Loathe or want all medical interventions?

- What judgments do you make about single moms? Mixed-race couples? Gender non-conforming parents? Same-sex couples? Or, for that matter, more traditional couples?

- Are you comfortable with and prepared for clients who are often larger than others?

- How will you help yourself deal with the possibility of perinatal injury or death?

- Do you frequently feel unprepared for or uninformed about clients' discomforts and concerns?

- Is your knowledge of maternity healthcare dated or your connection with younger generations inadequate?

- Do you feel "in over your head" or inadequately trained for the complexity of clients' needs?

All these attitudes and feelings manifest in our treatment room in one way or another. See Box 8.6 for ways to reduce their negative impact on your work.

Box 8.6
Overcome your obstacles

Once you identify what is getting in your way, here is how to turn your obstacles into advantages.

Do not assume. Be careful about pushing your own experiences onto your clients. Just because you have given birth, do not assume that you know how your client is feeling. Empathize while still honoring her uniqueness.

Acknowledge your ignorance. If you cannot, or do not want to, be a parent, use that lack of experience as a strength. You can approach each client with "beginner's mind" – eager to learn about each client's specific needs, without assuming that you know what they are going through.

Ask questions. Your training is useful only if you apply it to the exact needs of each client. Asking questions shows that you care, and that you are applying your knowledge in a way that is helpful.

Use your breath. Practice a slow, easy breathing as you work, to keep yourself calm and focused. When distracting thoughts or emotions arise, do not deny them or judge yourself. Instead, acknowledge them, focus on your next exhalation and return your awareness to your client.

Help yourself. Get more education, talk with a counselor or psychologist, or discuss your issues with a friend or practice supervisor. Look for mentoring and/or practice supervision in your bodywork community to help you work your way through these often complex and overlooked issues.

Align business with purpose. Engage in awareness activities, self-reflection or business coaching and mentoring that attune(s) your personal and professional goals with your business activities (Sohnen-Moe 2016; Bowers 2018).

Learn more. Remember to stay familiar with our profession's ethical standards (NCBTMB 2019). Know the laws applicable in your jurisdictions and the parameters of your professional organizations.

And even more. Seek the highest, most comprehensive hands-on education available for this specialized client population, and remember to stay current and to grow in your knowledge.

(See online resources for more ways to overcome obstacles.) 🌐

Ethics

The intensity of pre- and perinatal work can create many ethical gray areas. You can easily wander beyond your scope of practice when a client asks your advice about a medical procedure. Boundaries can become nebulous when a very needy person becomes your client, or in the fluid intensity of labor massage. The power imbalance inherent in our relationship can widen as a client's neediness increases, as can the potential for client transference and therapist countertransference of earlier familial relationships. The easy camaraderie of expectant people can cause you to blunder on confidentiality issues. And the dry wording of ethical guidelines and legal parameters can clash with a client's legitimate maternity needs.

When you identify any of these gray areas in your own work, take active steps to find clarity. Any of the ideas listed in Box 8.6, or the Benjamin/Sohnen-Moe Ethical Congruency Checklist in Box 8.7, can guide your way. In addition, we strongly urge you to seek professional, confidential support from a colleague, counselor or another professional. Schedule regular meetings where you can debrief when clients' situations are difficult for you or trigger your own personal experiences. This is particularly urgent after a client's difficult birth or a pregnancy or postpartum loss.

Box 8.7
Ethical congruence checklist

In practicing self-accountability, we strive for ethical congruence: making decisions that are congruent – consistent or in alignment – with the ethical values that apply to each situation. Whenever you are contemplating an action (or inaction) that you find questionable, you can use the following questions to test for ethical congruence. Ask yourself:

- What does your gut say?
- Do you get butterflies just thinking about the issue?
- Do you have doubts?
- Do you need to sacrifice any of your personal or professional values?
- Is it against the law, policies or a professional code of ethics?
- Is this fair to all concerned parties in the short term as well as the long run?
- How would it hold up to scrutiny if all the details were made public?
- How would you feel if the people you hold in high esteem knew your decision?
- How would you feel if your decision were emblazoned on the headline of your local newspaper?
- How would you feel about yourself when all is done?

If any of your answers suggest that you are facing an ethical conflict, use this information as a cue to step back and re-evaluate your options.

From Benjamin B, Sohnen-Moe C (2014) The Ethics of Touch, 2nd edn. Tucson: Sohnen-Moe Associates. Used with permission from the authors.

your chosen resources, honor your experience by unburdening yourself of those feelings to someone who can nurture your own healing.

From the treatment room

It's pretty inevitable that part way through a first session, a new pregnant client will say, "You know so much about pregnancy and babies! How old are your children?" For 10 years now I have been giving them the same answer: "I actually haven't been pregnant. I received incredible, extensive training and became a certified prenatal, postpartum and labor massage therapist, and that experience allows me to tailor each massage to my individual client's needs."

Many therapists decide to learn pregnancy massage when they are pregnant themselves, but I took a different path. My passion is orthopedic therapeutic massage and treating clients working through life transitions – and for many people there is no greater transition in life than becoming a parent! From the outside, some might assume that my personal inexperience is a hindrance, but I would disagree. Do I need to have had hip surgery to work with a postoperative client?

– Faith Davis, therapist

What would you do?

Review the obstacles to success with the pre- and perinatal market discussed in this chapter. Identify those that are relevant to you. What strategies can you develop to potentially dissolve those impediments? What are the first three steps you can take from among your strategies?

Practice supervision can also help you to honor your obligation to maintain professional boundaries with your client. Your work with her may provoke feelings in you that are not appropriate to share with her. Whatever

Male Therapists

Being a male therapist who works with pre- and perinatal clients can feel like an additional obstacle. Some maternity clients – just like some non-pregnant clients – will always prefer a female therapist. You just must accept this. Some people are hesitant to work with a male therapist, because they worry he will be inappropriate, that he will "mansplain" or work too deep, or because they have had a negative experience in the past. It is critical to work against these perceptions. Here is how to demonstrate that a male can be a marvelous maternity therapist:

- Be impeccably professional in every interaction.

- Listen carefully and do not assume you know what is wrong with potential clients or that you know how to fix them.

- Do not try to prove how strong you are or how deep you can work. Instead, see each client as unique, and be responsive to their particular needs and preferences.

- Make your treatment room, just like your demeanor, feel both warm and clinical.

- Stay well read and up to date on maternity trends. You cannot be pregnant, but you can be aware of the things your client may be concerned about.

- Teach partners simple massage techniques during pregnancy, birth and postpartum. This includes the partner in both the birth and the mother's therapy with you, and these lessons may help allay concerns that partner may have about you.

- If your client is single or having difficulties with her partner, be aware of potential ethical gray areas. Provide professional, nurturing and therapeutic care without acting like a substitute partner.

Sustaining Your Business

Some of the most successful prenatal and perinatal massage therapists are double- and triple-certified providers of other forms of maternity care. These additional skills, education and credentials can be reassuring to tentative clients and professionals alike. Your other offerings also benefit from the trusting relationship you build with your massage therapy client. When she needs a lactation consultant, for example, you are the obvious choice. You can market your other skills side by side with massage to aid your clients in multiple ways.

Areas to consider:

- birth and/or postpartum doula

- infant massage instructor

- pediatric massage therapist

- pre-conception massage therapist

- lactation consultant

- pre- and postnatal yoga teacher

- childbirth educator

- ultrasound technician

- belly caster (a person who molds a plaster cast of an expecting mother over her abdomen and breasts)

- prenatal photographer

- midwife or midwife's assistant

- nurse.

Individual practitioners often find additional success by expanding their businesses to directly collaborate with some of these other maternity-focused providers. Some therapists form maternity massage therapy and women's wellness centers. Others create, staff and/or coordinate hospital-based prenatal and postnatal massage therapy services (Kolakowski 2018). (See profiles in this chapter and online resources for guidance in working in hospitals.) 🌐

For perinatal career longevity, look to preventing burnout and managing your own self-care. Charge for and organize your time appropriately. Have proper equipment, practice the body mechanics in Chapter 3, and get help at the first signs of wear and tear niggling at your joints and soft tissues. Look back to Chapter 5 to review some of the critical issues of working with the long hours and intensity of labor and birth. Find sources for professional practice supervision, mentoring, and continued education and development.

From the treatment room

I think a lot about my "image" that I portray to new clients, trying to find the balance between caring, involved, focused and "professional" behavior, including what and when to share, and how I respond to client needs. I do sometimes go the extra bit for someone who may be needing special attention, especially postpartum – fitting her in somewhere, having a grandma volunteer come in to hold a baby for her, work an extra appointment in on Saturday because that feels right for me.

Reality here in my city is that pregnant people with money and/or benefits are usually working. We need to be available when they are if we want to attract this market. As they get closer to their due dates and begin their maternity leave, they will be available for the weekday daytime appointment times, but initially you need to meet them half-way.

I do believe "It takes a village," and I am proud and happy to step up and join the village. That helps me when I am tired or overbooked or need a holiday. Remembering that this is important work helps me as I strive to make it sustainable as I age.

– Linda Hickey, therapist

Developing a healthy maternity massage therapy business requires thorough theoretical and practical education, and persistent promotion. Active marketing brings the right people together to support your practice growth, in both clients and a solid referral network. A multifaceted focus – sound practice management, nuanced critical thinking and session design, and activities that educate your clients and the wider community – promotes the normal, healthy development of both you and your thriving pre- and perinatal business.

Stories of Successful Therapists

As you complete your study of this book, we suspect you might be wondering how all this knowledge and these skills come together in the workplace. What follows are stories to inspire and inform you as you grow *your* career. These tales are directly from the treatment room, filled with passion, purpose, determination, curiosity, creativity, setbacks and successes. These are the stories of us, your authors, and several other outstanding therapists who currently practice prenatal and perinatal massage therapy. We all also form the authorized teaching team for this body of knowledge (see online resources for more about us, and for a gallery of many additional tales from others). We have been refining this work for at least 10 years, most more than 20, and one for 39 of her 47 years in practice!

If you are just beginning your pre- and perinatal education or have only a few years of maternity massage experience, your future in this work can be somewhat unclear. Despite your idealism, ambitiousness and energetic enthusiasm, what lies ahead for you can be fuzzy, particularly when you peer past your first decade in the work. Every therapist's path is unique, but as highly experienced therapists, we think that our stories might provide a glimpse of where you might be heading.

From the Treatment Room of Margi Hadorn

"When training to be a massage therapist, prenatal bodywork was one of the skill sets that I had a strong desire to learn more about. It took me about 10 years to finally have the resources and time, and to find an in-depth course. The four days I spent in the Pre- and Perinatal Massage Therapy classroom turned out to be the starting point of a journey that has taken me through 20 years of practice.

Marketing has never been my strength, but with my enthusiasm intact, and my newly obtained knowledge, I set out identifying obstetricians near the massage office where I worked. I emailed and wrote letters detailing the wonderful benefits of massage for pregnancy, especially with issues that were out of a physician's primary areas of concern. Many of those patient complaints were the very same that I learned techniques to work with in the Pre- and Perinatal Massage Therapy workshop. I enclosed business cards offering small discounts for physicians, midwives and nurse practitioners in the hope of making connections with professionals who also served the pregnant population. I offered to do lunchtime meet-and-greets in their offices, allowing us to get acquainted and so they could ask me questions about exactly what prenatal massage therapy was all about. Making connections with like-minded professionals is helpful in this specialty, so I asked colleagues for marketing ideas. A co-worker gave me the name of a nurse-midwife who was a great connection for referring clients and who allowed me to advertise in the three offices where she worked.

In addition, I developed my ideas about how I would teach labor preparation for partners, and I took an infant massage class. Once I had prenatal clients come in for treatments, I had the opportunity to introduce more new ways for them to feel confident in their bodies and to look forward to their labors and births. Soon the connections were overlapping, and this was so exciting to me! Patients of my midwife connection shared my name in their prenatal yoga class. I told my own non-pregnant clients about how great a gift certificate for prenatal, postpartum or infant massage would be.

My practice is small. I work with six other therapists but independent of them. I have always maintained a practice where I massage many types of clients. I feel that this keeps me energized in many aspects of massage therapy. I am grateful for what I have learned from all the clients I have worked with and the professionals I have met along the way. I am a better therapist for my non-pregnant clients since learning to effectively, safely massage pregnant clients. Even after all these years, I still have so much to learn, from clients, healthcare professionals and students."

From the Treatment Room of Pam Guldi

"Just a year after being licensed as a massage therapist, one of my roommates, a midwifery student, invited me to a mini-course for doula training. I had never considered this before but was intrigued, went and loved every minute. Soon afterwards, one of my regular massage clients became pregnant and asked me to attend her birth. Watching this mother labor made me nervous at first, but it was empowering to see how much relief she received from massage between contractions. I quickly found myself encouraging her and teaching the father how to assist me with a double hip squeeze. The birth was magical! I left in awe and thinking deeply about mothers'

psychological and physiological needs during pregnancy, birth and postpartum.

Within a year I was pregnant for the first time. My son's home waterbirth transformed me into a "birth junkie," and I knew I wanted more.

After the birth of my second child, I began teaching infant massage for free at my local public library. This allowed me an outing with other adults as well to market my massage practice. (Side note: bringing your own baby to use as the demo has its benefits and disadvantages. It is lovely to demonstrate techniques on a child you know so well, but frustrating when said baby does not cooperate or has other needs.) These classes became an excellent opportunity to normalize motherhood for new moms needing reassurance that everything does not have to be perfect; they are not alone.

Wanting more education for prenatal clients, I first attended Pre- and Perinatal Massage Therapy specialization training in 2001. Later I became a certified doula through DONA.

I began to see more women in my practice. Often, I would massage a woman throughout her pregnancy, attend her birth and then teach the parents infant massage. Later I became certified through Birthing From Within childbirth education and offered classes to expecting mothers and couples.

Like most women, I realized that working and having young children is a constant juggling act. When my children were very young, it was often difficult to find reliable childcare while I left them to attend a birth. I gradually accepted fewer doula clients and sought more training in women's care. I studied under Rosita Arvigo (Maya Abdominal Therapy) in Belize in 2014, and I traveled to Kerala, India, in 2015 to study Ayurveda. Today, my practice is focused on the full range of women's health, from prenatal to postpartum, instruction in infant massage, and women's reproductive and digestive well-being throughout the cycle of life into elder years.

My pre- and perinatal training was the genesis for my career in care for women and has provided the basis for so much of my further learning. It has had the most impact on my knowledge and confidence as a therapist. Now that I am in my 28th year as a therapist, I am choosing to limit my private practice clients, but I continue to share my passion for working with women and their families. I teach other therapists the nuances of skilled palpation, the mind–body connection, the flexibility and strength needed to contribute to and not control when at a birth, and the dynamic relationship between therapist and client."

From the Treatment Room of Marjeanne Estes

"I have been practicing massage therapy for over 20 years. Prior to my massage career, I was a pharmacist. I have taught massage therapy for many years and really love helping students find their way, connect with the body and really understand anatomy, fascia and how strong body mechanics will preserve their career longevity. I also work in an integrated wellness center at a hospital. My pharmacy background really supports my massage work in this setting.

The center is open to the public, and we are available to treat patients in their rooms, should they choose to book a session. I see a wide variety of clients dealing with many physical as well as health challenges. I love my work there because it is constantly challenging me with something new. Many times, I have to use my critical thinking skills to figure out a complex issue that a client is presenting that I may not be familiar with. Even though I have been doing massage for 20 years, I am still learning, and I love that.

With one of my specialties being pre- and perinatal massage therapy, I often treat patients who are in the maternity hospital on bed rest. These patients may be there for a few days to a few months, and that can be incredibly challenging physically as well as mentally. Many times, I walk into one of their rooms for an appointment, only to find them on the phone, managing business or things at home, as well as other little ones visiting who do not understand why mom cannot come home. Then there is the stress of being in the hospital for constant medical intervention. Their stress levels are usually high. Next on the list is the physical discomforts of being in a hospital bed. I am thankful I have a treasury of techniques and training to work with their physical as well as their emotional needs. They tend to be the most grateful clients – so thankful for that one hour of relief and relaxation.

I once worked with a client who was expecting twins who was in the hospital for three months. She received a massage weekly. Her physician had thought they would need to do a C-section at about 31 weeks. Instead, they let her go home at 33 weeks, and she had the babies at 36 weeks. That is the power of massage and the work we do!"

From the Treatment Room of Sparrow Harrington

"I started Sparrow's Nest in 2014 with the specific intention of serving new and expectant families with skilled bodywork from fertility through postpartum. We are a team of five pre- and perinatal certified therapists, and roughly 80 percent of our clients are either pregnant or newly postpartum. We are committed to listening to our community and adding services where there are unfulfilled needs, especially in maternity care.

I have built this business from the ground up, which has been far from easy. My family of entrepreneurs has normalized many of the struggles I have faced. I have seen my own mother, a general contractor, work the notoriously long hours of a business owner, live with months of uncertainty, ride the waves of highs and lows, and come out the other side with a thriving business. Now, with 30-plus years under her belt, she will smile at me when I am feeling lost, and tell me, "Just keep going. It's worth it."

Originally, I thought maternity massage therapy would be a stepping-stone to my true desire to become a midwife. Although I was attending births as a doula and apprenticing as a midwifery assistant, ultimately, maternity massage therapy provided me with the deepest sense of purpose and gratification. I left my midwifery studies, but I am grateful for the valuable insight into birth culture and prenatal care those experiences offered.

I started working out of the birthing center where I was apprenticing. Relatively quickly, my private practice became full, and I knew I wanted to eventually multiply my hands by creating a team. Within two and a half years, that was a reality. The biggest challenge at that stage was client hesitancy to perceive us as a group practice. For a while, clients only wanted to see me, because I was the word-of-mouth referral from their friend. That resistance lasted for almost two years, but clients are finally accepting and embracing the wonderful therapists on my team easily. I adore my team. Part of the way we maintain camaraderie is to get together for four hours monthly to refine our skills, talk through unique or difficult cases, and recommit to our vision and collective purpose in this work.

Several factors helped create success for us. Undoubtedly, I have benefited from investing in mentoring with my teachers and in meeting regularly with a business coach. I have had both famous clients and influencers who were happy to provide social proof of the work's benefits. We also utilize social media to provide educational posts, answer questions, and show video clips of sample sessions. I have also had many tea dates with local practitioners, midwives, doulas, chiropractors, physical therapists and so on, to create a personal level of trust for referrals. In addition, we donate sessions to local charities, including Breastfeed LA, NARM "Jump Start" Program supporting Student Midwives of Color, and several local moms' groups. All these symbiotic relationships help to bolster trust and word-of-mouth referrals.

I have definitely had my share of challenges and disappointments on this journey so far: from a flaky business partner who left me stranded when it was time to sign a lease, to difficult landlords, to business copycats and outright website plagiarism. To a large degree, it is par for the course, as with any business. I am proud of everything we have built, and still feel there is lots of growing to do. My biggest personal challenge to date is learning how to navigate and trust that my business is sustainable as I step away to care for my own newborn. Being a new mother has already deeply shaped my continued commitment to this work, and how Sparrow's Nest will move forward into the future."

From the Treatment Room of David M Lobenstine

"I have long known that I wanted to be a father. I took the Pre- and Perinatal Massage Therapy specialization workshop soon after graduating from the Swedish Institute. I signed up mostly out of curiosity, eager to be more a part of the process of pregnancy. I had no idea of the depth to which that workshop would expand and alter my massage career. I have been massaging now for 15 years – in a wellness center, in too many spas to count, at the US Open Tennis Tournament, in a hospice,

and now in my own private practice. And I have been developing and teaching my own continuing education courses for almost as long.

Throughout, I have purposely not specialized my work – neither my teaching nor my massaging. I delight in the diversity of people on my table and in my classroom. I delight in the diversity of topics I can teach, and the ways to effect change with my clients.

But that said, my work with prenatal clients informs all the work that I do. Because it seems to me that the process of pregnancy is a particularly profound manifestation of what the human species is capable of; and our work with pregnant clients is a particularly profound manifestation of what massage is capable of! Our bodies are always changing, throughout our lives, in ways that are both beautiful and difficult. Nowhere is that change as massive as during pregnancy! And as therapists, our greatest possibility is to assist our clients through the unending transitions of life.

Working with pregnant clients is a perpetual reminder of how much our touch can accomplish – and of the real limits of our ability to effect change. Our specialized prenatal techniques can make a huge difference in the myriad difficulties of pregnancy. And just as important, our mindful care can help to calm and soothe, even with – especially with – those clients with severe conditions that limit what we are able to do. At the same time, working with pregnancy clients is humbling; we know that the aches and pains and burdens will likely return, or even grow worse, as pregnancy progresses. My sessions remind me that I cannot "fix" my clients. I cannot take away their problems. Instead, we can strive to facilitate whatever their body is able to do amidst these astounding changes.

Being a male therapist only crystallizes all that we are able and unable to do in our work. I will never feel the increased restriction of the breath as the growing belly constricts the ribcage. I will never know the ebb and flow of labor. I am an outsider, and I try to use that position to be a better therapist: my client is always the expert on her body. I try to listen closely, ask all the questions necessary and offer suggestions. But most importantly, I try to give each client space to come back to neutral: to let go as she is ready, to find ease as she is able.

And in that space, in each session, I try to demonstrate the perpetual possibility of change. With my techniques I remind each client that ease is always possible, even amidst pain. That their body can be both as strong as pregnancy demands, and as supple as labor requires. And that our work together can continue, however she needs and for as long as she needs – throughout the pregnancy, but perhaps even more important, into the new and beautiful difficulties of parenthood!"

From the Treatment Room of Michele Kolakowski

"I have been extremely blessed to have many diverse opportunities to follow my passions and be of service to childbearing women and infants. My private practice started in a professional office in 1992, moved to my home, to another professional office, and then back at home as my growing family's needs changed. In addition to a private practice, I looked for a variety of opportunities to teach maternity and infant massage to new mom and family support groups, social service agencies, spas, and at massage therapy schools.

My clients teach me, and they constantly remind me of the essential healing ingredients they need: caring, skillful touch, listening ears, and introspective questions to find their own answers and engage their intuition. It seems that when it comes to childbearing and babies, there is a staggering amount of information and advice (sometimes unsolicited!) to assimilate, and it can be overwhelming. I try to create a sanctuary for women and babies (and myself!).

For 12 years, I was fortunate to belong to Longmont United Hospital's BirthPlace Massage Therapy team. In private practice and in teaching, I mostly work with healthy women and babies. In the hospital setting, I see similar healthy people and babies and also the rest of the real world: the "underbelly" of the childbearing experience, as I call it. These include the following:

- women with little or no prenatal care
- patients with acute high-risk conditions and complications
- young teenagers who have been raped, including cases involving incest, and are birthing their first babies

- drug addicts who are withdrawing
- women who are incarcerated but out of jail long enough to labor and birth
- women who have been abused and whose babies are going into social service custody due to domestic violence
- people who live in poverty
- women whose babies have not survived.

As painful as these situations are, these are the very situations that also so desperately need our caring work. Not only has it been an exquisite practice in non-judgment and the need for bringing the same compassion and skill to each of these people and their infants, but it also has motivated me to take better care of myself. I love being outside in nature, practicing yoga, gardening and enjoying my family. I encourage you to find the "underbellies" in your local community and reach out to care for those women and children, and engage regularly in the self-care practices that nurture and sustain you.

In the second and third decades of my career, I remain curious and committed by adding related areas of study to my skills and services – pursuing more women's health massage therapy continuing education, becoming a birth and postpartum doula, and lactation consultant. With my exquisite postpartum doula group, Sanctuary Doulas, and sister non-profit, the Postpartum Abundance Project, my current mission is integrating more postpartum massage into our remarkable home visits for new and growing families. I want to blossom this business model beyond my local community to across the country."

From the Treatment Room of Carole Osborne

"My pre- and perinatal massage therapy career was sparked about 40 years ago by my own first pregnancy and an influx of pregnant clients and friends. This interest was a daring endeavor in the early 1980s, when pregnancy was considered a total contraindication for massage therapy. My intrigue and needs led me to extensive collaborations with colleagues and perinatal professionals. From those explorations, I developed my own system for meeting the physical and emotional needs of childbearing. This book conveys the ongoing maturation of that system.

My pre- and perinatal massage therapy practice grew along with my family. By the time my two were both in grade school, I had combined my commitment to somato-emotional integration with maternity-focused massage therapy to form two separate yet intimately entwined bodywork specializations. With passion, knowledge and artistry powering my work, I have always thrived in the freedom of a private practice. I also relished the expansive collaborations I had when I worked for many years in the office of an osteopathic physician, more briefly in a women's medical and wellness center, and frequently in close collaboration with mental health professionals.

My maternity clientele has primarily been people with complex prenatal or postpartum concerns. I have had many of my expectant massage therapy students on my treatment table. More recently, one client was a mother who was once a babe in my first infant massage class; another was my son's partner, while expecting my grandsons and in those early foggy postpartum months; and, just months ago, my own daughter with my first granddaughter swirling inside. I have yet to work with a mom who was once in utero under my hands; it seems my clients have had many more baby boys! But maybe someday. All my clients continue to inspire me and catalyze humility and profound respect.

My best practice successes have come with these realizations:

- Presence is crucial. I really do not have the answers, but I can be present and assist my clients in knowing their needs to make their own best choices.

- If I offer my skills, knowledge and awareness, they can maximize the best outcomes and most enjoyment of their childbearing experiences, no matter what those are.

- Pregnancy, labor, birth and parenting have only one constant, like life itself: change. I need to stay grounded, present, flexible, judicious and educated, and all will be well in our work together.

- Perhaps the most important aspect of my pre- and perinatal massage therapy career is knowing that each mother I touch will likely go on to touch her own child more fully. Those early experiences will create unbreakable bonds, a deep connectiveness in her child, her family, and that circle of unity will expand out into her community. With enough healthy touch in our families, our family of humanity becomes more peaceful, more connected. This gives me great comfort when society seems ever more fractured and violent, and our children and grandchildren will live in that future. As I look back on these decades and anticipate a close to my professional life within the next decade, I bask in the satisfying career that I have had."

Chapter Summary

So, with those stories told, our book is near its end. Before we close, take a few minutes to sift over the words of wisdom of these stories. Feel our professional passion and dedication in these many venues. Soften yourself by thinking of the thousands of people we have served. Then peer into your mind and your heart. Take a deep breath. Allow a vision to begin forming …

There you are in a massage therapy room in the setting where you most want to work. This room invites relaxation, exudes wisdom and competence, and is fully supplied to support your hands-on work. You are standing next to your table with a dear, round client whose gestational energy warms you and your room. She is comfortable and receptive as she lies tenderly and professionally draped, securely positioned. You have aligned your body to feel comfortable and grounded. Your hands are powerful, yet gentle, as they effectively soothe, encourage and guide her into relaxation and pain-free well-being. Your heart is open, compassionate and empathetic as you listen to what has heart and meaning for her, buoying her joys and hearing her difficulties. Your mind is clear of distractions, worries, advice and other chatter. You observe, assess, intuit and access all the information that you need to be safe and effective in your care of her.

A sense of connection and meaning begins to envelop you both. You realize that you are nurturing the birth of a mother and of her baby. You have become a prenatal and perinatal massage therapist.

Think it through

To deepen your knowledge, go to our online resources, answer the test questions for this chapter and explore further. 🌐

References and Further Reading

Allen L (2016) Nina McIntosh's The Educated Heart, 4th edn. Philadelphia: Lippincott, Williams & Wilkins.

AMTA (American Massage Therapy Association) (2019) State of the Massage Therapy Profession: 2019 Fact Sheet. Available at: https://www.amtamassage.org/globalassets/documents/src/2019-pdf.pdf [accessed July 13, 2020].

Andrade C (2013) Outcome-Based Massage: From Evidence to Practice, 3rd edn. Baltimore: Lippincott, Williams & Wilkins.

Benjamin B, Sohnen-Moe C (2014) The Ethics of Touch, 2nd edn. Tucson: Sohnen-Moe Associates.

Bowers K (2018) The Accidental Business Owner. Edinburgh: Handspring.

Chaitow L (2017) Palpation and Assessment in Manual Therapy, 4th edn. Edinburgh: Handspring.

Fogarty S, Barnett R, Hay P (2020) Safety and pregnancy massage: a qualitative thematic analysis. Int J Ther Massage Bodywork. 13(1):4–12.

Fulton B (2015) The Placebo Effect in Manual Therapy. Edinburgh: Handspring.

Gilbert E, Harmon J (2003) Manual of High-risk Pregnancy and Delivery, 3rd edn. St. Louis: Mosby.

Kolakowski M (2018) This is How to Start a Hospital-based Massage Program. Massage Magazine. Business tips, Online exclusives 267. Available at: https://www.massagemag.com/hospital-based-massage-therapy-90116/ [accessed July 2, 2020].

Massage Business Blueprint. Available at: https://www.massagebusinessblueprint.com/ [accessed March 1, 2020].

NCBTMB (National Certification Board for Therapeutic Massage and Bodywork) (2019) Code of Ethics. Available at: https://www.ncbtmb.org/code-of-ethics/ [accessed November 15, 2019].

Osborne C (2009) Pre- and Perinatal Massage Therapy: Survey of Massage Therapists. Available at: https://bodytherapyeducation.com/recommended-products-services-resources/graduates-survey/ [accessed January 1, 2020].

Osborne C (2011) How to network with fertility experts in the medical realm 31 Oct. Available at: https://bodytherapyeducation.com/how-to-network-with-fertility-experts-in-the-medical-realm/ [accessed January 1, 2020].

Osborne C (2013) Maternity Massage: The Benefits of Prenatal and Perinatal Touch. Available at: https://bodytherapyeducation.com/maternity-massage-of-prenatal-and-perinatal-touch/ [accessed July 2, 2020].

Sefton JM, Shea M, Hines C (2011) Developing, maintaining, and using a body of knowledge for the massage therapy profession. Int J Ther Massage Bodywork. 4(3):1–12. Available at: https://doi.org/10.3822/ijtmb.v4i3.141 [accessed July 15, 2020].

Sohnen-Moe C (2016) Business Mastery, 5th edn. Tucson: Sohnen-Moe Associates.

Thompson D (2018) Hands Heal, 5th edn. Baltimore: Lippincott, Williams & Wilkins.

Thompson D, Brooks M (2016) Integrative Pain Management: Massage, Movement and Mindfulness Based Approaches. Edinburgh: Handspring.

Turgeon R (2008) Massage Therapy on Trial: Dealing with the Legal System. Presentation to the AMTA National Convention, Phoenix, September 18.

Walton T (2011) Medical Conditions and Massage Therapy: A Decision Tree Approach. Baltimore: Lippincott, Williams & Wilkins.

Zulak D (2018) Clinical Assessment for Massage Therapy: A Practical Guide. Edinburgh: Handspring.

GLOSSARY

active labor
second phase of first stage of labor when cervix effaces and dilates fully from 6 to 10 centimeters.

active listening
listening in a way that helps others to feel heard; feeds back what one hears to confirm accuracy of understanding and to encourage further sharing and self-exploration.

acupressure
form of Asian bodywork therapy with theoretical roots in Chinese Medicine Theory for balancing body's energy by applying pressure to specific acupuncture points to release tension, strengthen weaknesses, relieve common ailments, prevent health disorders and restore body's vital life force.

amniotic fluid
fetal urea in which fetus floats in amniotic sac; consists of 98 percent water and 2 percent other organic matter excreted by fetus during gestation.

Apgar scores
measurement system of newborn health including activity, pulse, grimace, appearance and respiration measured one and five minutes after birth.

areolas
pink or brown area surrounding female breasts' nipples containing tiny sebaceous glands that lubricate and protect it during suckling.

aromatherapist
healthcare provider trained in use of volatile plant materials, also known as essential oils, with intention of improving an individual's health, mood or cognitive functioning.

arrested labor
also known as labor dystocia; when cervical dilation stops during active labor, or descent of baby is very prolonged or stops during labor's second stage.

assisted reproductive technology (ART)
also called artificial reproductive technologies; includes all fertility treatments in which either eggs or embryos are assisted; involves surgically removing eggs from a woman's ovaries, combining them with sperm in a laboratory, and returning them to client or surrogate gestational carrier, or donating eggs to another person; does not include treatments in which only sperm are handled (such as intrauterine insemination) or procedures in which a woman takes medications only to stimulate egg production without intention of having eggs surgically retrieved.

Aston Patterning
system of bodywork, ergonomic analysis and movement coaching designed by Judith Aston to restore natural alignment and dynamic well-being to individuals.

asynclytic presentation
oblique malpresentation of fetal head in labor; found during vaginal examination; may cause increased pain, stalled labor progress or Cesarean birth.

attachment
also known as bonding; a sense of connection and affection that unites humans in relationship and that develops with time and contact.

baby blues
temporary normal emotional adjustment in first two weeks after childbirth; new mothers feel anxious, irritable, emotionally oversensitive, erratic and overwhelmed, and may have difficulty with normal sleep and eating.

banner ad
advertisement that extends to side (usually top or right side) of a website.

bed rest
partial or total restriction of activity to conserve energy and reduce strain to maternal systems when complications or high-risk conditions threaten or occur.

birth doula
trained and experienced attendant who provides a laboring person with continuous non-medical, physical and emotional support to help her have the most satisfying birth experience as client defines it; other kind of doula is a postpartum doula who offers postpartum care.

birth plan
summary of a mother's priorities, concerns and preferences for her care while laboring and giving birth, written for self-clarification and to communicate clearly with providers.

birthing pool or tub
lightweight or installed tub of sufficient depth for a laboring woman to immerse herself to enhance relaxation and reduce painful sensations.

Bishop score
helps identify individuals who would be most likely to achieve a successful induction; assessed by a maternity healthcare provider's pelvic examination for five measurements – cervical position, consistency, dilation, effacement and pelvic station.

bloody show
lightly blood-tinged vaginal secretions, before active labor begins and during labor, that come from small capillaries in cervix opening during effacement and dilation.

bodyCushion™
positioning system of four main sections, each composed of layers of shaped foam that conform to and cradle body in a variety of positions.

body mechanics
organization and use of body's energy and structure to perform a task.

bonding
also known as attachment; sense of connection and affection that unites humans in relationship and that develops with time and contact.

bow stance
standing posture with one foot forward, with a shoulder's width and two to three foot lengths between feet, and with knees and hips flexed; modified from tai chi for massage and bodywork.

Braxton Hicks contractions
uterine contractions occurring prior to true labor; distinguished from true labor in their irregularity in length and frequency.

breast crawl
innate newborn reflexes with leg and arm movements to propel baby from mother's abdomen to chest, where head movements and mouth openings will cause baby to self-latch and initiate breastfeeding.

breech presentation
when fetal buttocks or feet (rather than head) present in maternal pelvis first; includes frank breech (buttocks at cervix), complete breech (both buttocks and feet down) and footling breech (only one or both feet down).

bulk mailing
larger quantities of mail prepared for mailing at reduced postage.

carpal tunnel syndrome
pain, numbness, tingling and/or weakness in thumb, index, middle and half of ring fingers; caused by irritation to median nerve, in pregnancy and postpartum, usually a result of edema primarily.

catecholamines
stress hormones including adrenaline (epinephrine), noradrenaline (norepinephrine), cortisol and others – counteract effects of oxytocin and endorphins during labor and birth.

ceiling side
side of your sidelying client's body that is more readily available to work with.

cerebral palsy
variety of central nervous system injuries usually incurred pre- or perinatally, or in early infancy; results in hyper- and hypotonic muscles, poor coordination and involuntary movements.

cervical insufficiency
weak, short or structurally defective cervix that can spontaneously dilate before term in absence of contractions, resulting in pregnancy loss.

cervical lip
section of an otherwise fully dilated cervix that has not retracted over fetal head, usually anterior cervical section.

cervical mucus plug
thickened mucus that fills cervical opening during pregnancy to prevent bacteria and any substances from entering uterus; releases from cervix in pre-labor or early labor phase.

Cesarean birth
surgical procedure through lower abdominal wall and uterus so that fetus can be removed from uterus rather than passed through vagina for birth.

childbirth education
courses that offer information, skills and experiential activities to prepare expectant people for childbirth.

chloasma
estrogen-induced brown or darker pigmentation forming a mask-like shape over a pregnant woman's nose, forehead and cheeks.

chorioamnionitis
inflammation of chorion and amnion, membranes that surround fetus; usually associated with bacterial infection.

chronic hypertension
gestational hypertensive disorder occurring prior to pregnancy or that develops before 20 weeks' gestation.

coccygodynia
tailbone-related pain that can occur when sitting on hard surfaces and can be result of high pressure on pelvis or breaking coccyx during childbirth.

colostrum
concentrated golden-colored, protein-rich, immunologically rich first breast milk created during second half of pregnancy and available through first few days postpartum before mature, more voluminous milk comes in.

complications
medical conditions that develop in pregnancy, labor and/or postpartum that may result in negative outcomes for mother, baby or both.

confidentiality
guarantee of privacy and protection of clients' information, session progress, health and other information.

cortisol
adrenal hormone produced in response to stress and anxiety that influences metabolism of proteins, increases blood pressure and blood sugar, and depresses immune system.

countertransference
projections of a therapist onto a client of emotional attitudes and/or past history.

cross-fiber friction
deep pressure with thumb or fingers across axis of muscle fiber, across specific lesions in muscle bellies, musculotendinous junctions, tendons, tenoperiosteal junctions or ligaments; created by James Cyriax, MD, and developed by Ben Benjamin and others.

cyanosis
bluish discoloration of skin due to poor circulation or inadequate oxygenation of blood.

cytomegalovirus
virus found in body fluids, spread through contact and fluid exchange, that can cause many prenatal complications; most common congenital and perinatal viral infection.

deep tissue massage
slow, specific strokes or compressions with thumbs, fingers or elbows through fascial planes and muscles to release myofascial tissue's habitual holding patterns; includes sculpting, structural balancing and integration, skin rolling, and other therapies based on principles of Ida P Rolf.

deep vein thrombosis (DVT)
formation or presence of a clot (thrombus) in a deep vein, usually iliac, femoral or deep saphenous veins.

de Quervain's syndrome
painful inflammation of thumb tendons resulting in thumb, wrist and sometimes forearm pain caused by overuse and injury in abductor pollicis and extensor pollicis brevis tendons.

diaphoresis
sweating.

diastasis recti
separation at midline of rectus abdominis at linea alba of three-fingerwidth or wider gap between left and right muscle bellies; caused by hormonal effects and structural stress of growing uterus pressure against these muscles, as well as strain from activity.

diethylstilbestrol syndrome
syndrome caused by medication used to prevent miscarriages that resulted in high percentage of offspring with reproductive organ anomalies and diseases that can complicate pregnancy and birth; widespread use of diethylstilbestrol discontinued in United States by 1971, when it was recognized as a teratogen.

dilation
opening of uterine cervix to 10 centimeters to allow passage of fetus into vagina during birth.

disseminated intravascular coagulopathy
complex hemorrhagic and tissue destructive condition, threatening fetal and maternal life.

diuresis
increased urine output.

dizygotic
also called fraternal twins; used to describe a multiple gestation pregnancy derived from two separate ova, where each fetus has its own placenta, amnion and chorion.

dysuria
difficult or painful discharge of urine.

early labor (latent phase)
beginning phase of first stage of labor; lasting until cervix has dilated to 6 centimeters.

eclampsia
a gestational hypertensive disorder with onset of seizure activity in woman with pre-eclampsia.

ectopic pregnancy
one of more dangerous causes of bleeding in first trimester, where zygote starts to develop outside of uterus in fallopian tube, ovary, cervix or abdomen.

edema
excessive fluid retention and swelling; may be dependent, normal accumulations in legs and feet, arms and hands; systemic or generalized throughout body; and/or pitting, where depression and blanching of tissue occur for several seconds to several minutes after pressed.

effacement
cervical changes of last weeks of pregnancy or early and active labor that shorten and flatten cervix.

electronic advertising
promotions done through websites, commonly in form of banner ads, e-mail blasts and social media (such as Twitter or Facebook).

electronic fetal monitoring
detecting fetal heartbeat continuously or intermittently to assess baby's well-being during uterine contractions; various types of medical equipment measure, record and display those readings; sometime done by external monitor on abdomen, or internal monitor is placed on fetal scalp.

e-mail blast
e-mail message sent to multiple recipients, intended to inform them of announcements, events or changes.

endometritis
infection of endometrium, decidua and adjacent myometrium of uterus.

engagement
also known as lightening or dropping; sign of readiness for labor when widest part of fetal head, or other fetal body part closest to cervix, descends into pelvis.

engorgement
painful distention of breast caused by increased blood and lymph circulation and milk production; usually occurs in early days postpartum and until breastmilk production and baby's needs synchronize.

epidural
administration of anesthetic into epidural space of spinal column to numb sensory and motor nerves leading to lower body; most common pharmaceutical pain management for labor and birth.

epinephrine
also known as adrenaline; adrenal hormone responsible for flight, fright or flight response to stress, and to increasing strength and stamina for demanding situations, such as second and third stages of labor.

episiotomy
enlargement of vaginal opening via surgical incision to perineum.

essential oils
highly concentrated essences of aromatic plants.

estimated due date
date that spontaneous onset of labor is expected to occur; estimated by adding 280 days (nine months and seven days) to first day of last menstrual period; accuracy depends on accurate recall by mother, assumes regular 28-day cycles, and occurrence of ovulation and conception on day 14 of cycle.

estrogen
reproductive hormone which promotes growth of breasts and uterus; increases vascularization, swells gums and other mucous membranes, and causes skin pigmentation changes in pregnancy and birth; works synergistically with relaxin and progesterone to soften connective tissue.

expansional balance
movement concept involving free extension of skeletal frame in all directions in space through cycling awareness of vertical and horizontal joint expansion; originated by Michael Nebadon and developed by Ed Maupin.

family-centered Cesarean birth practices
evolving practices including clear sterile drape for mother to view her baby's birth, as well as skin-to-skin contact and breastfeeding in operating room.

femoral venous pressure
force of blood against walls of femoral veins of legs.

fetal distress
problems with fetal heart rate or activity levels.

fetal position
also known as fetal lie; orientation of fetus relative to internal opening of cervix and pelvis; most common positions are occiput anterior and occiput posterior.

fibrinolysis
process by which fibrin, a blood protein that coagulates to form clots, is dissolved.

fibrosis
changes in soft tissue associated with chronic congestion, contraction of muscle, thickening of fascia and increased formation of fibrous tissue; usually palpable, painful and likely to produce areas of referred pain.

first stage of labor
when cervix effaces and dilates fully to 10 centimeters; divided into three phases – early (latent), active and transition phases.

forceps
obstetrical tong-like instrument sometimes used to assist fetus's descent during second stage of labor.

fourth stage of labor
also known as "golden hour"; final stage of labor in first one or two postpartum hours; time when feelings of love and attachment can flourish during eye and skin-to-skin contact and first breastfeeding.

fundus
upper uterine section between fallopian tubes.

gastric reflux
also known as heartburn; burning and pain caused by stomach (gastric) acid injuring and inflaming esophageal mucous linings.

gate theory of pain
concept that stimulation of nerves that perceive pleasure, pressure and temperature can inhibit amount of painful stimulus perceived in brain because these sensations travel on nerves that fire faster than those nerves perceiving pain.

genital herpes
viral infection causing painful blisters around red base, appearing periodically on genitals, thighs, buttocks or sacrum.

gestation
conception and development of baby/babies in utero.

gestational diabetes
glucose intolerance beginning and first detected during pregnancy near 24 weeks and associated with neonatal complications.

gestational hypertensive disorders
group of hypertensive disorders all characterized by high blood pressure that develops during pregnancy, birth or postpartum and can proceed from mild to severe and life-threatening in severity.

gestational trophoblastic disease
spectrum of disorders originating in placenta with abnormal hyperproliferation of trophoblastic cells that normally would develop into placenta; two most common types are molar pregnancy and choriocarcinoma.

grand multiparity
condition of a woman who has had five or more previous pregnancies; high-risk factor.

gravid
pregnant; carrying a developing fetus or fetuses.

gravidity
number of times that a woman has been pregnant; gravidity and parity are highly correlated; for example, a woman who is described as "gravida 3, para 2" has had three pregnancies and two births after 24 weeks.

HELLP syndrome
acronym for Hemolysis, Elevated Liver enzymes and Low Platelet count, life-threatening variant of pre-eclampsia/eclampsia syndrome.

hemoglobinopathies
inherited blood disorders with abnormal, variant form of hemoglobin or decreased production of hemoglobin; significantly complicate pregnancy and birth, and increase risk of infant mortality.

hemorrhage
more than normal vaginal bleeding during pregnancy, birth and postpartum; more than 2 cups of blood during third stage of birth, or more than normal lochia soaking more than one peripad an hour, or blood clots egg-sized or bigger; potentially life-threatening to mother and baby.

hemorrhoids
aching, swollen mass of dilated veins in anal tissue; can also occur vaginally, when known as vulvar varicosities.

high-order multiples
multiple gestation pregnancy of three or more babies.

high-risk factors
biophysical and psychosocial issues that women have currently or have a higher likelihood of developing during pregnancy, birth and/or postpartum, with resulting higher morbidity and mortality for mother and/or baby.

horse-riding stance
standing posture with feet parallel, shoulder-width apart and aligned with each other directly under flexed ankle, knee and hip joints.

human chorionic gonadotropin
hormone produced by placenta after implantation; its presence is detected in some pregnancy tests; maintains corpus luteum, which secretes progesterone during first trimester.

human placental lactogen
hormone responsible for metabolic processing of glucose, carbohydrate and other nutrients; prepares mammary glands for lactation.

hyperemesis gravidarum
pregnancy complication with persistent, uncontrollable nausea and vomiting beyond 20th week of pregnancy.

hysterectomy
surgical removal of uterus.

implantation bleeding
vaginal bleeding, typically light, caused by fertilized egg attaching to uterine lining at 6 to 12 days after fertilization; women often mistake implantation bleeding as normal period, which can lead to incorrect prediction of due date.

infertility
male or female condition resulting in inability to conceive after one year of normal, unprotected sexual intercourse, or inability to carry a pregnancy to term.

intake
process or form for collecting and/or recording fundamental facts about client, taken at first visit and updated with each subsequent session.

intrauterine growth restriction
growth of baby below normal rate inside uterus; most common cause is placental dysfunction; baby is at risk for low birth weight, low Apgar scores, decreased oxygen and sugar levels, meconium aspiration, trouble tolerating vaginal birth and maintaining body temperature after, and stillbirth.

intrauterine pressure
force of uterine contents, amniotic fluid, placenta and fetus exerted against interior muscular walls of uterus.

in vitro fertilization
most common assisted reproductive technology, which involves extracting client's eggs, fertilizing eggs in laboratory, and transferring resulting embryos into client's or surrogate gestational carrier's uterus.

involution
postpartum process of uterus contracting to pre-pregnancy size and location in pelvis, and resuming non-pregnant functioning.

kinesthetic awareness
simultaneous abilities to attend to one's inner state, coordinate movement (such as massage techniques) and maintain awareness of where one is in time and space.

lability
constantly changing and unstable emotional state.

labor
process of uterine muscle contractions to thin and dilate cervix and move fetus and placenta through and out vagina; has four stages of progress.

labor augmentation
medical intervention to sustain and enhance ineffective uterine contractions after labor begins.

labor dystocia
also known as arrested labor, dysfunctional labor or failure to progress; difficult or failed progress during labor.

labor induction
using medical or surgical interventions to stimulate uterine contractions before their spontaneous onset.

lactation
secretion of milk by breasts to feed an infant.

large for gestational age (LGA)
also known as macrosomia; used to describe newborns whose birth weight is above 90th percentile on growth chart and weigh more than 8 pounds 13 ounces (4 kg) at term due to accelerated overgrowth for length of gestation; often born by Cesarean to avoid maternal and fetal injury.

last menstrual period dating
starting date used to calculate estimated due date – date that spontaneous onset of labor is expected to occur; due date may be estimated by adding 280 days (nine months and seven days) to first day of last menstrual period.

lateral recumbent
lying on one's side; used to describe sidelying position.

lift table
massage table that adjusts to variable heights by either hydraulic or electrical power.

lightening
also known as engagement or dropping; sign of readiness for labor when widest part of fetal head, or other fetal body part closest to cervix, descends into pelvis in preparation for labor.

linea nigra
dark line of skin pigmentation appearing midline from sternum or umbilicus to pubis on pregnant abdomen during second half of pregnancy; baby's roadmap to breast.

lochia
normal vaginal discharge after childbirth consisting of blood, mucus and tissue.

lordosis
increased anterior curve of lumbar spine.

low birth weight
also known as small for gestational age; preterm, term or post-term infant weight usually less than 5½ pounds (2.5 kg) or less than 10th percentile on standard growth charts.

macrosomia
also known as large for gestational age; describes newborns whose birth weight is above 90th percentile on a growth chart and weigh more than 8 pounds 13 ounces (4 kg) at term due to accelerated overgrowth for length of gestation.

mastitis
inflammation of breast tissue; most common in first three weeks postpartum but can occur anytime in lactation; symptoms include breast redness, tenderness and warmth, and flu-like symptoms; results from milk stasis as result of insufficient drainage of breast, oversupply of milk, pressure on breast from poorly fitting bra, blocked milk duct, missed feedings, breakdown of nipple via fissures, cracks or blisters, and rapid weaning.

meconium
earliest infant stool, thick and sticky like tar, dark olive-green, and almost odorless; unlike later feces, meconium is composed of materials that infant ingests during intrauterine life; meconium aspiration is inhalation of stools passed in utero and can lead to further fetal compromise.

meralgia paresthetica
neurological disorder characterized by localized area of burning sensation, pain and/or numbness on anterolateral aspect of thigh.

midwifery
healthcare profession focused on providing prenatal care, attending births, and offering continuing care of new mother and her baby; midwives complete prescribed course of studies in apprenticeships, formal university programs, or combination, to become certified nurse midwives or direct-entry midwives.

miscarriage
also known as spontaneous abortion; loss of early pregnancy, usually before 20 weeks of gestation and usually resulting from natural causes; often happens early in a pregnancy that woman may not yet know about; heavy bleeding is most common sign, and is often accompanied by uterine cramping.

molar pregnancy
one of gestational trophoblastic diseases, when fertilized egg grows into abnormal mass or tumor as result of chromosomal issues; fertilized egg cannot survive and will often shed itself, with first-trimester bleeding being first symptom.

monozygotic
multiple gestation pregnancy, known as identical twins, which develops when single, fertilized ovum splits during first two weeks after conception; fetuses share one placenta and chorion, and usually one amnion.

morbidity
state of being diseased or unhealthy.

morning sickness
nausea and/or vomiting during pregnancy; primarily a response to rapidly increasing hormonal levels during first trimester and sometimes longer.

mortality
death.

multifetal reduction
in multiple gestations, the procedure for reducing the number of fetuses to minimize the risk of maternal and fetal complications later in pregnancy and birth.

multigravidas
women who have birthed more than one baby.

multiparous
having experienced one or more previous childbirths.

multiple gestations
the presence of two or more babies in the uterus during pregnancy.

muscle energy techniques (METs)
method of producing relaxation of a muscle prior to stretching it by having client use muscle or its antagonist with minimal strength against therapist's resistance to that action.

myofascial release
system of connective tissue manipulation involving non-gliding fascial traction and stretching to lengthen and soften fascia; sometimes used in combination with other deep tissue and osteopathic techniques; developed by John Barnes and others.

networking
marketing method used for expanding business and finding broader referral and communication network; created through associating with like-minded or related business people either in person in community groups (example: San Diego Birth Network) or through social media networking by building online communities through "groups" and "friends lists" that allow greater interaction on websites, as well as more connectivity and interaction between Web users (examples: Facebook, Twitter and LinkedIn).

newborn intensive care unit (NICU)
intensive care unit in a hospital designed for premature and medically fragile newborn babies requiring special care and equipment.

norepinephrine
also known as noradrenaline; stress hormone responsible for fight, fright or flight response to mobilize brain and body for action such as second and third stages of labor.

obstetrics
branch of medicine that cares for women during pregnancy, labor, birth and puerperium period; obstetricians are physicians who practice obstetrics.

occiput anterior
fetal position with fetal occiput facing mother's pubic bone.

occiput posterior
fetal position with fetal occiput facing mother's sacrum.

oligohydramnios
decreased amount of amniotic fluid between 32 and 36 weeks' gestation; results from any condition that prevents baby from making urine or blocks it from going into amniotic sac.

on-site massage chair
folding, adjustable specialty chair for performing massage with a client seated, in a variety of work, medical, therapeutic or recreational settings.

oxytocin
pituitary hormone of love and healing that stimulates uterine contractions, release of milk into milk ducts, and feelings of nurturing; synthetic version is called pitocin.

paradoxical breathing
situation when abdomen contracts with inhalation and expands with exhalation, which is opposite of normal breathing dynamics.

parasympathetic branch of the autonomic nervous system
part of nervous system that slows heart rate, increases intestinal and gland activity, and relaxes sphincter muscles; together with sympathetic nervous system that accelerates heart rate, constricts blood vessels and raises blood pressure, it constitutes autonomic nervous system.

parity
number of times woman has given birth to baby with gestational age of 24 weeks or more, regardless of whether child was born alive or was stillborn; a woman who has never carried a pregnancy beyond 24 weeks is nulliparous or para 0; parity and gravidity are highly correlated.

passive movements
movements of varying amplitude, intensity and speed, performed by therapist to gently move client's body or move specific joints; includes joint mobilizations, stretching, traction, rhythmic deep tissue blends, sensory repatterning, Trager™, strain–counterstrain and positional release systems.

pelvic floor exercises
variety of squeezing, lifting and releasing exercises to maintain and improve tone and relaxation of pelvic floor's sphincter and sling muscles; also known as Kegels after surgeon who first designed a biofeedback device to measure and guide strengthening of these muscles.

pelvic station
measurement of labor progress and baby's passage through pelvis; relationship of crown of baby's head to pelvic landmarks of bilateral ischial spines.

perforator veins
blood vessels that traverse deep fascia and form connecting channels between superficial and deep venous systems, carrying blood from superficial to deep veins and muscular veins.

perinatal
time surrounding childbirth, most specifically last five months and month immediately after birth.

perinatal mood and anxiety disorders
most common complication of childbearing years and leading cause of maternal morbidity and mortality; constellation of mental health issues, from depression and anxiety to psychosis.

perineum
external surface of pelvic floor between the vulva and the anus in the female body.

peripartum cardiomyopathy
disease affecting the heart muscle; leading cause of maternal morbidity, accounting for 23 percent of deaths in postpartum period; signs and symptoms include chest pain and shortness of breath or difficulty breathing without exertion.

physiological labor and birth
natural process powered by a woman's and her baby's innate capacities.

piriformis syndrome
pain, numbness and/or tingling in gluteal and posterior leg regions as a result of chronic piriformis tension entrapping and compressing sciatic nerve.

pitocin
synthetic form of oxytocin used to induce or augment labor by stimulating uterine contractions.

placenta
membranous and vascular organ that begins developing in pregnancy's pre-embryonic first seven days; attaches to inside wall of uterus, providing nourishment and waste removal for growing baby via umbilical cord; produces many pregnancy and labor hormones; at term, moves approximately 100 gallons of blood per day and weighs 2 pounds (0.9 kg).

placenta abruptia
premature separation of normally implanted placenta after 20th week of gestation and prior to birth, followed by concealed or apparent mild, moderate or severe hemorrhage.

placenta accreta, increta and percreta
defect in vascular attachment of placenta that allows it to attach directly or through uterine muscles rather than to innermost endometrium only; results in greater risk of hemorrhage and uterine rupture or inversion.

placenta previa
bleeding complication, literally "afterbirth first," when placenta implants in lower uterus covering or near cervical opening (os) rather than normal location closer to top of uterus or fundus.

polyhydramnios
when too much amniotic fluid surrounds baby between 32 and 36 weeks; associated with fetal developmental and chromosomal anomalies.

postpartum
time after birth of a baby, including puerperium period of first six to eight weeks of extensive adjustments; some timelines extend further.

postpartum doula
person who is trained to care for postpartum people and family in their homes.

post-term
used to describe pregnancy that goes beyond full term.

practice supervision
discussions and explorations with more experienced practitioner or instructor or small peer group that help improve client outcomes and practitioner self-awareness and development.

precipitous labor
labor and birth that occur in three hours or less.

pre-eclampsia
gestational hypertensive disorder characterized by hypertension, edema and proteinuria; multisystemic, pregnancy-induced syndrome resulting from endothelial cell dysfunction.

pregnancy-related pelvic girdle pain
discomfort during pregnancy and/or postpartum that causes pain, instability and limitation of mobility and functioning in any of three pelvic joints – bilateral sacroiliac joints and pubic symphysis; also known as perinatal pelvic pain syndrome (PPPS), which refers to pain in pelvic region that starts during pregnancy or within first three months after birth.

premature rupture of membranes
spontaneous opening or breaking of amniotic sac before onset of labor.

prenatal
period of time from conception to 37 to 42 weeks of pregnancy, when fetus is developing and growing.

presenting part
fetal part closest to cervix or born first by Cesarean birth.

preterm labor
also known as premature labor and/or birth; labor beginning early, between weeks 20 and 37 of pregnancy.

primary Cesarean birth
refers to Cesarean birth in woman who has not had a previous Cesarean birth.

primiparous
giving or having given birth for the first time.

progesterone
meaning "for pregnancy"; reproductive hormone that prepares and maintains uterine lining for implantation of fertilized egg, and supports its continued development; affects breast and cervical tissue and other smooth muscles; works synergistically with relaxin and estrogen to soften connective tissue.

prolactin
pituitary hormone that triggers and sustains milk production in response to tactile breast stimulation.

prone
lying face-down position.

prostaglandins
hormones that affect uterine smooth muscle, vasodilation and constriction; ripen cervix in preparation for labor.

proteinuria
sign of pre-eclampsia and eclampsia where urine contains an abnormal amount of protein; sign of kidney dysfunction with damaged filtration that allows proteins to leak from blood into urine.

protracted labor
slower than normal cervical dilation during active first stage of labor.

puerperium
time from birth of placenta to six weeks postpartum.

rebozo

traditional Central and South American shawl often used in pregnancy, birth and postpartum to provide comfort and labor support.

reflexive techniques

massage techniques directed to cutaneous or neurological referral zones to effect either systemic change or local change at distant "referred" sites; vary from light to very deep pressure; include many Asian bodywork techniques, connective tissue massage (*Bindegewebsmassage*), reflexology or zone therapy of feet or hands, and trigger point (neuromuscular) therapies.

reflexology

also known as foot reflexive zone therapy, type of reflex massage descended from ancient natural therapies that accesses subtle energy of feet; uses thumbs or fingertips to compress undifferentiated nerves in skin against bone at specific sites to create a distant specific effect and to balance and harmonize body towards health and well-being; also performed on hands.

relaxin

placental hormone that works with progesterone to maintain pregnancy; works synergistically with estrogen and progesterone to soften connective tissue.

restless leg syndrome

movement disorder which causes urge to move legs and is associated with uncomfortable or unpleasant sensation, such as pulling, drawing, crawling, wormy, tingling, pins and needles, prickly; sometimes sudden muscle twitches may also occur.

Rh incompatibility

blood disease resulting from conflicting maternal and fetal blood Rh (Rhesus) factors that cause an antigen–antibody reaction.

rubella

also known as German measles; viral infection resulting in fever, swollen glands, rash and possible congenital defects in a fetus if mother is infected during first half of pregnancy.

search engine optimization

various techniques to improve a website ranking in Internet data analysis systems in hopes of attracting more visitors.

second stage of labor

time from full cervical dilation through fetal descent through pelvis, as measured by pelvic station and until birth of baby; characterized by mother's active pushing and passive descent or laboring down using positions for gravity, pelvic opening and rest to facilitate baby's passage.

semireclining

also known as semi-recumbent; partially seated, partially lying position on massage table with tilt-top table or other equipment on regular massage table; in pregnancy, 45- to 75-degree angle elevation from client's hip to head; ideal postpartum when baby is held or fed during sessions.

sidelying

also known as lateral recumbent; client position on table supported on either left or right side.

Side Lying Positioning System

six-part grouping of cushions engineered specifically to ergonomically support client while lying on her side; can be adapted to semireclining position as well.

small for gestational age (SGA)

preterm, term or post-term infant weight usually less than 5½ pounds (2.5 kg) or less than 10th percentile on standard growth charts; SGA infants are different from preterm infants, who often have underdeveloped respiratory systems; SGA infants often have developed respiratory systems, but require frequent observations for hypoglycemia because of inadequate glycogen stores, leading to need for frequent feedings.

somatic practices

educational and health-enhancing methods of massage and therapeutic bodywork addressing whole body through touch and/or movement, and often with attention to emotional connections as well.

spider veins

also called spider angioma or telangiectasias, or vascular nevi; tiny, visible capillaries with wavy, spider-like patterns, primarily on legs or small blood vessels and appearing superficially on neck, thorax, face and arms, which usually disappear after giving birth.

spontaneous abortion
also known as miscarriage; loss of early pregnancy, usually before 20 weeks of gestation and usually resulting from natural causes.

stillbirth
also known as intrauterine fetal demise; loss of a fetus after 20th week of gestation and up to and during labor and birth.

strain–counterstrain
type of osteopathic passive movement that seeks to relieve "tender points" in soft tissues by positioning client in maximal comfort position and holding; created and developed by Lawrence Jones, DO.

stress incontinence
involuntary leakage of urine and/or fecal matter with physical activity, increased intra-abdominal pressure such as coughing, sneezing or lifting baby, or inadequate pelvic floor sphincter function; occurs during pregnancy and after birth secondary to perineal trauma; can be severe enough to impact quality of life, including social or hygiene issues; benefits from referral to women's health physical therapy for specialized treatment.

striae gravidarum
reddish or darkened lines where growing uterus and expanding underlying tissues have stretched and torn components of skin; particularly common on abdomen, hips or breasts.

subchorionic hemorrhage
pregnancy and birth complication where blood gathers between uterus and chorion membrane; can happen during first trimester but more common in second trimester; associated with poor outcomes for both mothers and babies.

supine
lying face-up position.

supine hypotensive syndrome
decreased blood pressure caused by uterus compressing inferior vena cava sufficiently to reduce venous return; symptoms include uneasiness, dizziness, weakness, nausea, shortness of breath or other discomforts when lying flat on back, although some report no symptoms.

surrogacy
also known as use of gestational carrier; laboratory fertilization of embryos that are transferred to another person's uterus for remainder of gestation.

sympathetic branch of autonomic nervous system
nerve network that increases heart rate, and constricts blood flow to viscera and skin while increasing it in skeletal muscle; prompts production of stress hormones epinephrine and norepinephrine.

symphysis pubis dysfunction
also known as symphysis pubis separation; instability and/or misalignment of articular structures at anterior junction of two halves of pubic bone.

table side
side that client is lying on when laterally recumbent on table.

tai chi chuan
martial art and exercise and meditation system based on interplay of polarities of movement, stance and energy; originated in ancient China and developed by many modern masters of various schools of instruction and practice.

target market
defined group of potential customers who have similar characteristics (age, location, interests and so on), on whom promotional efforts can be focused.

tarsal tunnel syndrome
pressure on tarsal nerve as it passes ankle due to extra fluid, resulting in foot pain and/or numbness.

tee stance
standing posture with feet shoulder-width apart and one foot, empty of weight, about a foot length ahead of other weighted foot.

teratogens
substances that can cause fetal defects in utero.

term
also known as full term; normal gestational period of pregnancy to 37 to 42 weeks, when baby is ideally born.

third stage of labor
time from birth of baby through birth of placenta.

thoracic outlet syndrome
compression of brachial plexus, with pain, numbness or tingling in entire hand and along arm.

thrombi
blood clots; singular blood clot is thrombus.

thromboembolism
obstruction of blood vessel by blood clot carried by circulation from site of origin; often migrating to lungs, thereby creating pulmonary embolism.

thrombophilias
blood disorders characterized by imbalance in naturally occurring blood-clotting proteins or clotting factors, increasing risk of developing blood clots; significantly complicate pregnancy and birth, and increase risk of maternal and infant mortality.

thrombophlebitis
inflammation of blood vessel caused by blood clot (thrombus) within vessel.

tidal volume
amount of air exchanged with each breath cycle.

tilt-top table
massage table that features top surface that is manually or electrically adjustable to various angles and heights off flat line of most standard tables.

toxoplasmosis
parasitic infection carried in cat feces, contaminated soil or undercooked meat that has a high likelihood of infecting fetus, causing congenital damage and other complications.

Trager™
movement education approach and mind/body integration using rhythmic active and passive movements to help release deep-seated physical and mental patterns and facilitate deep relaxation, increased physical mobility and mental clarity.

transference
psychological reaction in which client displaces her thoughts, feelings or behaviors about a significant other onto her therapist.

transition phase
first stage of labor's third and final phase of cervical dilation from 8 to 10 centimeters.

trigger point
hypersensitive and hyperirritable spot, most often found in taut bands and nodules in skeletal muscle; when pressed, often creates local and distant pain referred in characteristic patterns; the variety of systems for working with these points originate in the work of Dr Janet Travell and Dr David Simons.

trimester
40 weeks of pregnancy with three phases of 13–14 weeks each: first trimester 1–13 weeks, second trimester 14–27 weeks and third trimester 28–40 weeks and up.

trizygotic
high-order multiple gestation pregnancy derived from three separate ova, where each fetus has its own placenta, amnion and chorion.

tubal ligation
surgical cutting and tying of fallopian tubes to prevent conception.

twin-to-twin transfusion syndrome
complication of multiple gestation pregnancy involving transfusion of blood from one twin to other twin.

umbilical cord prolapse
occurs when umbilical cord protrudes into birth canal ahead of baby during birth, causing cord compression that compromises blood and oxygen supply to baby; more likely to occur with premature rupture of membranes, preterm birth, polyhydramnios, breech birth, multiple gestations birth, or unusually long umbilical cord.

uterine atony
lack of uterine muscle tone that can result in excessive perinatal blood loss and postpartum hemorrhage.

uterine competence
normal structure and functioning of uterus for maintaining pregnancy and birthing a baby.

uterine ligaments
thickened areas of connective tissue surrounding uterus that support and position uterus, fallopian tubes and ovaries within pelvis and also connect it to rectum and bladder; each ligament has unique pain patterns.

uterine rupture
tearing of uterine wall, usually at site of previous surgical scar or placenta accreta, increta and percreta; potentially life-threatening for mother and baby.

vacuum
obstetrical intervention sometimes used to assist fetus's descent during second stage of labor.

varicose veins
weakened areas where valves in vein have collapsed, allowing pooling of blood.

vasodilation
increased blood flow to area by expansion of blood vessels.

zone therapy
also known as reflexology; type of reflex massage from ancient natural therapies that accesses subtle energy of feet; uses thumbs or fingertips to compress undifferentiated nerves in skin against bone at specific sites to create distant specific effect and to balance and harmonize body towards health and well-being; also performed on hands.

INDEX

Note: Page number followed by *italic* indicates figure.

A

Abdominal
  diastasis recti   19, 20, 75, 115, 203, 211
  effleurage   48, 110, 112, 127, *127*, 187
  healing   *212*
  kneading   223, *223*
  massage   51–53, *51*, 177, 179, 182, 183, 187, 206
  postpartum   206, 208, 211–212, 219
  precautions   23, 41, 48, 51–53, 104
  tapotement   2*24*
  trigger points   *224*
  vibration   *224*
Abnormal fetal growth/movement   244–245
Abuse
  post-traumatic stress syndrome   155, 169, 254, 259–261
  sexual   260
  spousal   237
Active listening   184
Active stage labor, *see* labor
Acupressure   15, 148
American College of Obstetricians and Gynecologists (ACOG)   44, 76, 174, 199
Amniotic fluid   43
  imbalances and infections   245
Anterior Hip Deep Tissue Sculpting   107, 142, *142*
Apgar scores   25
Arm Swedish Massage   146, *146*
Arm techniques   145–147
Aromatherapy   62
Asian bodywork therapies   58–59
Assessment   273–274
Assisted reproductive technology   6, 236–238
Asthma   245–246
Aston patterning   220
Autonomic sedation sequence   14, 100–101, 106–107, 121, 122, *122*, 158, 160, 173, 179, 191, 207, 215, 217, 246, 276, 278

B

"Baby blues"   205, 207, 256
Back pain, *see* musculoskeletal system
Bed rest   54, 57, 65, 111, 116, 146, 240, 242–244, 248–249, 256, 258–259, 269–270, 281, 288
Benefits of massage therapy   29
Birth doulas   5, 177
Birthing pool (tub)   176
Birth plan, benefits of   162
Blood clots, *see* thrombi *and* circulatory system
Body mechanics, mother's   215–219
Body mechanics, therapist's   *91, 93, 94*
  alignment principles   90–95
  bow stance   90
  breathing   90, 95
  expansional balance   90
  horse-riding stance   90
  in labor   170
  tai chi chuan   89–90
  tee stance   90
Braxton Hicks contractions   171
Breast
  changes postpartum   204
  changes prenatally   26
  engorgement   123, 213
  feeding   13, 29, 167, 182, 200, 202, 204, 210
  massage   213–214, *213*
  mastitis   213, 250
Breathing   14, 95, 107, 118, 123, *123*, 137, 148, 155, 207, 209, 211, 212, 215, 219, 246

C

Calf cramps   54, 76, *110*, 112, 118, 142, 226
Cardiovascular disease and hypertensive disorders   246–248
Carpal tunnel syndrome   12, 14, 22, 75, 92, 111, 119, 216
Catecholamines   167
Cautionary areas   50–60, 220

Cervical lip   180
Cervical Transverse Rocking   107, 124, *124*, 207, 215
Cervix and Pelvic Floor Relaxation   188
Cesarean birth   183–185
  family-centered   183
  healing   209–210
  incision   9, *184*
  scar massage   *184*, 210–212, 225–226, *225*
  vaginal birth after Cesarean   183
Charting   277, 278
Childbirth education   4, 24, 115, 154, 155, 270
Chloasma   16
Chorioamnionitis   245
Chronic hypertension   64, 246, 247
Chronic tension   19
Circulatory system
  benefits of massage therapy for   11–14
  chronic hypertension   64
  deep vein thrombosis (DVT)   54, 55, 58
  eclampsia   246, 247, 248
  fibrinolysis   13
  gestational hypertension   246
  heart-rate variability   14
  HELLP syndrome   246
  hemorrhage   13, 181, 202, 204, 228, 229
  hypertensive disorders   12, 14, 65, 109, 116, 145, 239, 246–248
  perforator veins   54, 110
  peripartum cardiomyopathy   246
  postpartum clotting factors   204
  spider veins   12, 13
  thrombi   13, 65, 243, 244, 248
  thromboembolisms   54
  thrombophlebitis   54
  varicose veins   12, 57–58, 65, 80, 111
  vasodilation   12
Client education and presentations   271–272
Coccygodynia   219

Complications   5, 40, 46, 52, 63–64,
        237, 238–240, 241, 242, *243*,
        244–256
    bed rest for   242–243
    labor, *see* labor complications
    prenatal, *see* prenatal complications
    signs and symptoms of   239
Confidentiality   259
Contraction Distraction   188, *189*
Countertransference   163
COVID-19   xviii, 64, 237, 251
Craniosacral techniques   119, 142
Critical thinking   275–276
Cross-fiber friction   23, 57, 134, *135*,
        147, *147*
Cyanosis   64
Cytomegalovirus   251

D

Decision trees   277
Deep tissue massage   14, 23–24,
        26, 48–49, *55*, 57, 107, 155,
        172–173, 191, 209, 212–214,
        217–219
    anterior hip   107, 142, *142*
    lateral pelvis   107, 112, 117, 128, *129*,
        177, 212, 217, 219
    paravertebral   107, 118, 130, *131*
    pectoral girdle   112, 118, 132–134,
        133–134, 219
    ribcage   137–138, *137*
    sacroiliac joint rhythmic   112, 138–139,
        138–139, 140, 175, 177, 180,
        191, 209
    wrist and flexors   119, 146, *146*, 190,
        214, 217
Deep vein thrombosis (DVT)   54, 58,
        see also thrombi *and* circulatory
        system
De Quervain's syndrome   216
Diabetes   7, 64, 116, 244, 248, 249
Diastasis recti   19, 20, 75, 115, 203, 211
Disseminated intravascular
        coagulopathy   258

Diversity   4, 89, 103, 163, 199–200
Draping
    breasts   *87*
    ceiling-side hip and leg   *85*
    seated   86
    semireclining   83
    sidelying   84

E

Eclampsia   246, 247, 248
Edema   12, 14, 22, 29, 55, 64, 78, 80, 82,
        110, 113, 247, *247*
Electronic fetal monitoring   155
Emotional expression   50
Endocrine system   10, 202
    estrogen   10, 11, 15, 16, 102, 109, 166,
        202, 246
    oxytocin   10, 167, 170, 171, 201, 202
    postpartum endocrine changes   4, 20,
        27, 64, 66, 72, 202
    prenatal endocrine activity   *11*
    progesterone   11–17, 102–103, 166,
        202, 206, 246
    relaxin   10, 61, 81, 103, 108, 166,
        206, 276
Endometritis   250
Epidural   9, 25, 170, 177–179, 181, 183,
        189–190, 192, 200, 218, 220, 239,
        245, 250
Episiotomy   159, 203, 239, 250
Equipment and environment
        recommendations   73–75
Essential oils   62
Estrogen, *see* endocrine system
Ethics   101, 283–284

F

Fetal distress   258
Fetal origins hypothesis   7
Fetal position   21, 46, 136, 187–188
    optimal   9
Fibrinolysis   13
First stage labor, *see* labor

First trimester massage   41, 101–107
Foot Reflexive Zone Therapy   58, 112, 124,
        124, 148, 215, 226
Full-Body Integration   121–126

G

Gastric reflux   15
Gastrointestinal system   15, 204
    benefits of massage therapy for   15
    discomforts   15, 145
    heartburn (gastric reflux)   15, 46,
        77, 87, 112, 115, 118, 148, 171,
        242, 244
    hemorrhoids   13
    hiatal hernia   115, 118, 130, 147, 148
    "morning sickness"   10, 15, 101, 145
Gate theory of pain   23
Gestational diabetes   248–249
Gestational hypertensive disorders   12, 14,
        109, 116, 246
Grounding hold   189, *189*

H

Heart-rate variability (HRV)   14
Hemorrhage   13, 181, 202, 204,
        228, 229
High-risk
    factors   44, 53, 58, 64
    pregnancies   46, *63*, 237–261
Hip joint   19, 22, 75–76, 81, 90
    decompression   112, 144, *144*,
        209, 219
    infinity mobilization   112, 117, 143, *143*,
        179, 191, 209, 219
    internal rotation and rocking   144, *144*
Hospital   154, 155, 161, 163, 165, 169,
        170, 174, 175, 176, 178, 180, 182,
        227, 237
Hydrotherapy   62, 165, 176, *176*, 226
Hyperemesis gravidarum   249–251, 255
Hypertensive disorders   12, 14, 65, 109,
        116, 145
Hysterectomy   204

I

Iliopsoas Structural Balancing   209, 212, 219, *226*

Infant
  carrying and nurturing   215
  massage   220
  positioning during massage   218
  preventing strain from care   43, 170, 216

Infections   250–251

Infertility   236

Intake forms   4, 64, 273–274

Integumentary system   16, 204
  benefits of skin stimulation   16
  chloasma   16
  linea nigra   16
  striae gravidarum   16, 204

Internet marketing   269–270

Intrauterine pressure   42, 44, 47, 61, 76, 82, 104, 106

In vitro fertilization (IVF)   236–238

J

Joints, *see* musculoskeletal system

K

Kinesthetic awareness   23, 29, 89, 104, 121, 123

L

Labor   5
  active   174–176, *176*
  arrested   181
  attending labor and birth as massage therapist   160–166
  "back labor" birth sensations   *168*
  birth positions   *156*
  dystocia   181, 251
  epidurals   9, 25, 177–178
  epinephrine   167
  facilitation   25
  first stage of   172
  fourth stage of   182, *182*

heat and cold therapy   175, 180, 181, 189–190
hormones in labor   166–169
induction   60
massage techniques   26, 155–193, *158*
occiput anterior (OA) position   177
occiput posterior (OP) position   177
pelvic station   174
physiological labor and birth   154
pre-labor   171–172
precipitous   251, 252
preparation for   23–24
protracted   181
second stage of   160, 180–181
stimulation points   190, *190*
stress hormones in labor   167–168, *167*
Technique Manual   187–193
third stage of labor   181–182
touch in labor   24–26, 169
transition phase   179

Labor complications
  induction and augmentation   116, 170
  labor dystocia   181–182, 251–252
  rapid labor   115

Labor Progress Handbook   169

Laminar Groove Inching   127, *128*, 191, 209, 219

Last menstrual period dating   236

Lateral Pelvis Deep Tissue Sculpting   107, 112, 117, 128, *129*, 177, 212, 217, 219

Lateral recumbent position   46

Leg precautions   54, *55*, 80, 105, 112, 113, 119, 127, 129, 142–145, 181, 189

Leg Swedish Massage   54, 145

Leg techniques   142–145

Liability   279–280

Localized massage (labor)   190–191

Log roll technique   201

Low birth weight   5, 7, 207, 257–258

Lumbar Lengthening   107, 111, 129, *129*, 219

Lumbosacral Joint Decompression   112, 130, *130*, 177, 181, 209, 212

Lymph drainage therapy   13, 179, 247, 248

M

Male therapists   285

Marketing   268–270, 286–287

Mastitis   213, 250, 251

Meconium   245

Meralgia paresthetica   115

Miscarriage   41, 44, 51, 53, 60, 110, 131, 253

Molar pregnancy   249

Multifetal reduction   237

Multiple gestation   64, 77, 110, 237, 244, 255, *255*

Muscle energy techniques   23

Muscular Tension and Joint Pain Relief (labor)   175, 180, 191

Musculoskeletal system   17–22
  back pain   17–23, 43, 45, 53, 114, 116, 131, 156, 177, 218, 226–227, 239
  calf cramps   54, 76, 112, 118
  coccygodynia   219
  de Quervain's syndrome   216
  joints   22
    hormonal effects on   22
    most stressed by pregnancy   22, 155
    precautions   50, 52, 55, 56
    sacroiliac joints   20, 80
    symphysis pubis dysfunction   118, 127, *141*, 142
  meralgia paresthetica   115
  pregnancy-related pelvic girdle pain (PPGP)   19, 148, 155, 206, 218
  referred pain   20, 21
  restless leg syndrome   22
  ribcage pain   22
  ribcage trigger points   137–138, *138*
  sacroiliac joints   20
  sciatica and piriformis syndrome   21, 114
  structural imbalance   19
  symphysis pubis dysfunction   20, 61, *61*, 110
  tarsal tunnel syndrome   12, 22, 142

Myofascial release   23

Myofascial restriction   15

N

Neonatal intensive care unit (NICU)   240
Nervous system   23, 101, 104, 154, 208, 238
    autonomic nervous system   8–9, 14, 16, 189
    nerve compression in pregnancy   114–115
Networking   269
Norepinephrine   167

O

Oakworks Side Lying Positioning System   73, 76, 78, 79, *80*, 81, 89, 200
Obstacles to business success   280–284
Occiput anterior (OA) position   177
Occiput posterior (OP) position   177
Occiput Traction and Rocking   107, 125, *125*, 191
Oligohydramnios   245
Osteopathic soft tissue treatments   23
Oxytocin   10, 167, 170, 171, 201, 202

P

Pain and pressure   48–50
Pain control   17–19, 22–23, *26*, 29
Parasympathetic activation   23, 104
Paravertebral Deep Tissue Sculpting   107, 118, 130, *131*
Pectoral Girdle Cross-Fiber Friction   134, *135*, 217, 219
Pectoral Girdle Deep Tissue Sculpting   112, 118, 132, *133–134*, 219
Pectoral Girdle Mobilizations   107, 112, 131, *132*
Pelvic Alignment Education   107, 112, 135–136, *136*
Pelvic floor
    incontinence   17, 147
    Kegel exercises   17
    massage (perineal massage)   159
    postpartum healing   159, 200

Pelvic Girdle Decompressions   107, 112, 136, *136*
Pelvic station   174
Perforator veins   54
Perinatal mood and anxiety disorders (PMADs)   28, 256
Perinatal pelvic pain syndrome (PPPS)   19, 148, 155, 206, 218, 302
Perineal massage   159
Peripartum cardiomyopathy   246
Piriformis syndrome   *18*, 19, 21, 105, 114, 127, *129*, 142, 209
Placenta
    abnormalities of   237, 257
    function of   16, 65
Polyhydramnios   245
Positioning
    chair   156
    checklists   75
    prone   42
    semireclining   45–46, 77–78, *78*
    sidelying   46–48, 79–82, *80*, 83, *84*, 89, 200
        advantages   46–48, *47*, 78, 79, *80*, 83, *84*
    side-to-side switches   88
    supine/prone switches   87
    supine/semireclining/sidelying switches   87
    supine   45, 47, 76, 77, 130, 141
    symphysis pubis dysfunction, positioning for   118
    trimester guidelines   12, *21*, 65–66, 101, 103, 105, 107, 109, 111, 113, *113*, 115, 119
Postpartum   27–28, 198–229
    Technique Manual   223–229
Postpartum clotting factors   204
Post-traumatic stress disorder (PTSD)   155, 254, 259
Pre-eclampsia   7, 131, 216, 245, 246
Pregnancy   6, 159
    first trimester of   41, 102–107
    second trimester of   108–112, *108*
    third trimester of   113–119, *113*
Pregnancy-related complications, *see* prenatal complications

Pregnancy-related pelvic girdle pain (PPGP)   19, 148, 155, 206, 218
Prenatal complications   63–64, 238–262
    abnormal fetal growth or movement   244–245
    amniotic fluid imbalances   245
    antepartum bleeding   255, 258
    biophysical factors for   237
    environmental factors for   162
    general guidelines   255, 257
    gestational diabetes   248–251
    gestational hypertensive disorders, degrees of   12, 14, 109, 145, 239, 246
    hyperemesis gravidarum   249–250
    infections   xviii, 64, 237, 250–251
    miscarriage and stillbirth   253–255
    pitting edema   247, *247*
    pre-eclampsia symptoms   246–247
    preterm labor/prematurity   258
    signs and symptoms of pre-eclampsia   239–240
    warning signs of   116
Prenatal massage tables   74
Prenatal postural changes   114, *114*
Prenatal Technique Manual   121–148
Preterm labor and births   5, 44, 52, 245, 258
Print advertising   272
Print marketing   270
Progesterone   10, 12, 15, 109, 166, 202
Prostaglandins   166
Proteinuria   246
Protracted labor   181
Puerperium   198
"Pump and dump"   13

R

Rapid eye movement (REM) sleep   205
Referrals   269
Reflexive techniques   15, 17, 28, 52, 110, 210, 213, 241, 251
Relaxin   7, 8, 10–11, 13, 20
Respiratory system   12, 204, *see also* breathing
    benefits of massage therapy for   9, 12, 14, 29

Ribcage
  Deep Tissue Sculpting   107, 112, 118,
    137, *137*, 217, 219
  prenatal changes   127
  trigger points   20, 22, 107, 112, 118,
    137, *138*, 217, 219

S

Sacral counterpressure   20, 59, 105, 122,
    158, 169, 175, 191, *192*
Sacroiliac Joint Decompression   112,
    138–139, *138–139*, 175
Sacroiliac Joint Rhythmic Deep Tissue   112,
    139–140, *139–140*, 175, 177, 180,
    191, 209
Safety guidelines   41–66
Second stage labor, *see* labor
Sensory-motor system   24
Sidelying positioning, *see* positioning
Skin-to-skin contact   202
Sleep   4, 5, 22
Smells   61
Somatic practices   48
Spa treatments and settings   61–62
Spider veins   12, 13
Spinal Rocking   107, 112, 140, *140*, 207, 215
Spinal Seated Fascia Stretching   209, 217,
    219, 227–228, *227–228*
Spontaneous abortion   53
Stillbirth   206, 238, 253–254
Stress   5–6, 8, 25, 50, 62, 166, 205,
    208, 258
Stress incontinence   17, 109, 159,
    204, 212

Striae gravidarum   16, 204
Structural Balancing Education   106, 111,
    125, *125–126*, 141, 218–219
Supine hypotensive syndrome   45, *45*, 47,
    76, 111, 130, 141, 255
Supine positioning, *see* positioning
Surrogacy   238
Swedish massage   13, 15, 23, 48, 64, 141,
    144, 213
Symphysis pubis dysfunction   20, 61, *61*,
    110, *118*, 127, 141
Symphysis Pubis Rebalancing   141,
    141–142, 209, 212

T

Tai chi chuan   89
Tarsal tunnel syndrome   12, 21, 141, 144
Thai massage techniques   61
Thigh Adductors Passive Relaxation   112,
    193, *193*
Third stage labor, *see* labor
Thoracic outlet syndrome   22, 74, 114,
    118, 122
Thrombi   13, 54–57
Thromboembolisms   54, 204, 237, 244
Thrombophlebitis   54, 57
Torso Techniques   127–142
Toxoplasmosis   251
Transference   163
Traumatic birth   259–261
Trigger point therapy   14, 23
Trimester   12, 17, 19, *see also* pregnancy
Tubal ligation   204
Twin-to-twin transfusion syndrome   255

U

Umbilical cord prolapse   245
Urinary system   17, 145
  frequency   17
  incontinence   17, 109, 212
  urinary tract discomforts   145
Uterus
  competence   44
  contractions   171
  fundal massage   228, *228*
  growth   21
  intrauterine pressure   42, 44, 61, 76, 82
  involution   182, 198, 202, *203*
  ligaments   21, *21*, 42, 80, 117, 205
  positioning   229, *229*

V

Vaginal birth after previous Cesareans
    (VBAC)   183
Vaginal bleeding   261
Varicose veins   12, 54–58, 65
Vasodilation   12

W

Wrist Acupressure   107, *148*, *250*
Wrist and Flexors Deep Tissue
    Sculpting   119, 146, *146*, 190,
    214, 217
Wrist Passive Movements   119, 146–147,
    147, 190, 214, 217
Wrist Retinaculum Cross-Fiber
    Friction   147, *147*, 217